MUTATIONS IN HUMAN GENETIC DISEASE

Edited by **David N. Cooper** and **Jian-Min Chen**

Mutations in Human Genetic Disease
http://dx.doi.org/10.5772/2912
Edited by David N. Cooper and Jian-Min Chen

Contributors

M. Yavuz Köker, Hüseyin Avcilar, Tina V. Hellmann, Joachim Nickel, Thomas D. Mueller, Mathilde Varret, Jean-Pierre Rabès, Suad AlFadhli, Mihaela Tica, Valeria Tica, Alexandru Naumescu, Mihaela Uta, Ovidiu Vlaicu, Elena Ionica, Akl C. Fahed, Georges M. Nemer, Afig Berdeli, Sinem Nalbantoglu, George Seki, Shoko Horita, Masashi Suzuki, Osamu Yamazaki, Hideomi Yamada, Daniel Frías-Lasserre, Paweł Krawczyk, Tomasz Kucharczyk, Kamila Wojas-Krawczyk, Yu Wang, Nanbert Zhong, Biao Li, Predrag Radivojac, Sean Mooney, A. Sassolas, M. Di Filippo, L.P. Aggerbeck, N. Peretti, M.E. Samson-Bouma, Musaffe Tuna, Christopher I. Amos

Published by InTech
Janeza Trdine 9, 51000 Rijeka, Croatia

Publishing Process Manager Oliver Kurelic
Technical Editor InTech Prepress, Novi Sad
Cover InTech Design team

Additional hard copies can be obtained from orders@intechopen.com

Mutations in Human Genetic Disease, Edited by David N. Cooper and Jian-Min Chen
p. cm.
ISBN 978-953-51-0790-3

For EU product safety concerns:
IN TECH d.o.o., Prolaz Marije Krucifikse Kozulić 3, 51000 Rijeka, Croatia,
info@intechopen.com or visit our website at intechopen.com.

Meet the editors

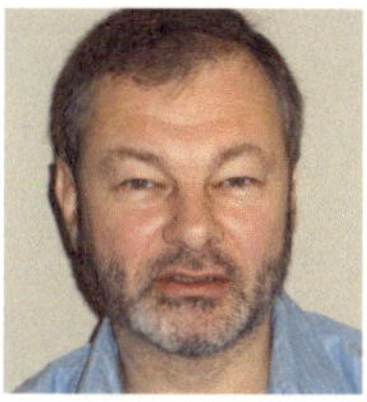

David N. Cooper is Professor of Human Molecular Genetics at Cardiff University in the UK. His research interests are largely focused upon elucidating the mechanisms of mutagenesis underlying human genetic disease, but include genotype–phenotype relationships in various inherited conditions, as well as human evolutionary and population genetics. He has published over 350 papers in the field of human molecular genetics and curates the Human Gene Mutation Database (http://www.hgmd.org), a comprehensive database of mutations causing human inherited disease. Professor Cooper is European Editor of Human Genetics and Editor of the Genetics & Disease section of Wiley's Encyclopedia of Life Sciences.

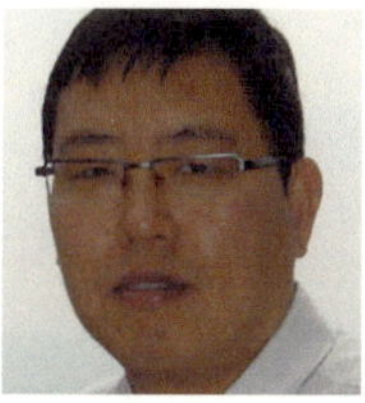

Jian-Min Chen is Director of Research at the Etablissement Française du Sang-Bretagne, Brest, France. He obtained his M.D. in 1993 from the Academy of Military Medical Sciences, Beijing, China and his Ph.D in 2002 from the Université de Bretagne Occidentale, Brest, France. He joined the INSERM team headed by Prof. Claude Férec in 1998 and took up his present position in 2008. He is interested in the genetic basis of chronic pancreatitis and cystic fibrosis as well as the mechanisms of mutagenesis underlying human genetic disease.

Contents

Preface

Just over 30 years ago, the first heritable human gene mutations were characterized at the DNA level: gross deletions of the human α-globin and β-globin gene clusters giving rise to α- and β-thalassaemia (1978) and a nonsense mutation in the human β-globin (*HBB*) gene causing β-thalassaemia (1979). With the number of known germline mutations in human nuclear genes either underlying or associated with inherited disease now exceeding 125,000 in ~5,000 different genes (Human Gene Mutation Database; http://www.hgmd.org; October 2012), the characterization of the spectrum of human germ-line mutations is proceeding apace. Such information is beginning to shed new light on longstanding questions such as the nature of disease predisposition, the determinants of the genotype-phenotype relationship, the molecular basis of reduced penetrance and the measurement of the human gene mutation rate, as well as posing profound questions pertaining to how we conceptualise genetic disease. Thus, from data generated by the 1000 Genomes Project, it has become clear that an average human genome typically contains ~100 loss-of-function variants, with ~20 genes being completely inactivated. In addition, even apparently healthy individuals harbour many tens or even hundreds of potentially deleterious variants in their genomes whose impact on the phenotype is usually still unknown.

Mutations are also likely to play a role in many complex genetic diseases (such as heart disease, neuropsychiatric disease or diabetes). These are conditions that do not display simple Mendelian patterns of inheritance even although genes may exert an important influence; hence close relatives of individual patients will often have an increased risk of developing the condition. These disorders are thought to be due to the combined effects of genetic variants at multiple gene loci, interacting with the environment. Complex disease has a very significant impact on human health because of the high population incidence of these conditions (unlike most Mendelian disorders which tend to be individually rare).

The advent of next-generation sequencing has also made possible the detailed characterization of whole cancer genomes, allowing for the first time a comprehensive assessment of the lexicon of somatic mutations driving tumorigenesis in a given cell or tissue. It has become clear that cancer genomes often constitute an intricate patchwork of clustered, or even overlapping, somatic lesions. Next-generation sequencing has the major advantage of being capable of simultaneously detecting genome/exome-wide, deletions, insertions, copy number alterations and translocations as well as nucleotide substitutions (including hot-spot mutations in known cancer-related genes). Such studies are transforming our knowledge of oncogenic pathways and providing novel molecular targets of use in diagnosis, prognostic and therapeutic contexts. The ultimate goal is to provide a personalized treatment regime for both solid tumours and hematologic malignancies by tailoring health care to the individual patient using their own genetic information. Significant challenges remain to be addressed, such as the dissection of intra-tumoral DNA sequence heterogeneity and the development of powerful new bioinformatic tools with which to differentiate reliably between driver and passenger mutations.

It should be abundantly clear from the above that the study of mutation is relevant to all of us, not just the minority of individuals who may be afflicted in a very immediate way by inherited disease or cancer. In this volume, the interested reader will find 14 chapters on different aspects of mutation as it impacts human genetic disease. It is hoped that this book will not only be of practical assistance to those scientists and clinicians already working in the field but will also serve to encourage others to make their own unique contribution to understanding the nature and pathological consequences of mutation in the human genome.

David N. Cooper
Department of Medical Genetics, Haematology and Pathology, Cardiff University School of Medicine, Institute of Medical Genetics Building Heath Park, Cardiff, Wales

Jian-Min Chen
Directeur de Recherche, Institut National de la Santé et de la Recherche Médicale (INSERM), U613, Brest, France;
Etablissement Français du Sang (EFS)- Bretagne, Brest, France

Chapter 1

Missense Mutation in AR-CGD

M. Yavuz Köker and Hüseyin Avcilar

Additional information is available at the end of the chapter

http://dx.doi.org/10.5772/35758

1. Introduction

Chronic granulomatous disease (CGD) is an inherited disorder of the innate immune system characterized by impairment of intracellular microbicidal activity of phagocytes. Mutations in one of four known nicotinamide adenine dinucleotide phosphate (NADPH) -oxidase components preclude generation of superoxide and related antimicrobial oxidants, leading to the phenotype of CGD. Defects in gp91-phox, encoded by *CYBB* gene, lead to X-linked CGD and have been reported to be responsible for approximately 65% of all CGD cases. The autosomal gene in CGD are *CYBA*, encoding p22-phox, *NCF2*, encoding p67-phox, *NCF1*, encoding p47-phox, and *NCF4*, encoding p40-phox (figure 1) (1,2). The mutation in these genes, respectively, abolishes the activity of the oxidase and leads to autosomal recessive chronic granulomatous disease (AR-CGD) which is approximately 35% of all CGD cases (table 1).

2. Phenotype- genotype correlation in CGD

Identification of specific mutations in CGD patients may help to clarify some of the variability in clinical severity seen in this disorder and shows genotype-phenotype correlation. In general, X-CGD patients follow a more severe clinical course than patients with an AR-CGD and exhibit in the first years of life. AR-CGD patients follow a milder clinical course, especially p47-phox defect, and mostly seen in first and second decade of life. AR-CGD patients with missense mutations usually exhibit a mild clinical course, associated with a residual activity of p47-phox and also p22 and p67-phoxs. However, the level of superoxide generation does not always correlate with the clinical course. Some patients suffer from severe and recurrent infections despite having neutrophils with 10–20% of normal oxidase activity (1). Within our study with 40 AR-CGD families, we could not define a direct correlation between the molecular defect and the clinical course of the disease. Either truncations (nonsense and frameshift mutations) or missense mutations could have resulted in severe influence on phenotype.

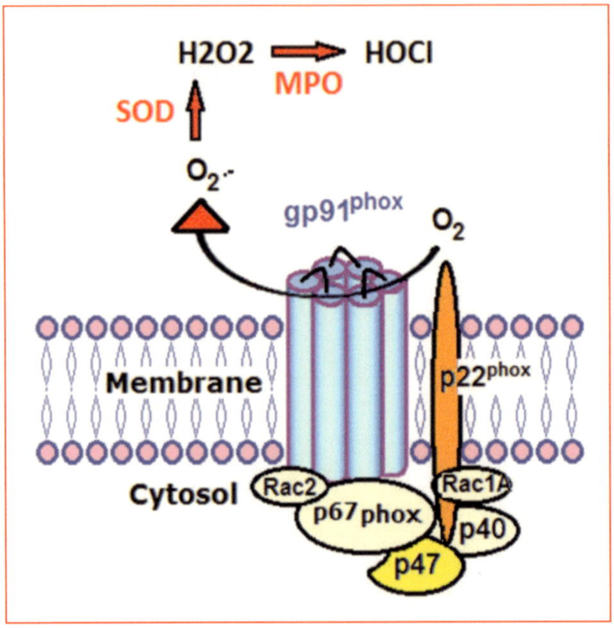

Figure 1. NADPH oxidase enzyme subunits and complex in activation phase.

Components	**gp91 phox**	**p22 phox**	**p47 phox**	**p67 phox**
Gene	CYBB	CYBA	NCF1	NCF2
Chromosome	Xp21.1	16q24	7q11.23	1q25
Number of Exon	13	6	11	16
The length of bp	30kb	8.5kb	15.3kb	40kb
Genotype	X91, X-linked R	A22, OR	A47, OR	A67, OR
Incidence %	%60	%5	%30	%5
The length of aa. chain	570	195	390	526
Localization	membrane	membrane	cytosol	cytosol

Table 1. The molecular characteristic of NADPH Oxidase components.

3. *CYBA* (cytochrome *b* alfa chain) gene

Cytochrome *b* is comprised of a light a-chain and a heavy b-chain. This gene encodes the light, alpha subunit which has been proposed as a primary component of the microbicidal oxidase system of phagocytes. Mutations in this gene are associated with AR-CGD that is characterized by the failure of activated phagocytes to generate superoxide, which is important for the microbicidal activity of these cells. http://www.genecards.org/cgi-bin/carddisp.plgene=*CYBA*.

In about 5% of the CGD patients, the disease is caused by mutations in the cytochrome *b* alfa chain *(CYBA)* gene. The *CYBA* gene encoding p22-phox which contains 195 amino acid, is localized on chromosome 16q24, has a size of about 8,5 and contains six exons and transmembrane and proline rich domains [3, 4]. *CYBA* gene encoding p22-phox has 19 different missense mutations in 65 mutated alleles and has more missense mutation than other NADPH oxidase subunit genes (table 2a) (figure 2). Mutations in the *CYBA* gene have been updated by [Roos et al., (2)] and are reviewed in Human Gene Mutation Database, (HGMD; http://www.hgmd.cf.ac.uk/ac/all.php).

P22-phox has a key role in the interaction of NADPH-oxidase subunits and any difference in amino acid pattern of this phox protein may change the globular conformation of this protein due to the difference in the electrophoretic characteristic of new amino acid, which prevents the complex formation with other subunits.

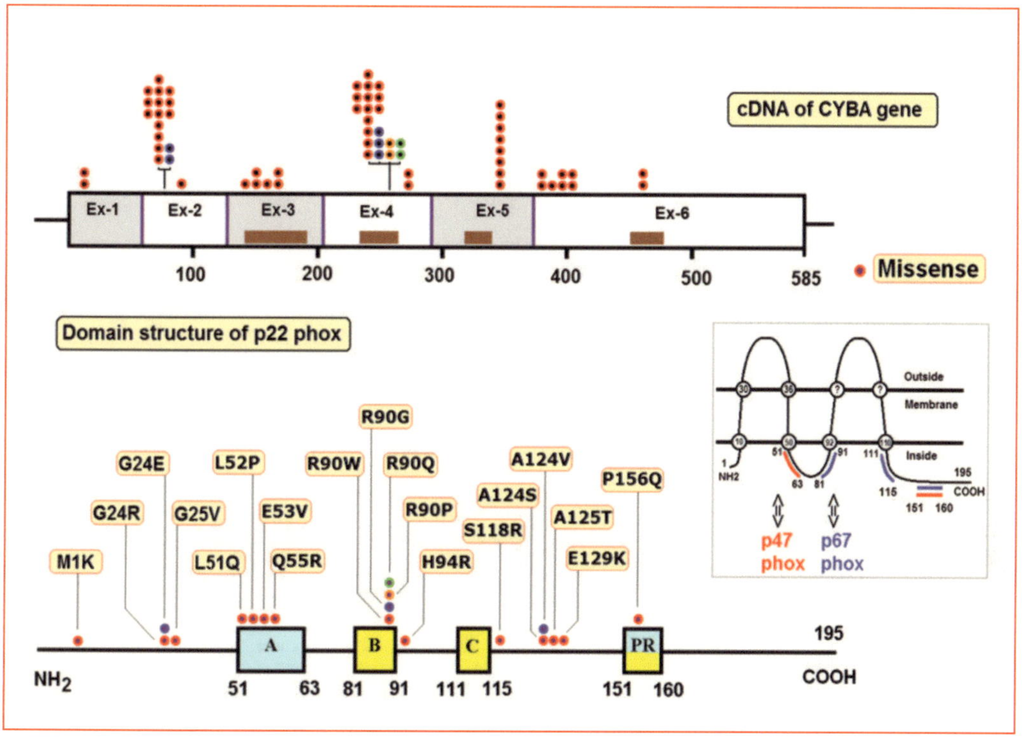

Figure 2. Missense mutations in *CYBA* gene, encoding p22-phox; *CYBA* gene contains 6 exons. P22-phox contains trans-membrane and proline rich domains. Missense mutation points in *CYBA* gene and change in encoded 195 aa. of p22-phox represented in the figure (2).

Missense mutation points may have an important role in the interaction with other subunits, so the amino acid change in that regions may change the property of interactions and prevents or decreases the complex formation, so the activity of NADPH oxidase was abolished.

Total numbers of alleles which have missense mutations are 65 of 173 mutated alleles in *CYBA* gene and the percentage of missense mutations in that mutated alleles are %37,5 (table 2a) (2). Percentage of missense and all mutations of *CYBA* gene in the overall mutations of AR-CGD is %6.3 and %16.8, respectively (table 3 and 4). Most prevalent missense mutations points in *CYBA* gene are c.70G>A, c.268C>T and c.354C>A which cause p.Gly24Arg, p.Arg90Trp and p.Ser118Arg in p22-phox, respectively (table 5).

4. *NCF1* (Neutrophil Cytosolic Factor 1) gene

In about 25% of the CGD patients, the disease is caused by mutations in the neutrophil cytosolic factor 1 (*NCF1*) gene on chromosome 7q11.23, which encodes p47phox, one of the structural components of the NADPH oxidase and has a size of about 40 kb and contains 11 exons (5, 6). The protein encoded by this gene is a 47 kDa cytosolic subunit of neutrophil NADPH oxidase and is required for activation of the latent NADPH oxidase and contains 390 amino acids and PX, SH3a, SH3b and polybasic domains (figure 3).

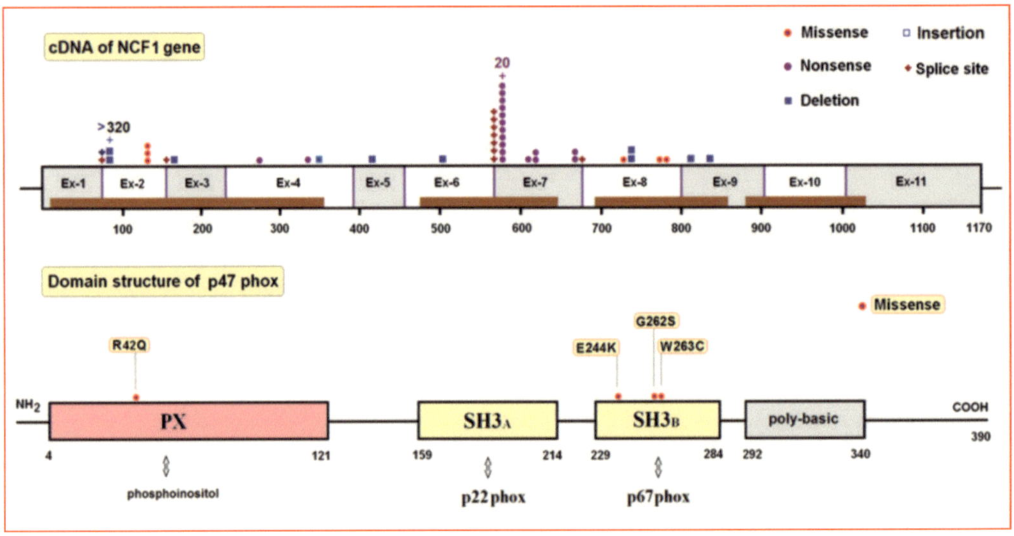

Figure 3. Missense mutations in *NCF1* gene, encoding p47-phox; *NCF1* gene contains 11 exons. p47-phox contains PX, SH3a, SH3b and polybasic domains. Mutation points in *NCF1* gene and change in encoded 390 aa. of p47-phox represented in the figure (2).

A very common mutation found in these patients is a GT deletion in a GTGTrepeat sequence at the beginning of exon 2 of NCF1 (c.75_76delGT) gene (5, 7). *NCF1* gene encoding p47-phox has only 4 different missense mutation in 6 alleles (table 2b) (figure 3) (2). P47-phox has an important role in the interaction of cytoplasmic NADPH-oxidase subunits and any difference in amino acid pattern of this phox protein may abolish the complex formation with other subunits.

Total numbers of alleles which have missense mutations are 6 of 63 (other than delta-GT mutation in exon 2, in more than 620 alleles) mutated alleles in *NCF1* gene and the percentage of missense mutations in that mutated alleles are %9,5. The percentage of missense and all mutations (including delta-GT mutation) of *NCF1* gene in the overall mutations of AR-CGD is %0.6 and %66.4, respectively (table 3 and 4). So, this high percentage due to the high number of delta-GT mutation in exon 2 of *NCF1* gene and is more than all the mutations in AR-CGD (table 5). This deletion points is hot-spot mutation region for *NCF1* gene.

5. *NCF2* (Neutrophil Cytosolic Factor 2) gene

The neutrophil cytosolic factor 2 (*NCF2)* gene encoding p67-phox is localized on chromosome 1q25, has a size of about 40 kb and contains 16 exons and TRP1-4, AD, SH3a, PB1 and SH3b domains (figure 4) (7, 8). *NCF2* gene, encoding p67-phox, has 41 different missense mutations in 171 mutated alleles (table 2c) (2, 4, 5, 6). Mutations in the *NCF2* gene have been published by [Roos et al., (2)] and are reviewed in Human Gene Mutation Database, (HGMD; http://www.hgmd.cf.ac.uk/ac/all.php). P67-phox has a major role in the interaction of NADPH-oxidase subunits in cytoplasm and any difference in amino acid pattern of this phox protein may prevent the complex formation with other subunits (figure 1).

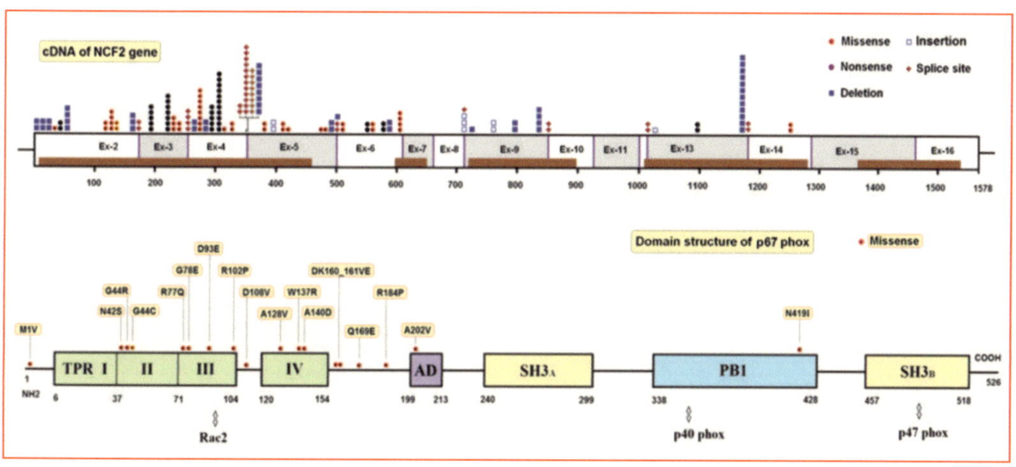

Figure 4. Missense mutations in NCF2 gene, encoding p67-phox; *NCF2* gene contains 16 exons. P67-phox contains TRP1-4, AD, SH3a, PB1 and SH3b domains. Mutation points in *NCF2* gene and change in encoded 526 aa. of p67-phox represented in the figure (2).

Total numbers of mutated alleles leading AR-CGD in *NCF2* gene are 171 and 41 of them are missense and percentage of missense mutations in that mutated alleles are %24 (table 2c) (2). Percentage of missense and all mutations of *NCF2* gene in the overall mutations of AR-CGD is %4 and %16.6, respectively (table 3 and 4). Most prevalent missense mutations points in *NCF2* gene is c.279C>G which causes p.Asp93Glu in p67-phox (table 5).

Nucleotide change	Amino acid change	Amino acid	# of families (alleles)
c.2T>A	p.Met1Lys	**M1K**	1(2)
c.70G>A	p.Gly24Arg	**G24R**	**9(14)**
c.71G>A	p.Gly24Glu	**G24E**	1(2)
c.74G>T	p.Gly25Val	**G25V**	1(1)
c.152T>A	p.Leu51Gln	**L51Q**	1(1)
c.155T>C	p.Leu52Pro	L52P	1(2)
c.158A>T	p.Glu53Val	E53V	1(1)
c.164C>G	p.Pro55Arg	Q55R	1(2)
c.268C>T	p.Arg90Trp	R90W	**8(14)**
c.268C>G	p.Arg90Gly	**R90G**	1(2)
c.269G>A	p.Arg90Gln	R90Q	2(3)
c.269G>C	p.Arg90Pro	R90P	1(2)
c.281A>G	p.His94Arg	**H94R**	1(2)
c.354C>A	p.Ser118Arg	**S118R**	**4(8)**
c.370G>T	p.Ala124Ser	**A124S**	1(2)
c.371C>T	p.Ala124Val	**A124V**	1(1)
c.373G>A	p.Ala125Thr	**A125T**	1(2)
c.385G>A	p.Glu129Lys	**E129K**	1(2)
c.467C>A	p.Pro156Gln	**P156Q**	1(2)
19 different alleles			65 alleles

(a)

Nucleotide change	Amino acid change	Amino acid	# of families (alleles)
c.125G>A	p.Arg42Gln	**R42Q**	**3(3)**
c.730G>A	p.Glu244Lys	**E244K**	1(1)
c.784G>A	p.Gly262Ser	**G262S**	1(1)
c.789G>C	p.Trp263Cys	**W263C**	1(1)
4 different alleles			6 alleles

(b)

Nucleotide change	Amino acid change	Amino acid	# of families (alleles)
c.1A>G	p.Met1Val	**M1V**	1(1)
c.125A>G	p.Asn42Ser	**N42S**	1(2)
c.130G>C	p.Gly44Arg	**G44R**	2(4)
c.130G>T	p.Gly44Cys	**G44C**	1(2)
c.230G>A	p.Arg77Gln	**R77Q**	3(3)
c.233G>A	p.Gly78Glu	G78E	1(2)
c.279C>G	p.Asp93Glu	D93E	**4(8)**

c.305G>C	p.Arg102Pro	R102P	1(1)
c.323A>T	p.Asp108Val	D108V	1(2)
c.383C>T	p.Ala128Val	**A128V**	1(2)
c.409T>A	p.Trp137Arg	W137R	1(2)
c.419C>G	p.Ala140Asp	A140D	1(1)
c.[479A>T; 481A>G]	p.AspLys160_161ValGlu	**DK160_161VE**	1(1)
c.505C>G	p.Gln169Glu	**Q169E**	1(2)
c.551G>C	p.Arg184Pro	**R184P**	1(2)
c.605C>T	p.Ala202Val	**A202V**	2(4)
c.1256A>T	p.Asn419Ile	**N419I**	1(2)
17 different alleles			41 alleles

(c)

Table 2. (a) Missense Mutation in *CYBA* gene. (b) Missense Mutation in *NCF1* gene. (c) Missense Mutation in *NCF2* gene.

Autosomal Gene	Alleles with missense mutations		Alleles with mutations&		In the all mutations of AR-CGD	
	#	%	#	%	Missense %	Total mutations %
CYBA	65	37,5	173	100	6.3	16.8
NCF1	6	9,5*	63 +620*	100	0.6	66.4
NCF2	41	24	171	100	4	16.6
NCF4	1	50	2	100	0.1	0.2
In AR-CGD	113	27.6	409+620*	100	11	100

*: (delta-GT mutations in exon 2, not included)

&: Including nonsense, missense, splice site, deletion and others.

Table 3. Distribution of number and percentage of missense and all mutations in genes (*CYBA, NCF1, NCF2* and *NCF4*) of AR-CGD.

Autosomal Gene	# of different missense mutations	Total # of different mutations&	Different missense / different all mutations in that gene
CYBA	19	55	%34.6
NCF1	4	23	%17.4
NCF2	17	54	%31.5
NCF4	1	2	%50
In AR-CGD	41	134	%30

Table 4. Number and percentage of different missense mutations in genes (*CYBA, NCF1, NCF2* and *NCF4*) of AR-CGD.

Autosomal Gene	Nucleotide change	Aa change	Number of family (alleles)
CYBA	c.70G>A	p.Gly24Arg	9(14)
"	c.268C>T	p.Arg90Trp	8(14)
"	c.354C>A	p.Ser118Arg	4(8)
NCF1	c.125G>A	p.Arg42Gln	**3(3)**
NCF2	c.279C>G	p.Asp93Glu	4(8)

Table 5. Most prevalent missense mutation in the genes of AR-CGD.

6. *NCF4* (Neutrophil Cytosolic Factor 2) gene

NCF4 gene encoding p40-phox with 339 amino acids is localized on chromosome 22q13.1 has a size of about 4,4 kb and contains 10 exons. P40-phox interacts primarily with p67-phox. Up to know, the first mutation in *NCF4* gene was founded in a family with compound heterozygote mutations and one of the mutations was a missense with c.314G>A in one allele, which causes change in p.Arg105Gln amino acid in the structure of p40-phox (2, 9).

7. Conclusion

19 different alleles in *CYBA* gene, 4 different alleles in *NCF1* gene, 17 different alleles in NCF2 gene and one allele in *NCF4* gene have missense mutations which cause change in amino acid patterns of NADPH oxidase subunits and results in AR-CGD. The percentage of missense mutations in the overall mutations of AR-CGD is %11 (table 3). One of the most prevalent missense mutations in AR-CGD is in *CYBA* gene with c.70G>A, in 14 alleles of 9 families, which causes p.Gly24Arg in p22-phox (table 5).

In p22-phox the first interaction with p67-phox occur in B part (domain) which is located between 81-91 amino acids in p22-phox. There are 4 different missense mutations (in 21 alleles of *CYBA* gene) change amino acid (arginine) at position 90. So, this position is highly susceptible to any conformational changes which may prevent the interaction with p67-phox. So, the change in the molecular structure of this part may abolish the stability and function of p22-phox and latent NADPH oxidase could not be activated leading to AR-CGD. P22-phox has more different missense mutation than other NADPH oxidase components. The ratio of the number of different missense mutation and the number of amino acid in the chain is approximately 19/195 (%9.74). The different missense mutation to overall amino acid chain length in p67-phox is 17/526 (%3.23). But, the ratio in p47-phox is 4/390 (%1). This result shows that p67-phox has 3 times and p22-phox has approximately 10 times high incidence of different missense mutations than p47-phox in their primary amino acid structure. The underlying reason for this may be the highly specific interaction and function of p22-phox which is vulnerable to any change in the globular structure of protein.

Author details

M. Yavuz Köker
Erciyes BM Transplant Centre, Division of Immunology, University of Erciyes, Kayseri, Turkey

Hüseyin Avcilar
Kökbiotek Company, Kayseri, Turkey

Acknowledgement

This study is kindly supported by TÜBİTAK with project number 110S252.

8. References

Roos D, Kuijpers TW, Curnutte JT. Chronic granulomatous disease. In: Primary Immunodeficiencies, 2nd edition (Editors: Ochs HD., Smith CIE., Puck JM.), New York: *Oxford University Press*, 2007; 37: 525–49.

Dirk Roos, Doug Kuhns, Anne Maddalena, Jacinta Bustamante, Caroline Kannengiesser, Martin de Boer, Karin van Leeuwen, M. Yavuz Köker, Baruch Wolach, Joachim Roesler, John I. Gallin and Marie-José Stasia. Hematologically Important Mutations: The Autosomal Recessive Forms of Chronic Granulomatous Disease (Second Update). *Blood Cells, Molecules, and Diseases*, 44: 291-299, (2010).

Dinauer MC, Pierce EA, Bruns GAP, Curnutte JT, Orkin SH. Human neutrophil cytochrome b light chain (p22phox): gene structure, chromosomal localization and mutations in cytochrome-negative autosomal recessive chronic granulomatous disease. *J Clin Invest* 1990;86:1729–37.

M.Y. Köker, K. van Leeuwen, M. de Boer, F. Çelmeli, A. Metin, T.T. Özgür, İ. Tezcan, Ö. Sanal, D. Roos. Six Different *CYBA* Mutations Including Three Novel Mutations in Ten Families from Turkey, Resulting in Autosomal Recessive Chronic Granulomatous Disease. *Eur J of Clin Invest*, 39(4): 311-319, (2009).

Roos D, de Boer M, Koker MY, Dekker J, Singh-Gupta V, Ahlin A, Palmblad J, Sanal O, Kurenko-Deptuch M, Jolles S, Wolach B. Chronic granulomatous disease caused by mutations other than the common GT deletion in *NCF1*, the gene encoding the p47 (phox) component of the phagocyte NADPH oxidase. *Hum Mutat*, 27(12):1218-1229, (2006).

Roos D, de Boer M, Kuribayashi F, Meischl C, Weening RS, Segal AW, Ahlin A, Nemet K, Hossle JP, Bernatowska-Matuszkiewicz E, Middleton- Price H. Mutations in the X-linked and autosomal recessive forms of chronic granulomatous disease. *Blood* 87:1663–1681. (1996)

Franke U, Hsieh CL, Foellmer BE, Lomax KJ, Malech HL, Leto TL. Genes for two autosomal recessive forms of chronic granulomatous disease assigned to 1q25 (NCF2) and 7q11.23 (NCF1). *Am J Hum Genet* 1990;47:483–92.

M.Y. Köker, Ö. Sanal, K. van Leeuwen, M. de Boer, A. Metin, Türkan Patıroğlu, T.T. Özgür, İ. Tezcan, , D. Roos. Four Different *NCF2* Mutations in Six Families from Turkey and an Overview of *NCF2* Gene Mutations. *Eur J of Clin Invest,* 39(10): 942-951, (2009).

J.D. Matute, A.A. Arias, N.A.M. Wright, I. Wrobel, C.C.M. Waterhouse, X.J. Li, C.C. Marchal, N.D. Stull, D.B. Lewis, M. Steele, J.D. Kellner, W. Yu, S.O. Meroueh, W.M. Nauseef,, M.C. Dinauer, A new genetic subgroup of chronic granulomatous disease with autosomal recessive mutations in p40phox and selective defects in neutrophil NADPH oxidase activity. *Blood* 114 (2009) 3309–3315.

Chapter 2

Missense Mutations in GDF-5 Signaling: Molecular Mechanisms Behind Skeletal Malformation

Tina V. Hellmann, Joachim Nickel and Thomas D. Mueller

Additional information is available at the end of the chapter

http://dx.doi.org/10.5772/35195

1. Introduction

Members of the large transforming growth factor β (TGF-β) superfamily of secreted growth factors initiate cellular signal transduction via binding to and oligomerization of two different types of membrane bound serine/threonine kinase receptors termed type I and type II (Carcamo *et al.*, 1994, ten Dijke *et al.*, 1996, Massague, 2000). They execute important functions in early (e.g. gastrulation) as well as in later stages (e.g. patterning) of embryonal development, but are also essential for regulation of tissue homeostasis and repair in the adult organism (Rosen & Thies, 1992, Kingsley, 1994, Hogan, 1996, Reddi, 1998, Massague, 2000). A characteristic feature of this protein family is the high degree of promiscuity in the ligand-receptor interaction (for review see (Sebald *et al.*, 2004, Nickel *et al.*, 2009)). This is exemplified by the numeral discrepancy of a likewise large number of ligands - more than 30 ligands are known in mammals to date – and a comparably small number of receptors available for binding and signaling (Miyazawa *et al.*, 2002). Only 12 receptors exist in the TGF-β superfamily of which seven belong to the type I and five to the type II receptor subclass (Newfeld *et al.*, 1999). This implies that a given receptor typically binds more than one TGF-β member, but we usually see that even a particular TGF-β ligand binds more than one receptor of either subtype (for review see (Sebald *et al.*, 2004, Nickel *et al.*, 2009)). Noteworthy, another seemingly reduction in the signaling output is due to the fact that principally only two primary pathways are activated by all TGF-β members (Hoodless *et al.*, 1996, Nakao *et al.*, 1997). After ligand-dependent oligomerization of the single transmembrane receptors, the intracellular kinase domain of the type II receptor activates the type I receptor kinase domain by transphosphorylation of a type I receptor exclusive membrane-proximal glycine/serine-rich region, termed GS-box (Shi & Massague, 2003). This phosphorylation unleashes the binding site for a group of transcription factors called SMADs whose naming derives from their homology to *Drosophila's* mothers against decapentaplegic (MAD) and the *C. elegans* protein Sma (Derynck *et al.*, 1996). Dependent on the nature of the type I receptor present in the TGF-β ligand-receptor signaling complex R-SMAD proteins (for receptor-regulated SMADs) either belonging to the so-called SMAD1/5/8 or the SMAD2/3 family become phosphorylated. Subsequently, the so activated SMAD1/5/8 or SMAD2/3 proteins form heteromeric SMAD complexes comprising one R-SMAD of either of the aforementioned subfamilies and the common mediator SMAD protein SMAD4. This heteromeric SMAD complex then translocates into the nucleus where it regulates gene transcription by functioning as a transcription or co-transcription factor (see Fig. 1) (Heldin *et al.*, 1997, Miyazono, 2000, Massague *et al.*, 2005).

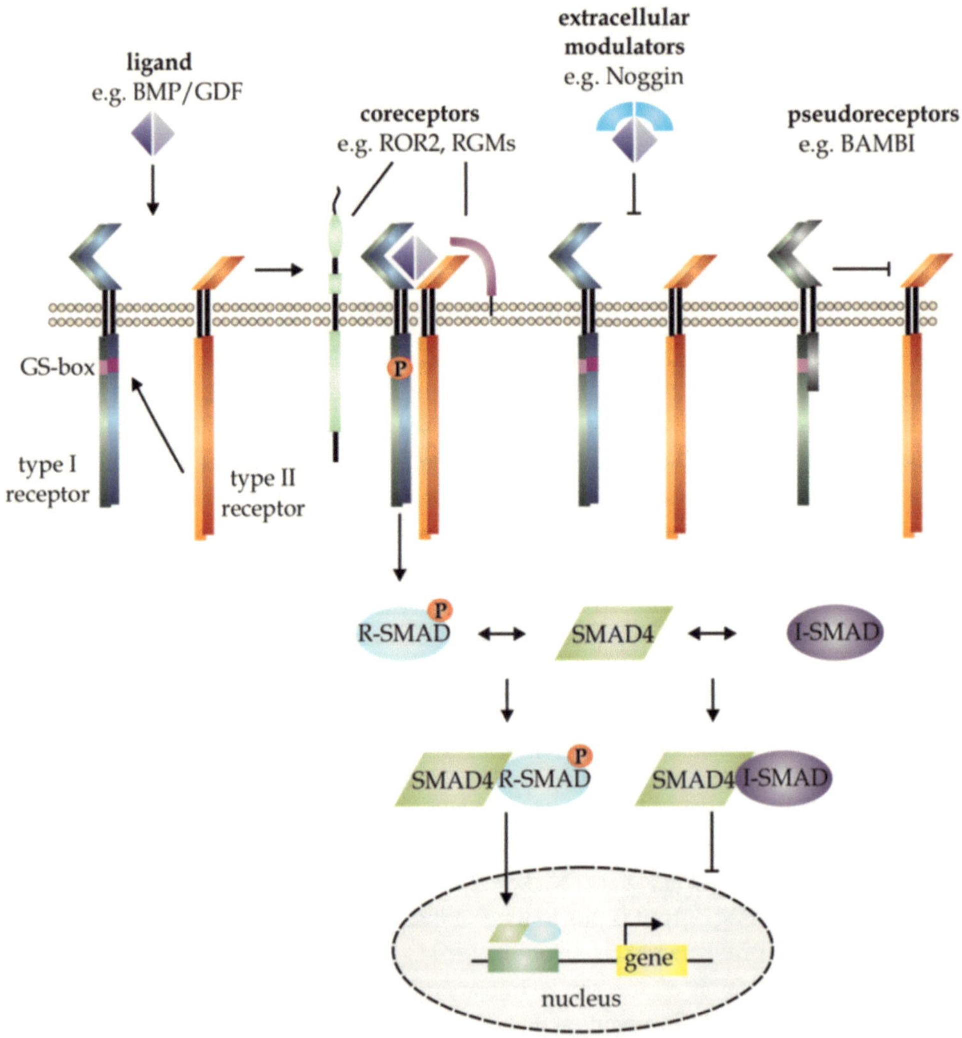

Figure 1. Signal transduction of BMPs and GDFs. Signal transduction is initiated by binding of the dimeric ligand to two types of transmembrane serine-/threonine kinase receptors termed type I and type II. Upon ligand binding the receptor chains oligomerize and the type II receptor transphosphorylates the type I receptor at the so-called GS-box thereby activating the kinase domain. Consequently, intracellular

downstream signaling components termed receptor-regulated SMADs (R-SMADs) are activated by phosphorylation. These R-SMADs then oligomerize with the common mediator SMAD (co-SMAD), SMAD4, translocate into the nucleus and in concert with other transcriptional modulators regulate target gene transcription. Regulation of this signaling pathway can occur at multiple levels as indicated. Thus, extracellular signaling modulators (e.g. Noggin, Follistatin) can bind to BMP/GDF ligands thereby preventing the interaction with their signaling receptors. On the membrane level coreceptors like ROR2 or members of the repulsive guidance molecule (RGM) family are thought to interact with the receptors and/or the ligands thereby amplifying the BMP/GDF signal. On the contrary, the pseudoreceptor BAMBI is an inhibitor of BMP as well as Activin signaling. The extracellular domain resembles the ligand binding interface of the type I receptors, while an intracellular kinase domain is lacking. The inhibitory function of the pseudoreceptor is potentially due to the formation of complexes with type I and/or type II receptors, thereby interfering with regular signal transduction. Amongst others, signal transduction can also be modulated intracellularly by the so-called inhibitory SMADs (I-SMADs), SMAD6 and SMAD7, where the I-SMADs compete with activated R-SMADs for interaction with SMAD4.

1.1. The multitude of biological functions of TGF-β members is established by a highly complex regulatory "cross-reactive" signaling network

Analysis of the patterning function of TGF-β members showed that they act as classical morphogens, i.e. the factors form a concentration gradient across the developing tissue and a specific cellular response is triggered dependent on the morphogen concentration (for review see (Wu & Hill, 2009)). A precise morphogenic function of an individual ligand can therefore only be explained in that either distinct tempero- and/or spatial distribution patterns of this ligand and its respective receptor(s) exist, which provide for specific signals at individual sites of action or in that the signaling event is tightly controlled by additional regulatory mechanisms. In the past years various studies identified a multitude of different components modulating the signal transduction of TGF-β members either outside the cell through secreted antagonists/modulator proteins (Ueno *et al.*, 1987, Smith & Harland, 1992, Francois *et al.*, 1994, Merino *et al.*, 1999b, Shimmi & O'Connor, 2003), at the cell surface level via activating coreceptors or deactivating pseudoreceptors or extracellular matrix components (Lopez-Casillas *et al.*, 1993, Onichtchouk *et al.*, 1999, Gray *et al.*, 2002, Wiater & Vale, 2003, Babitt *et al.*, 2005, Samad *et al.*, 2005, Lin *et al.*, 2007), or in the cell interior through proteins interacting with the receptors, SMAD components or via influencing receptor turnover or degradation (see Fig. 1) (Zhu *et al.*, 1999, Wotton & Massague, 2001, Chen *et al.*, 2006). The majority of these modulating mechanisms again involve proteins, which themselves exhibit promiscuous binding to several partners, thus resulting in a highly complex regulatory "cross-reactive" network. It thus seems logical that attempts or incidents, which *in vitro* seem to manipulate individual interactions by a defined mechanism, will *in vivo* inevitably lead to a massive intervention in an interweaved signaling network with established equilibrium of cross-interacting partners.

1.2. What can be learned from individual gene deletions?

Due to the morphogen's inherent coupling of ligand concentration and signaling activity it is therefore expected, that mutations causing an alteration in signaling capacities become visible in a broad variety of different phenotypes. Consistently, a vast number of mutations could be correlated with inherited diseases (see OMIM database). Although often a clear correlation between mutation and phenotype can be drawn, in most of the cases the molecular mechanism translating the individual mutation into the corresponding phenotype remains unclear. An alternative strategy to identify functions of individual signaling components in the above-described signaling network is to eliminate their signaling input or function by null mutations. In the past decades a large number of knockout mice have been generated (TGF-β ligands, receptors, modulator proteins, etc.) and the loss of individual or combinations of genes of the TGF-β signaling network were analyzed in detail in hetero- as well as in homozygous situations (Zhao, 2003). Surprisingly, given the importance of TGF-β members for embryonic development and organogenesis, deletion of some genes of this superfamily did not result in prominent phenotypes (e.g. BMP-6) indicating that others can maximally compensate for a loss of these signaling components. On the other extreme some individual gene deletion resulted in embryonic lethality (e.g. BMP-2 or BMPR-IA) indicating that these components might occupy invariable key signaling positions, but thereby also impeding a detailed elucidation of gene function during development. In these situations, gene function was often further analyzed using conditional knockout mice to overcome lethality or to allow a cell- or tissue-specific deletion of the target gene to study the gene function in a more restricted environment. For some of the genes investigated it could be demonstrated, that a multitude of biological functions are strongly connected to the presence of one gene product in a strict temporal and spatial manner. For instance, it could be demonstrated for the receptor BMPR-IA that this receptor is essential for the formation of mesoderm during embryogenesis, (Mishina *et al.*, 1995) but also for the differentiation and proliferation in postnatal hair follicles (Andl *et al.*, 2004). However, these examples should emphasize the main problem of identifying individual relations between the factors and their biological function in such regulatory signaling networks. For the analysis of such mutation/function relations it is essential that a particular mutation translates into a visible phenotype and that this mutation does not result in embryonic lethality.

2. The role of GDFs in limb development

Astonishingly, within the complex machinery of TGF-β signaling only a few components seem to fulfill these criteria and for those a collection of mutations have been identified in the past years. One of these genes encodes for growth and differentiation factor 5 (GDF-5), which – like the other members of the TGF-β superfamily – binds as secreted signaling molecule to a defined subset of type I and type II receptors and initiates the activation of downstream signaling cascades. The biological role of GDF-5 *in vivo* became first apparent from the genetic analysis of the *brachypodism* mice (*bp*) (Storm *et al.*, 1994), which also finally led to the discovery of GDF-5, -6 and -7. In *brachypodism* mice length and number of bones in the limbs are altered, but the axial skeleton does not seem to be affected (Gruneberg & Lee, 1973). It has already been suggested in the early 1980's that the *bp* mutation very likely disrupts a signaling event, which naturally leads to mesenchyme aggregation and chondrogenesis in the limb (Owens & Solursh, 1982). Initially three independent *bp* mutations have been described, which were all mapped to the *GDF5* locus on chromosome 2 all resulting in a frame-shift of the open reading frame and thus basically representing *GDF5* null mutations (Storm *et al.*, 1994). As a result of the *bp* mutations several long bones show reduced length and the first two phalanges in the digits II-V are replaced by a single bony element in all four extremities (Gruneberg & Lee, 1973). It is important to note that despite *GDF5* mRNA expression was reported to occur in a variety of non-skeletal tissues, e.g. the uterus, placenta, brain, heart, lung, kidney, etc., *bp* mice are fertile and do neither show behavioral abnormalities nor do they exhibit any morphological changes outside a few defined limb elements.

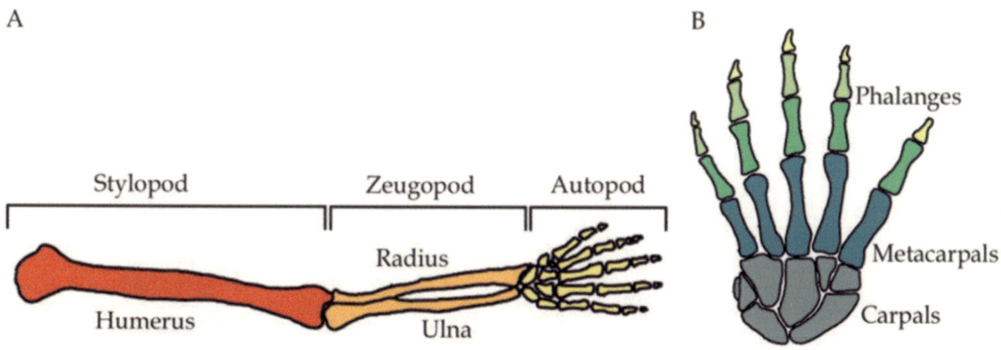

Figure 2. Schematic representation of the skeletal elements of a human limb and autopod.
A) Skeletal elements of a human limb. The stylopod gives rise to the humerus, the most proximal element of the limb skeleton, followed by the bony elements of radius and ulna, which derive from the zeugopod. Most distally, the autopod forms the bones of the hand.
B) Representation of the bony elements of the human autopod subdivided into the bones of the wrist (carpals), palm (metacarpals) and digits (phalanges).

The elements of the vertebrate limb originate from mesenchymal cells that first condense and subsequently initiate a differentiation program leading to the production of cartilage and bones in a highly defined fashion. These skeletal elements develop from single condensations in a proximal-to-distal sequence, which first grow and then branch and segment starting with the condensation forming the humerus at 10.5 days post coitus (dpc) (Wanek *et al.*, 1989, Storm & Kingsley, 1996, Francis-West *et al.*, 1999). The humerus aggregate then branches distally at 11.5 dpc thereby forming the condensations for the radius and the ulna (for nomenclature see Fig. 2). The digits develop as continuous structures called digital rays, which lengthen distally during further outgrowth. In order to build regular hands or feet the rays will then (13.5 - 15.5 dpc) be further separated in a sequential segmentation process to form the metacarpals and the phalanges. In mice *GDF5* mRNA is first detectable in the developing forelimb at 11.5 dpc in the proximal and distal region that will later form the shoulder and the elbow (Storm & Kingsley, 1996, Francis-West *et al.*, 1999). At 12.5 dpc GDF-5 is additionally expressed within the developing digital ray at a site that likely forms the future joint between the metacarpals and proximal phalanges. One day later at 13.5 dpc *GDF5* mRNA is expressed in the developing rows of carpals and in an additional stripe across the digital rays, with the sites coinciding with developing joints in the wrist and the first interphalangeal joint (Storm & Kingsley, 1996). At 14.5 dpc the segmentation process seems completed, an additional stripe of GDF-5 expression separates the developing intermediate and distal phalanges and now all elements of a mice forelimb are defined and undergo chondrogenesis (Fig. 3) (Storm & Kingsley, 1996).

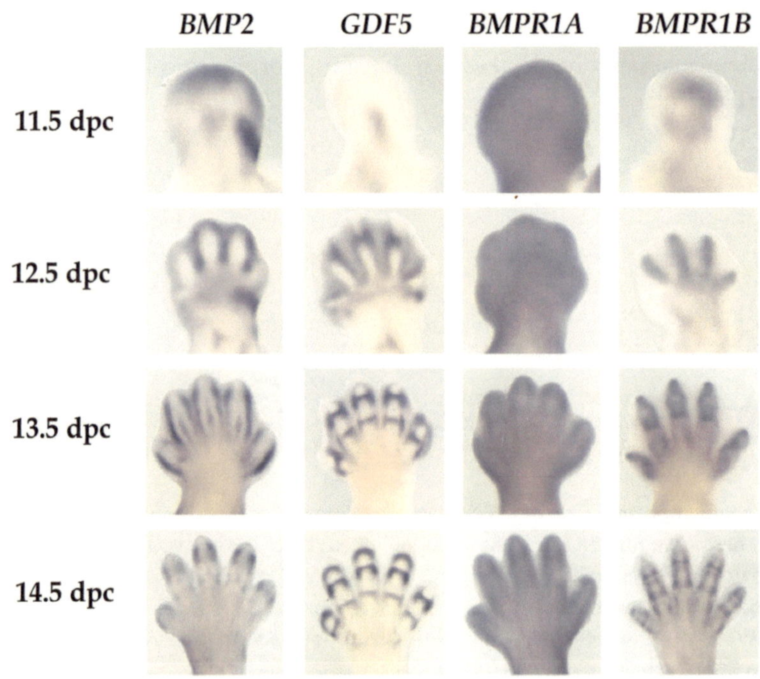

Figure 3. Expression pattern of *BMP2*, *GDF5*, *BMPR1A* and *BMPR1B* in the developing mouse fore limb.
Whole-mount in situ hybridization of *BMP2*, *GDF5* and their receptors *BMPR1A* and *BMPR1B* in a mouse fore limb at different embryonic stages. *GDF5* expression marks the developing cellular condensations. At 11.5 dpc *GDF5* is expressed in regions later forming shoulder and elbow. At 12.5 dpc *GDF5* is additionally visible in the future joints between the metacarpals and proximal phalanges. Later it is expressed in a stripe of the digital ray corresponding to the future interphalangeal joints separating the proximal from the intermediate (13.5 dpc) and the intermediate from the distal phalanges (14.5 dpc). *BMP2* expression is seen in the apical ectodermal ridge, the underlying mesenchyme and at the posterior side of the limb at 11.5 dpc. One day later, *BMP2* expression is mainly restricted to the interdigital mesenchyme as well as to the posterior wrist forming region, the wrist and the distal joints of radius and ulna. At 13.5 dpc *BMP2* expression can be localized to a region surrounding the cartilage condensations of the dorsal tendons, whereas at 14.5 dpc it is mainly found around the regions of future interphalangeal joints. *BMPR1A* shows a more or less uniform expression throughout the whole developing mouse limb at all stages depicted above. In contrast, *BMPR1B* expression at 11.5 dpc is restricted to developing condensations of the digit anlagen. Later, at 13.5 dpc 14.5 dpc, *BMPR1B* expression can be found in regions of the future interphalangeal joints.
Reprinted from The American Journal of Human Genetics (2009) *84*, 483-492, K. Dathe et al., "Duplications involving a conserved regulatory element downstream of *BMP2* are associated with Brachydactyly type A2", Copyright 2011, with permission from Elsevier.

The full process of joint formation occurs in three steps: First, special regions with high cell densities so-called interzones are formed corresponding to the stripes across the developing cartilage elements. Second, apoptosis leads to the removal of cells in the center of this interzone. Together with changes in the extracellular matrix on neighboring cells this creates a three-layered structure characteristic for the developing joint. Third, at both extremes of the interzone differentiation of the articular cartilage takes place leading to a fluid-filled gap between the (now segmented) skeletal elements (Haines, 1947, Mitrovic, 1978, Craig *et al.*, 1987). The above observations highlight GDF-5 as one of the earliest markers for joint formation, whose mRNA can be detected in the developing joint 24 to 36h prior to visible morphological changes in the interzone and its expression continues for 2 to 3 days (for details see Fig. 4). The reduction of the number of phalanges in the *brachypodism* mouse, which is basically a *GDF5* knockout mouse, is likely due to a failure in the segmentation in the digital rays (Storm *et al.*, 1994). In *bp* mice limb-bud development as well as the condensations for the initial digital rays seem normal, but during segmentation of the digital rays during 12.5 to 14.5 dpc the formation of an interzone leading to the separation of proximal and intermediate phalanges is absent in *bp* mice. However, as GDF-5 is expressed in all synovial joints in wildtype mice and not just in the first interphalangeal joints of digits II to V it seems apparent that GDF-5 cannot be the sole factor for the formation of all joints in the whole limb (Storm & Kingsley, 1996). Without knowing the nature and molecular functions of GDF-5 Hinchliffe and Johnson in 1980 already suggested that the *brachypodism* phenotype might be caused by the disruption of a **pattern** (of various factors) that determines the location of joints in the limb (Hinchliffe & Johnson, 1980). As GDF-5 shares between 80 and 86% amino acid sequence identity in its C-terminal mature part with GDF-6 and GDF-7 and the latter factors are also expressed during limb development it seemed logical to assume that these factors might compensate for the loss of *GDF5* in the *brachypodism* mutations (Storm & Kingsley, 1996). This hypothesis whether the two GDF-5 family members GDF-6 and GDF-7 can either substitute in case of a loss of *GDF5* or act in a synergistic manner was again tested by generating knockout animal models.

Both genes *GDF6* and *GDF7* are expressed in and around the developing joint (Hattersley *et al.*, 1995, Wolfman *et al.*, 1995), furthermore the mRNA expression pattern does not strictly overlap with that of *GDF5* (Wolfman *et al.*, 1997). Strong mRNA levels of *GDF6* can be observed in elbow and the carpal joints as well as the perimeter of the digital ray, whereas *GDF7* expression is restricted to the proximal interphalangeal joint (Settle *et al.*, 2003). Indeed, studies on *GDF6* knockout mice show fusions in joints different from those seen in the *brachypodism* mice - in *GDF6*$^{-/-}$ mice fusions of specific bones in the wrist and ankle correlate with the strongest *GDF6* expression in wildtype mice - possibly suggesting that a particular member of the GDF-5/6/7 family might be responsible for the formation of a subset of joints in the limb system (Settle *et al.*, 2003). Expression analysis using other joint markers such as *GDF5* (Storm & Kingsley, 1996), *PTHRP* (Parathyroid hormone-related protein, (Lanske *et al.*, 1996, Vortkamp *et al.*, 1996)) or *DELTAEF1* (a zinc-finger homeobox transcription factor, (Takagi *et al.*, 1998)) shows that the earliest stages of joint formation also occur in the absence of *GDF6* expression, but similar to the *brachypodism* mutations these morphological changes do not proceed and thus segmentation of these skeletal elements is

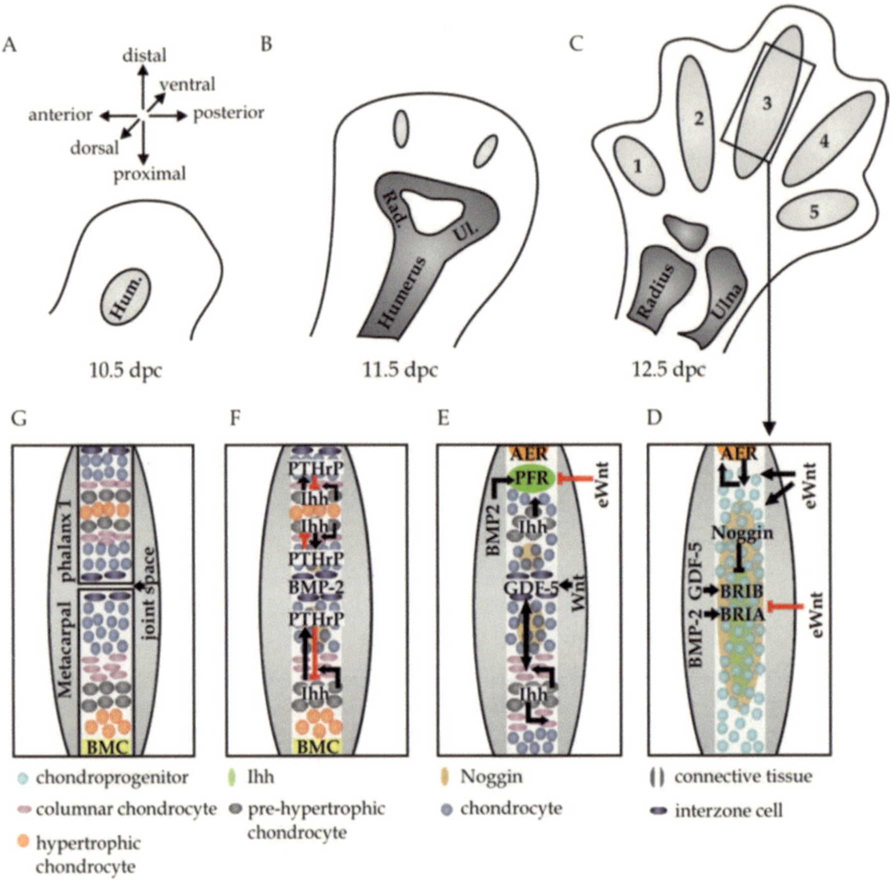

Figure 4. Schematic representation of limb bud outgrowth and determination of digit identities. A-C) Limb bud outgrowth. During limb bud initiation morphogen gradients determine the three main axes of the limb: proximo-distal, antero-posterior and dorso-ventral. Development of these gradients is under control of specific signaling centers such as the apical ectodermal ridge (AER) providing a proximo-distal gradient, the zone of polarizing activity (ZPA) producing an anterior-posterior gradient and the dorsal and ventral ectoderm establishing a dorso-ventral signal, thereby generating a morphogenic field inheriting the information for skeletal pattern formation (for review see Tickle, 2003 & 2006; Zeller, 2009). Skeletal elements of the vertebrate limb originate from mesenchymal cells that condense to form the cartilage anlagen, which develop in a proximo-to-distal manner starting with the condensation forming the humerus at 10.5 dpc. The humerus aggregate then branches distally at 11.5 dpc thereby forming the condensations of radius and ulna. The digits develop as continuous structures termed digital rays, which lengthen distally during further outgrowth. In order to build regular hands the rays will then (13.5 - 15.5 dpc) be further separated in a sequential segmentation process to form the metacarpals and the phalanges. D) Formation of the initial condensation in the human autopod. Distal mesenchymal cells under control of fibroblast growth factors (FGFs) derived from the AER and ectodermal Wnts (eWnts) remain in an undifferentiated, proliferative state. As cells escape from AER signaling they start to differentiate into prechondrogenic cells and later into chondrocytes, whereas chondrogenesis is negatively regulated by eWnt/β-catenin signaling. Mesodermally derived BMPs as well as GDF-5 positively influence differentiation by signaling via type I receptors BMPR-IA and BMPR-IB expressed in the chondrogenic precursor cells. E) Elongation and segmentation of the digit

condensations. Directed outgrowth of the condensations is achieved by BMP signaling in a region termed phalanx-forming region (PFR). This process is negatively regulated by eWnt signaling. Within the condensation pre-hypertrophic chondrocytes arise expressing Ihh, which positively influences PFR located BMP signaling. At the side of the future joint locally acting Wnt signals derived from the surrounding mesenchyme induce the differentiation of chondroprogenitor cells into flatened interzone cells expressing GDF-5. This process is encouraged by Ihh signaling from pre-hypertrophic condrocytes. Furthermore, GDF-5 and Ihh positively influence proliferation of columnar chondrocytes. F-G) Cavitation of the joint and growth of the digit. Ihh induces parathyroid hormone-related peptide (PTHrP) expressed in proliferative columnar chondrocytes underneath the future joint. PTHrP itself is a negative regulator of Ihh expression, thereby forming a negative feedback loop with Ihh. Interzone cells express BMP-2, which has a role in regulating apoptosis of these cells, thereby forming the joint cavity. The establishment of the so-called growth plate initiates further growth of the digit. This region is composed of zones of progressively differentiated chondrocytes: proliferating, columnar chondrocytes, followed by pre-hypertrophic chondrocytes expressing Ihh and finally hypertrophic chondrocytes eventually undergoing apoptosis thereby giving rise to the formation of the bone marrow cavity (BMC).

halted (Settle *et al.*, 2003). In contrast to *GDF5*$^{-/-}$ mice, which had fusions restricted to synovial joint, *GDF6*$^{-/-}$ mutants also showed defects in the cartilage and ligament structures of the middle ear and the coronal suture (a non-synovial joint) in the skull (Settle *et al.*, 2003). Analysis of the *GDF5/GDF6* double knockout mouse showed additional skeletal defects with many bones being strongly reduced in length or even being absent. As these defects are not observed in either one of the single knockout mice and are also observed in synovial joints outside the limbs it suggests that GDF-5 and GDF-6 act synergistically during the formation of specific joints (Settle *et al.*, 2003).

For GDF-7 function the effects in *GDF7*$^{-/-}$ mice are subtler and no changes in the skeletal patterning have been observed (Settle *et al.*, 2001). The phenotypes described comprise abnormal vesicle development in male mice (Settle *et al.*, 2001), smaller cross-sectional diameter of various long bones (Maloul *et al.*, 2006) and minor differences in tendon and ligament structures (Mikic *et al.*, 2006). A possible explanation for the very mild phenotype seen in *GDF7*$^{-/-}$ mice might be due to the upregulation of *GDF5* and *GDF6* mRNA expression above levels seen in wildtype mice leading to a partial compensation in the absence of *GDF7* (Mikic *et al.*, 2006). The above-described effects seen upon single or double deletion of GDF members indeed underline that GDF-5 alone, despite its patterning structure throughout the skeleton, does not induce the joint forming process in all joints of the developing limb. Moreover, it rather acts only on specific joints or might address additional ones throughout the limb in combination with GDF-6 or other factors (possibly in varying ratios) giving rise to the hypothesis that additional morphogens, e.g. members of the BMP superfamily, contribute to joint formation *in vivo*.

This idea that GDF-5 possibly acts via a defined combination with other factors to induce and maintain joint formation is supported by overexpression studies applying either locally ectopically GDF-5 protein (Storm & Kingsley, 1999) or by expressing GDF-5 systemically via retroviral transfection (Francis-West *et al.*, 1999). Interestingly, implantation of agarose beads soaked with recombinant GDF-5 into the limbs of chicken embryos did not lead to the development of additional ectopic joints. Instead, GDF-5 stimulated cartilage growth of existing cartilage, which - dependent on the location of the implantation - could even interfere with joint development (Storm & Kingsley, 1999). Studies using developing limbs of mice show similar results, implanting recombinant GDF-5 in hind limbs at 12.5 or 13.5 dpc showed that GDF-5 stimulated growth of currently present cartilage cells whereas the interdigital mesenchyme did not respond to GDF-5 treatment after 12.5 dpc. This different response of both cell types could also be seen when different cartilage differentiation markers such as Collagen2 and Indian hedgehog *(IHH)* were analyzed with both markers being induced upon GDF-5 treatment in the existing cartilage but not in the interdigital mesenchymal cells (Storm & Kingsley, 1999). This suggests that the different cells present in the developing joints lose their GDF-5 responsiveness at different times. GDF-5 can thus be considered as a pro-chondrogenic factor that acts in a stage-dependent manner and is required but not sufficient for joint formation.

3. Disorders in limb development

A group of skeletal malformation diseases observed in humans, i.e. brachydactyly, symphalangism and chondrodysplasia, exhibits similar limb deforming phenotypes as observed in *brachypodism* mice suggesting that similar mechanisms and factors are affected in humans (for review see (Temtamy & Aglan, 2008, Mundlos, 2009)). All phenotypes describe skeletal malformations of extremities – especially of the phalanges – caused by abnormalities in cartilage development. Typically all the brachydactyly-causing mutations affect the formation of synovial joints due to a deregulation of chondrocyte proliferation and/or differentiation. The classification of the different diseases has initially been done by examining the skeletal malformation phenotype (Bell, 1951). Genetic analyses later revealed disease-causing mutations not only in GDF-5, but also in other TGF-β ligands, receptors or modulator proteins as well as in other differentiation factors. Nowadays the different brachydactyly phenotypes are classified into eight different forms (BDA1-3, BDB1-2, BDC, BDD, BDE), which show clear differences regarding affected phalanges (see Fig. 5).

Of those the brachydactylies BDA1, BDD and BDE are caused by genes that are seemingly unrelated to the TGF-β/BMP signaling pathway. In BDA1, which is characterized by shortened intermediate digits in all phalanges, inactivating mutations in the gene encoding for the secreted morphogen of the Hedgehog family Indian hedgehog (*IHH)* seem to be the molecular cause (Gao *et al.*, 2001, Liu *et al.*, 2006). Indian hedgehog is regulating chondrocyte proliferation and is also required for ossification of endochondral bones (St-Jacques *et al.*, 1999, Karp *et al.*, 2000). The skeletal malformation phenotype resembles that of the *IHH*$^{-/-}$ knockout mice (St-Jacques *et al.*, 1999) and suggested that binding to the receptor Patched (PTCH) and its subsequent activation is impaired in patients suffering from BDA1. Modelling of a potential receptor interaction of IHH on the basis of the crystal structure of Sonic hedgehog bound to the hedgehog antagonist HHIP indicates that the four missense mutations at position Gly95, Asp100, Glu131 and Thr154 inactivate IHH via two different mechanisms (Bosanac *et al.*, 2009). The mutations of Gly95, Asp100 or Glu131 disrupt the conserved calcium coordination site present in hedgehog proteins, which was shown to be

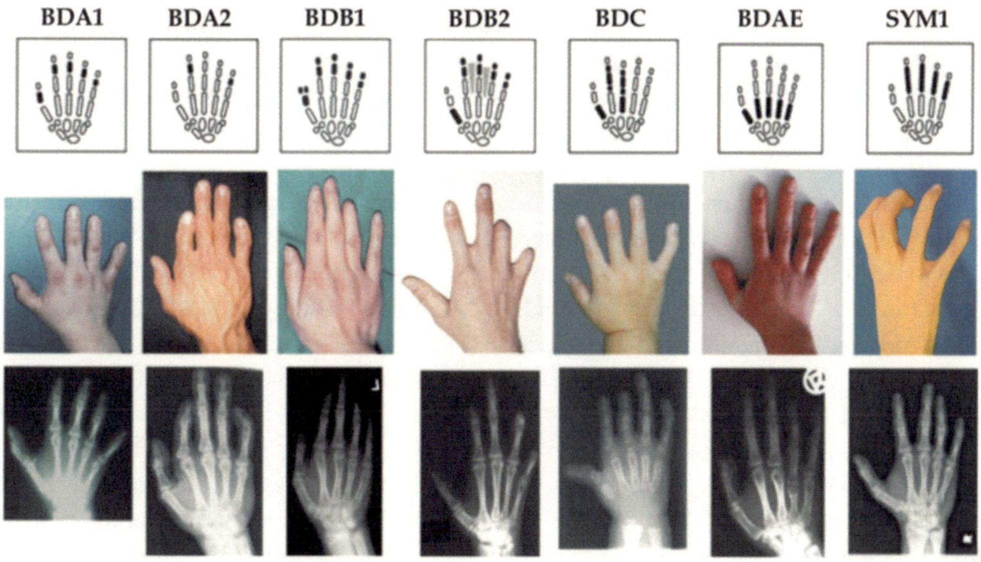

Figure 5. Clinical features of non-syndromic brachydactylies. In the top row, schematic representations of human hands depict specific phalanges and interdigital tissue affected in each skeletal malformation disease. Typical clinical features of hands are shown in the middle, corresponding X-rays underneath. Reprinted from Clinical Genetics (2009) 76, 123-136, S. Mundlos, "The brachydactylies: a molecular disease family", Copyright 2011, with permission from John Wiley and Sons.

required for high-affinity receptor binding (McLellan *et al.*, 2006, Gao *et al.*, 2009, Guo *et al.*, 2010). For the fourth mutation - T154I - identified recently no clear mechanistic explanation can be given, however based on the IHH 3D model Thr154 is located in close proximity to the other BDA1-associated missense mutations (Liu *et al.*, 2006) and thus possibly also interferes with receptor binding. Although neither IHH nor its receptors directly bind to TGF-β signaling components, BMP and IHH signals interact at various stages to regulate chondrocyte development. First of all, it has been shown that treatment of limb explants with the BMP antagonist Noggin leads to a decreased expression of *IHH* message (Minina *et al.*, 2001). Later Seki and Hata found that the *IHH* gene is a direct target of the BMP/SMAD signaling pathway due to the fact that GC-rich boxes in the promoter region of *IHH* confer binding of SMAD4 (Seki & Hata, 2004). This allows an upregulation of *IHH* expression in response to BMP signals. In the GDF-5 implantation experiments performed by Storm and Kingsley the GDF-5 dependent increase in the *IHH* mRNA message was used as a marker for chondrocyte differentiation (Storm & Kingsley, 1999). Secondly, there also seems to be a positive feedback loop as in chicken ectopic expression of IHH leads to an increased expression of BMP-2 and BMP-4 and similar results could be obtained in mice using transgenic animals in which the *IHH* gene expression is driven by a *COL2* promoter (Pathi *et al.*, 1999, Minina *et al.*, 2001). However, the effects of the deactivating IHH mutations in BDA1 are not exclusively transmitted via its direct regulatory roles on the BMP signaling pathway, besides the above described feedback loop between IHH and BMP pathways, both factors also exhibit independent functions in chondrocyte development (Minina *et al.*, 2001).

The brachydactylies BDD and BDE are characterized by a shortened distal phalanx in finger I and shortened metacarpals in fingers I to V, respectively. In both diseases mutations in the *HOXD13* gene seem to be the molecular cause (Caronia *et al.*, 2003, Johnson *et al.*, 2003). HOXD proteins represent homeobox transcription factors and disruption of the 5′ *HOXD* genes *HOXD11, HOXD12*, and *HOXD13* in mice have shown that these transcription factors exhibit important position-specific functions during limb development (Davis & Capecchi, 1996, Villavicencio-Lorini *et al.*, 2010). Two of three mutations described, I314L and Q371R seem to disrupt binding of the HOXD transcription factor to its target DNA site as deduced from structural modeling of the protein:DNA complex (Johnson *et al.*, 2003, Zhao *et al.*, 2007). Although the amino acid replacement is rather conservative, the leucine sidechain seems to introduce a steric hindrance to a neighboring pyrimidine base of the bound target DNA possibly altering the specificity for DNAs containing either a thymine or a cytosine in this sequence. For the second mutation, serine 308 to cysteine, it is difficult to deduce a molecular mechanism explaining the skeletal phenotype. Serine 308 located in the homeobox domain of HOXD13 is not in contact with the DNA and placed in a less conserved region, thus misfolding of the HOXD13 protein due to the different sidechain size and polarity of the introduced cysteine residue might explain the altered HOXD13 function. The effect of both mutations on DNA binding was however confirmed experimentally by electrophoretic mobility shift assays (EMSA) (Johnson *et al.*, 2003). Similar to BDA1 a direct regulatory or physical interaction of HOXD proteins and members of the TGF-β/BMP pathway is not apparent and thus it seems unclear at first sight whether the skeletal malformation phenotype of the HOXD13 mutants results from an independent parallel disturbed signaling pathway involved in limb development or whether HOXD13 might be an upstream or downstream target of the TGF-β/BMP signaling cascade. Suzuki *et al.* have found that both HOXA13 and HOXD13 transcription factors can enhance transcription of the *BMP4* promoter and may thus increase BMP expression (Suzuki *et al.*, 2003). Recently the group of Stefan Mundlos investigated the effect of the *HOXD11, -12, -13* and *HOXA13* genes on joint formation in mice and discovered that HOXD13 can directly bind and regulate the *RUNX2* promoter, whose activation is crucial for formation of cortical bone (Villavicencio-Lorini *et al.*, 2010). Studies using mice with defective *HOXA13* revealed that upon loss of *HOXA13* function mRNA expression for *GDF5* is downregulated, whereas mRNA for *BMP2* is upregulated (Perez *et al.*, 2010). As HOXA and HOXD proteins might form regulatory complexes, BDE initiating mutations in *HOXD13* may thus act via altering a defined concentration balance between GDF-5 and BMP-2 in the developing joint.

3.1. Disrupted GDF-5 signaling correlates with impaired joint formation

The other brachydactyly forms are caused by mutations in either *GDF5*, or other *BMP* genes, BMP receptors or modulator proteins thereby highlighting the central regulatory role of the GDF/BMP signals for proper joint formation. Mutations in the *GDF5* gene are found in brachydactylies of the type BDA1, BDA2 and BDC, but also in symphalangism and multiple synostosis syndrome phenotypes as well as in chondrodysplasias of the Grebe, Hunter-Thompson and DuPan type, which are more severe skeletal malformation diseases possibly due to the fact that in the latter syndromes the mutations in *GDF5* are homozygous or compound heterozygous (see Table 1). Mutations in the BMP type I receptor BMPR-IB as well as a duplication of an about 6kb element in the 3′ regulatory untranslated domain of the *BMP2* gene also lead to brachydactyly of the type BDA2 (Lehmann *et al.*, 2003, Lehmann *et al.*, 2006, Dathe *et al.*, 2009). Mutations in the orphan tyrosine receptor kinase ROR2, which might possibly act as a GDF-5 specific coreceptor thereby influencing receptor activation of this TGF-β member, lead to brachydactyly of the type BDB1 (Oldridge *et al.*, 2000, Schwabe *et al.*, 2000). Amino acid exchanges in the BMP modulator protein Noggin are observed in patients suffering from brachydactyly type B2 (BDB2) (Lehmann *et al.*, 2007). As there is a wealth of structural and functional data available for almost all of the above-mentioned factors a more in-depth analysis can be performed to analyze the molecular mechanism behind these disease-causing mutations.

3.2. Mutations interfering with BMPR-IB kinase activity and signaling

So far three mutations in the BMP type I receptor BMPR-IB could be correlated with brachydactyly BDA2. In the BMP/GDF signaling pathway three type I receptors, BMPR-IA (Alk3), BMPR-IB (Alk6) and ActR-I (Alk2) can be addressed by the different ligands for binding and signaling (Sebald *et al.*, 2004). *In vitro* interaction analyses show that GDF-5 can bind only to BMPR-IA and BMPR-IB with affinities in the nano-molar range (Nickel *et al.*, 2005), whereas it shows no measureable interaction with the type I receptor ActR-I (Heinecke *et al.*, 2009). These and other *in vitro* studies also showed that GDF-5 interacts preferentially with BMPR-IB exhibiting a 10 to 15-fold higher affinity for BMPR-IB than for BMPR-IA (Nickel *et al.*, 2005, Heinecke *et al.*, 2009). Furthermore, performing a more *in vivo*-like radioligand binding assay in order to analyze the interaction of radiolabeled GDF-5 via chemical crosslinking to cells that were either transfected with the different type I and type II receptors or endogenously express BMP receptors, an exclusive binding of GDF-5 to BMPR-IB could be detected (Nishitoh *et al.*, 1996). Despite this rather strong binding specificity of GDF-5 to BMPR-IB on whole cells measuring transcriptional activation in mink lung cells transfected with different combinations of BMP type I and type II receptors showed that GDF-5 can activate SMAD signaling via BMPR-IB **and** BMPR-IA with almost identical efficiency (Nishitoh *et al.*, 1996). However, BMPR-IA cannot substitute for BMPR-IB in all GDF-5 initiated signals, e.g. induction of the osteogenic marker alkaline phosphatase (ALP) by GDF-5 is observed in the murine pro-chondrogenic cell line ATDC5, which does not express BMPR-IB and thus in this case BMPR-IA can functionally replace BMPR-IB. Furthermore, in this cell line the concentration for half-maximal ALP induction is about 10-fold lower than for BMP-2, which correlates very nicely with the difference in BMPR-IA affinity of both BMP factors (Nickel *et al.*, 2005). In contrast, the mouse osteoblastic cell line MC3T3 or the mouse myoblastic cell line C2C12, which express BMPR-IA but not BMPR-IB, do not respond to GDF-5 in the alkaline phosphatase expression assay (but at the same time respond to BMP-2) (Nishitoh *et al.*, 1996). Besides the fact that in the context of the developing joint BMPR-IA might not be the correct signaling receptor for GDF-5, the spatially highly defined expression pattern of GDF-5 and the two BMP type I receptors in the junction between the growth plate and the developing joint suggests that at sites of high GDF-5 concentration only BMPR-IB is highly expressed whereas BMPR-IA expression is rather low (see Fig. 3) ((Wolfman *et al.*, 1997, Zou *et al.*, 1997, Sakou *et al.*, 1999, Storm & Kingsley, 1999, Yi *et al.*, 2001, Settle *et al.*, 2003, Minina *et al.*, 2005) for review see (Pogue & Lyons, 2006)).

All BDA2 causing BMPR-IB mutations are located in the cytoplasmic kinase domain. One exchange - isoleucine 200 to lysine (I200K) - is placed within the so-called GS (glycine/serine-rich) box, which is phosphorylated upon ligand binding and hetero-oligomerization of the type I and type II receptors (see Fig. 6A-C). Structural analysis of the kinase domains of the

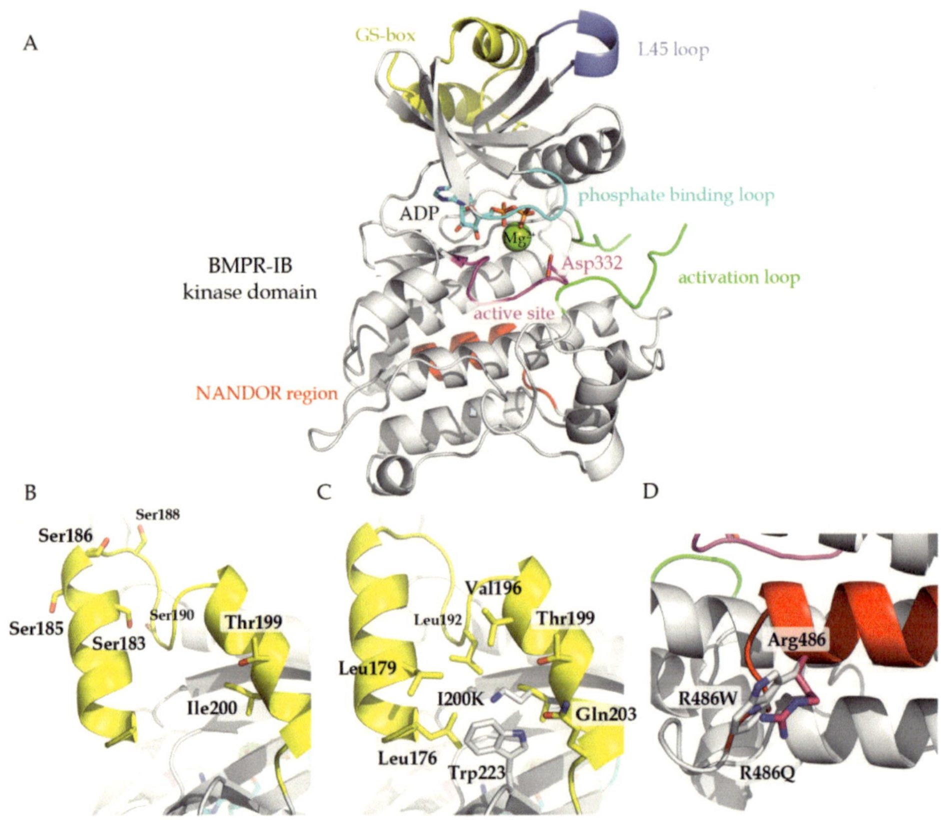

Figure 6. The kinase domain of the BMP receptor IB. A) Ribbon representation of a model of the BMPR-IB kinase domain (adapted from PDB entry 3MDY, (Chaikuad *et al.*, 2010a)). The elements important in kinase activity and or BMP signaling are indicated. Glycine/serine-rich (GS-)box: yellow; L45-loop for SMAD subgroup specificity: purple; phosphate binding loop: cyan; activation loop: green; active site with Asp332 in stick representation: magenta; NANDOR-region regulation downstream signal activation: red. B) Magnification of the GS-box with the relevant serine and threonine residues that become phosphorylated during BMP type I receptor activation shown as sticks. The location of Ile200 mutated in BDA2 is indicated. C) Isoleucine 200, mutated to lysine in BDA2, is surrounded by hydrophobic residues. Threonine 199, which is required to become first phosphorylated to allow for further phosphorylation events in the GS-box, is located in close proximity, suggesting that mutation

I200K might also act via abrogating the initial activating phosphorylation at Thr199. D) Magnification into the NANDOR domain of BMPR-IB. The mutated residue Arg486 is located at the solvent-accessible surface, thus mutations R486W and R486Q (shown in grey) very likely do not cause conformational alterations. This suggests that the NANDOR domain constitutes a binding interface for so far unknown proteins involved in the receptor activation.

BMP receptor BMPR-IB (PDB entry 3MDY, (Chaikuad *et al.*, 2010a)), of the TGF-β receptor TGFβR-I (Huse *et al.*, 1999) or the Activin type I receptor ActR-I (PDB entry 3H9R, (Chaikuad *et al.*, 2010b)) show that the GS-box domain in the inactivated state consists of two antiparallel α-helices. Functional analysis of the TGFβR-I receptor kinase revealed that phosphorylation of all conserved serine and threonine residues in the consensus motif (T/S)SGSGSG placed in the loop between the two helices is absolutely required for downstream signaling (Wieser *et al.*, 1995) and SMAD protein binding (Huse *et al.*, 2001). More importantly, threonine residue Thr200 in TGFβR-I (equivalent to Thr199 in BMPR-IB) adjacent to this consensus motif is absolutely conserved between TGF-β type I receptors and is crucial for ligand-dependent receptor activation. Mutagenesis showed that phosphorylation of this particular threonine residue is a pre-requisite for further phosphorylation of the GS-box motif located N-terminally of this residue (Wieser *et al.*, 1995). In the BDA2 associated mutation I200K in BMPR-IB the direct neighbor of Thr199 is exchanged from a hydrophobic isoleucine to a polar lysine residue. As the isoleucine is rather buried in this motif, the exchange might lead to local unfolding or the Ile to Lys substitution is such drastic that the recognition by the kinase responsible for phosphorylation of Thr199 and thus subsequent receptor activation is impeded (see Fig. 6A-C). *In vitro* kinase assays indeed revealed a complete loss of kinase activity of BMPR-IB carrying the I200K mutation (Lehmann *et al.*, 2003).

The other mutations in BMPR-IB associated with BDA2, R486Q or R486W, are located in the so-called NANDOR region (for non-activating non-down-regulating) (see Fig. 6A/D). This region at the C-terminus of the kinase domain is highly conserved between TGF-β type I receptors but placed quite distantly from the regulatory important regions such as the GS-box or the L45-loop, which mediate binding to R-SMAD proteins upon receptor activation or the active site of the kinase domain. Studies on the TGF-β receptors TGFβR-I (Garamszegi *et al.*, 2001) and TSR-I (Alk1) (Ricard *et al.*, 2010) show that mutations within this domain abrogate type I receptor endocytosis and signal transduction as R-SMAD proteins are not phosphorylated by these receptor mutants. In BMPR-IB the exchange of the surface-accessible arginine 486 by either glutamine or tryptophan diminished not only SMAD1/5/8 phosphorylation, but also led to strongly decreased expression of alkaline phosphatase in C2C12 cells transfected with BMPR-IB. This signaling-impaired phenotype could also be confirmed in a more physiological assay measuring chondrocyte differentiation in virally transduced chicken limb-bud micromass cultures (Lehmann *et al.*, 2003, Lehmann *et al.*, 2006). The effects of these mutations on downstream SMAD-dependent and SMAD independent signaling pathways as well as receptor endocytosis suggests that this region likely constitutes a binding site for not yet identified signaling components required for general receptor activation.

Skeletal malformation diseases have also been linked to mutations in the BMP signaling modulator Noggin, which directly binds to various BMP as well as GDF ligands and, when harboring mutations interfering with ligand binding, can cause skeletal malformations of the brachydactyly type. Noggin initially identified as a dorsalizing factor expressed in the Spemann organizer (Smith & Harland, 1992) was found to be an efficient BMP antagonist, which - by binding to the BMP ligands in the extracellular space with extremely high affinity in the picomolar range - can completely abrogate receptor binding and thus BMP signaling (Holley *et al.*, 1996, Zimmerman *et al.*, 1996). Despite its role in establishing a long-range BMP-4 morphogen gradient for dorsal-ventral patterning during gastrulation, Noggin also has functions later in development of the embryo (for a recent review see (Krause *et al.*, 2011)). Noggin knockout mice are embryonically lethal and show a complex phenotype (McMahon *et al.*, 1998), however it is important to note that mice being heterozygous for the Noggin null mutation develop normally (Brunet *et al.*, 1998). This suggests that the defects seen upon Noggin deletion do not result from gene dosage effects. Due to its expression in the ectoderm, loss of Noggin resulted in a severe neural tube phenotype with a failure of neural tube closure and a dramatic reduction in the amount of posterior neural tissue. As Noggin seems essential for ventral cell fates in the CNS development, motor neurons and ventral interneurons were lacking (McMahon *et al.*, 1998). Besides the neural abnormalities Noggin knockout mice showed also a drastically altered skeletal development (Brunet *et al.*, 1998, Tylzanowski *et al.*, 2006). All skeletal elements are affected with the severity of the axial defects increasing towards the posterior direction. However, analysis for ossification shows that the time point for ossification in these elements seems unchanged. These observations suggest that the loss of Noggin in the knockout mice affects cartilage development. The ablation of Noggin also affects limb development, with null mice having shorter limbs and fusions of various joints. By the use of a heterozygous transgene, where the Noggin gene has been replaced by *lacZ*, expression of Noggin in the developing limb could be analyzed in detail (Brunet *et al.*, 1998), showing that Noggin is strongly expressed in cartilage zones later forming bone, but is expressed at low levels or is absent in hypertrophic cartilage or joint cavities where GDF-5 expression is usually high. Analysis of the $NOG^{-/-}$ mice shows a massive overgrowth of cartilage in the limb, indicating that in wildtype mice Noggin represses the growth of these tissues in a negative feedback loop manner. It is known that in addition to GDF-5 a number of other BMPs, e.g. BMP-2, BMP-4, BMP-6 and BMP-7 are expressed in the limb and even the developing joints (Lyons *et al.*, 1989, Brunet *et al.*, 1998). Differential signaling of these different BMPs is required to induce apoptosis in interdigital tissues (Macias *et al.*, 1997) and in *Drosophila* sharp zones of activity of the fly BMP-homolog DPP, which do not necessarily correlate with the local DPP concentration, trigger local cell death to define joints (Manjon *et al.*, 2007). The locally highly variable expression of Noggin in the developing limb could provide for such a BMP activity modulating mechanism as *in vivo* Noggin inhibition of BMP signaling has distinct BMP specificity profiles (Zimmerman *et al.*, 1996, Seemann *et al.*, 2009, Song *et al.*, 2010). The important regulatory role of Noggin as an BMP antagonist is also highlighted by the fact that the Noggin gene is a mutational hotspot in several skeletal malformation diseases of the brachydactyly type BDB as well as the more severe multiple synostosis syndrome (SYNS1), proximal symphalangism (SYM1), tarsal-carpal coalition (TCC) or SABTT (stapes ankylosis with broad thumbs and toes) syndromes (for a recent review see (Potti *et al.*, 2011)).

3.3. Noggin a BMP interacting hub during limb and joint formation

Structure analysis of the complex of BMP-7 bound to Noggin provided insights into the molecular mechanism how Noggin antagonizes BMP signaling (Groppe *et al.*, 2002). The homodimeric Noggin embraces the BMP ligand and simultaneously blocks type I and type II receptor binding via its C-terminal four-stranded β-sheet structure resembling a finger-like structure as found in BMPs itself and a N-terminal peptide segment called clip (see Fig. 7). Whereas the type II receptor-binding epitope of BMP-7 is blocked by the large and structured C-terminal part, type I receptor binding is only inhibited by the small clip segment (Gln28 to Asp39 of human Noggin). Very few polar interactions, mainly between the polar main chain atoms of the Noggin clip and residues from BMP-7, stabilize this interaction. In addition to the polar interactions, Pro35 of Noggin, which is found mutated in several skeletal malformation diseases (Gong *et al.*, 1999, Dixon *et al.*, 2001, Mangino *et al.*, 2002, Lehmann *et al.*, 2007, Hirshoren *et al.*, 2008), points into a hole in the type I receptor-binding epitope of BMP-7 formed by hydrophobic residues thereby mimicking a key interaction in the BMP ligand-type I receptor interaction (Hatta *et al.*, 2000, Kirsch *et al.*, 2000, Kotzsch *et al.*, 2009).

The disease-causing mutations in Noggin known today can be clustered into three regions: the mutations located in the clip (P35A/S/R, A36P, P37R, P42A/R; (Gong *et al.*, 1999, Dixon *et al.*, 2001, Mangino *et al.*, 2002, Debeer *et al.*, 2004, Lehmann *et al.*, 2007, Hirshoren *et al.*, 2008, Oxley *et al.*, 2008)), the β-sheet domain (E48K, P42A;P50R, R167G, L203P, R204L, W205C, W217G, I220N, Y222D/C, and P223L; (Gong *et al.*, 1999, Dixon *et al.*, 2001, Takahashi *et al.*, 2001, Kosaki *et al.*, 2004, van den Ende *et al.*, 2005, Weekamp *et al.*, 2005, Dawson *et al.*, 2006, Lehmann *et al.*, 2007, Oxley *et al.*, 2008, Emery *et al.*, 2009)) or the dimerization domain (C184Y, P187S, G189C, M190V, and C232Y; (Gong *et al.*, 1999, Takahashi *et al.*, 2001, Lehmann *et al.*, 2007, Oxley *et al.*, 2008, Rudnik-Schoneborn *et al.*, 2010)). The molecular mechanisms by which these mutations disrupt proper function of Noggin can be classified in part. Mutations of prolines or from other residues to proline, e.g. P42R, P50R, P187S, L203P, or P223L, will potentially lead to misfolding of the Noggin mutant, such that local structures cannot be maintained leading to a secondary loss of other Noggin-BMP interactions or to lower dimer stability (and hence to decreased secretion) if these exchanges occur in the dimerization domain (see Fig. 7) (e.g. P187S, (Lehmann *et al.*, 2007)). Some mutations in Noggin involving proline residues and occurring in the clip region disrupt BMP-Noggin hydrogen bonds, e.g. A36P, P37R or introduce steric hindrance by replacing the proline residue for geometrically non-fitting amino acids, e.g. P35A, P35S, or P35R. Various amino acid exchanges observed in the β-sheet domain substituting a hydrophobic residue for a polar, e.g. I220N, or replacing a large hydrophobic amino acid in the hydrophobic core with a smaller one, e.g. W205C, W217G, Y222C, probably cause local unfolding and thus weaken the Noggin:BMP binding. The amino acid residues Glu48, Arg167 and Arg204 together form a hydrogen bond network, thus mutation of any of these

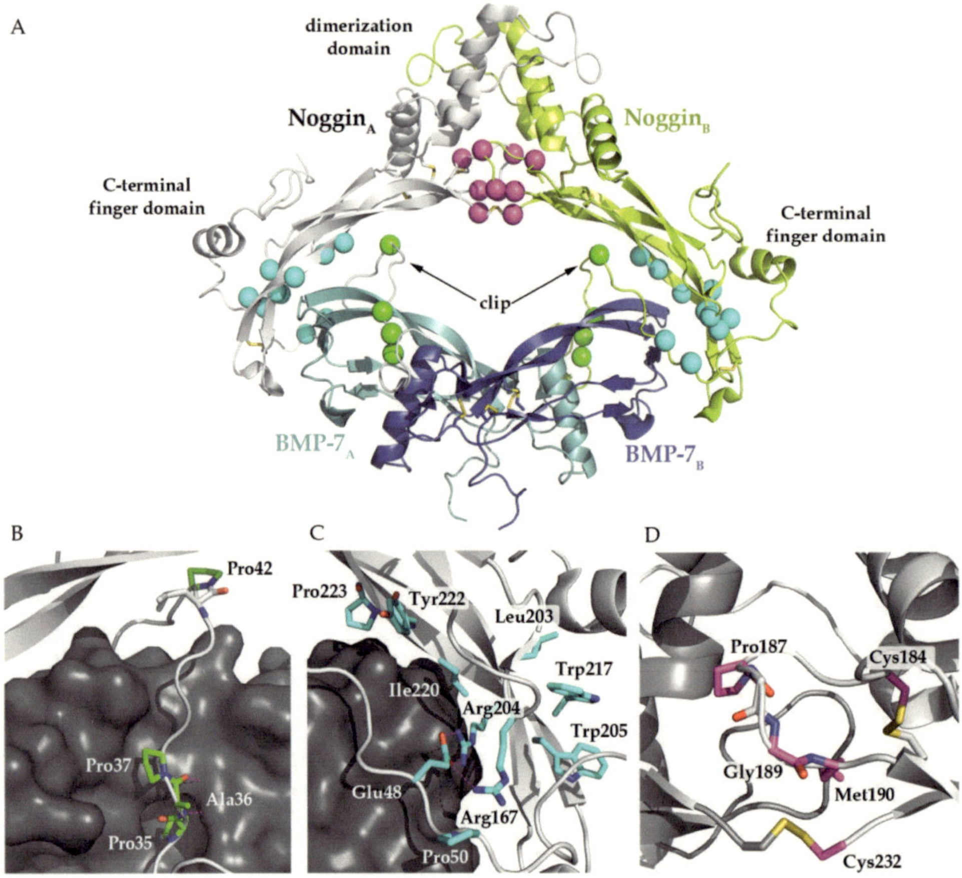

Figure 7. BMP inhibition by the modulator Noggin. A) Ribbon representation of the BMP-7:Noggin complex (PDB entry 1M4U, (Groppe *et al.*, 2002)). The dimeric Noggin (grey and light green) consists of three domains: the clip region located at the N-terminus, the C-terminal finger or β-sheet domain and a dimerization domain. By embracing the BMP ligand through the clip region and the C-terminal finger domain Noggin effectively blocks binding of type I and type II receptors thereby antagonizing BMP signaling. Mutations in Noggin identified in skeletal malformation diseases are shown as spheres color-coded according to their location in the aforementioned domains (green: clip region; cyan: finger/⊚-sheet domain; magenta: dimerization domain). B) Magnification into mutationally affected interactions between residues of the Noggin clip region and BMP-7 (shown as grey van der Waals surface representation). Mutation of the indicated residues (Pro35, Ala36, Pro37, and Pro42 are shown as stick representations with C-atoms in green) likely alters the conformation of the Noggin clip or disrupts polar interactions (indicated by stippled magenta lines) between Noggin and BMPs. C) Magnification into the interface between the Noggin finger domain and BMP-7. Residues in Noggin involved in skeletal malformation diseases upon mutation are shown as sticks (C-atoms are colored in cyan). Most mutations likely affect local folding of the finger domain thereby attenuating or disrupting Noggin binding to BMPs. D) Magnification into the dimerization domain of Noggin. Residues involved in disease-causing mutations are shown as sticks with the C-atoms colored in magenta. Mutation of most of the residues displayed will likely interfere with dimerization of Noggin, e.g. mutation of either Cys184 or Cys232 will directly disrupt the intermolecular disulfide bond or possibly shuffle the disulfide bond pattern in the dimerization domain.

three residues will disrupt this network likely causing local structure changes in the β-sheet domain of Noggin. Furthermore, all three charged residues are buried upon binding to BMP ligands, thus mutations resulting in unbalanced charges will probably lead to electrostatic repulsion upon ligand binding. The mutations in Noggin's dimerization domain, e.g. C184Y, P187S, G189C, M190V, or C232W, all will very likely disturb efficient dimerization either by disrupting the intermolecular disulfide bond through the formation of non-native intramolecular disulfide pairs or through interfering with the homodimer interface (see Fig. 7D) (Marcelino *et al.*, 2001, Lehmann *et al.*, 2007).

Interestingly, mutations in Noggin represent a rather heterogeneous picture of skeletal malformations with different digits being affected and from a mild phenotype, e.g. BDB2 to more severe traits, e.g. SYM1 or SYNS1 (Lehmann *et al.*, 2007, Potti *et al.*, 2011). A direct correlation between the location of the mutation in Noggin and the severity of the malformation seems not apparent although mutations in the clip domain are diagnosed more frequently with BDB2 and mutations in the dimerization domain usually result in SYM1 or SYNS1 disease (Potti *et al.*, 2011). From a structural point of view these possible differences might be explained due to the fact that destabilizing changes in the clip region of Noggin might affect only certain BMPs. Analysis of *in vitro* binding of BMP-7 to the Noggin mutant P35R showed a rather small 7-fold decrease in BMP binding affinity (Groppe *et al.*, 2002). For BMPs that exhibit high affinities for their type I receptors, e.g. BMP-2, BMP-4 or GDF-5 the weakened binding of the clip of Noggin to these ligands might allow for a competition mechanism in which the receptor binding to a Noggin:BMP complex subsequently strips off the antagonist. For those BMPs that have low binding affinities to their type I receptors, e.g. BMP-5, BMP-6 and BMP-7 even the decreased binding of the Noggin clip to the ligand is still sufficient to block receptor binding and hence signaling of these BMPs. The mutations in the β-sheet region of Noggin, however, should affect all BMP ligands similarly and the severity of the phenotype should principally correlate with the loss of BMP binding affinity. The amino acid substitutions in the Noggin dimerization domain are expected to exhibit the strongest phenotype as these mutations strongly affect dimerization and secretion efficiency of the Noggin protein. Even if a monomeric Noggin variant protein might be secreted, its binding to BMPs as a monomer will be severely impaired due to the loss of avidity. Thus the mutations in the clip of Noggin might only affect a subset of the different BMPs present in the developing joint thereby causing a distinct phenotype, whereas the other Noggin mutations more likely resemble the phenotype of a Noggin null mutation. With respect to the direct effect of Noggin on GDF-5 it is important to note that in mice even though the strongest expression of *GDF5* mRNA is found in the joint, Noggin mRNA here is absent at these late stages of joint development. Thus it is unclear at which timepoints the BMP antagonist Noggin directly modulates GDF-5 during joint formation *in vivo* (Brunet *et al.*, 1998). Furthermore, it has been shown that the loss of Noggin in homozygous null mice leads to a strong downregulation of the *GDF5* mRNA message (Brunet *et al.*, 1998), which would be compatible with the observed effect in loss-of-function Noggin mutants.

3.4. GDF-5: A key molecule in joint development and maintenance

Besides Noggin, the *GDF5* gene has been identified as a mutational hotspot in skeletal malformation diseases. To date, 14 missense mutations as well as a multitude of frameshift mutations have been identified in the translated region of the *GDF5* gene. Furthermore single nucleotide polymorphisms (SNPs) in the 5′ and 3′ untranslated region of the *GDF5* gene, three of which could be linked to enhanced susceptibility of developing osteoarthritis (OA), suggest that tempero-spatially highly defined gene expression of GDF-5 is required throughout life and is not limited to limb and joint development during embryogenesis (see Table 1 and Fig. 8).

Two SNPs in the 5′ untranslated regions (UTR) of *GDF5*, rs143383 and further downstream rs143384, share both a T-to-C transition in the *GDF5* core promoter. Functional studies using RNA extracted from the articular cartilage of OA patients harboring the SNP rs143383 revealed a significant, up to 27% reduced expression level of the osteoarthritis-associated T-allele relative to the C-allele, a phenomenon termed differential allelic expression (DAE) (Southam *et al.*, 2007). This allelic expression imbalance of *GDF5* could be extended to other soft tissues of the whole synovial joint, emphasizing that the single nucleotide

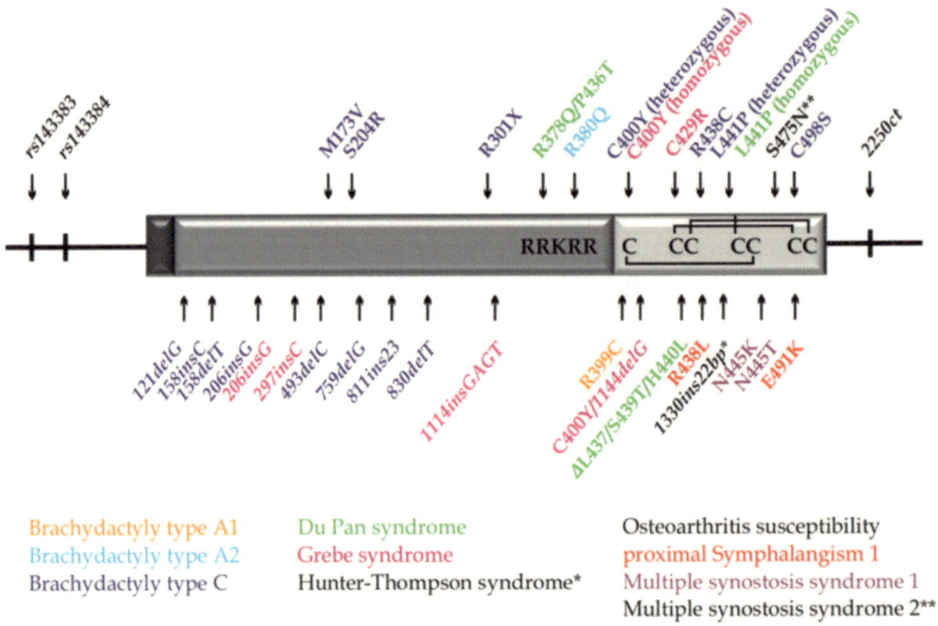

Figure 8. Localization of *GDF5* mutations. Arrowheads indicate the location of all currently known mutations linked to human skeletal malformation diseases affecting the limb. The specific inherited disease caused by each mutation is displayed in the legend underneath.
A GDF-5 monomer consists of an N-terminal signal peptide domain (black box), a prodomain (dark grey box) and the C-terminal mature part (light grey box) containing six highly conserved cysteine residues forming the cystine knot motif, whereas the seventh cysteine connects two monomers via an intermolecular disulfide bond. Italic type indicates nucleotide nomenclature; normal type represents single amino acid nomenclature. For references see Table 1.

mutation	location	hetero-/homozygous	disease	OMIM #	reference
rs143383	5´UTR *gdf5* gene	heterozygous	Osteoarthritis susceptibility	# 612400	(Miyamoto *et al.*, 2007)
rs143384	5´UTR *gdf5* gene	heterozygous	Osteoarthritis susceptibility	# 612400	(Rouault *et al.*, 2010)
2250ct	3´UTR *gdf5* gene	heterozygous	Osteoarthritis susceptibility	# 612400	(Egli *et al.*, 2009)
121delG	prodomain *gdf5* gene	heterozygous	Brachydactyly type C	# 113100	(Polinkovsky *et al.*, 1997)
158delT	prodomain *gdf5* gene	heterozygous	Brachydactyly type C	# 113100	(Everman *et al.*, 2002)
158insC	prodomain *gdf5* gene	heterozygous	Brachydactyly type C	# 113100	(Everman *et al.*, 2002)
206insG	prodomain *gdf5* gene	heterozygous	Brachydactyly type C	# 113100	(Polinkovsky *et al.*, 1997)
206insG	prodomain *gdf5* gene	homozygous	Chondrodysplasia, Grebe type	# 200700	(Stelzer *et al.*, 2003)
297insC	prodomain *gdf5* gene	homozygous	Chondrodysplasia, Grebe type	# 200700	(Faiyaz-Ul-Haque *et al.*, 2002a)
493delC	prodomain *gdf5* gene	heterozygous	Brachydactyly type C	# 113100	(Galjaard *et al.*, 2001)
M173V	prodomain *gdf5* gene	homozygous	Brachydactyly type C	# 113100	(Schwabe *et al.*, 2004)
S204R	prodomain *gdf5* gene	heterozygous	Brachydactyly type C	# 113100	(Everman *et al.*, 2002)
759delG	prodomain *gdf5* gene	heterozygous	Brachydactyly type C	# 113100	(Polinkovsky *et al.*, 1997)
811ins23	prodomain *gdf5* gene	heterozygous	Brachydactyly type C	# 113100	Everman, D. B. et al. 2002)
830delT	prodomain *gdf5* gene	heterozygous	Brachydactyly type C	# 113100	Everman, D. B. et al. 2002)
R301X	prodomain *gdf5* gene	heterozygous	Brachydactyly type C	# 113100	(Polinkovsky *et al.*, 1997)
1114insGAGT	prodomain *gdf5* gene	homozygous	Chondrodysplasia, Grebe type	# 200700	(Basit *et al.*, 2008)
R378Q/P436T	prodomain *gdf5* gene; processing site / mature domain	compound heterozygous	Acromesomelic dysplasia, DuPan syndrome	# 601146	(Douzgou *et al.*, 2008)
R380Q	prodomain *gdf5* gene; processing site	heterozygous	Brachydactyly type A2	# 112600	(Ploger *et al.*, 2008)
R399C	mature domain	heterozygous	Brachydactyly type A1	# 112500	(Byrnes *et al.*, 2010)
C400Y	mature domain; no processing/secretion	heterozygous	Brachydactyly type C	# 113100	(Thomas *et al.*, 1997)
C400Y	mature domain; no processing/secretion	homozygous	Chondrodysplasia, Grebe type	# 200700	(Thomas *et al.*, 1997)
C400Y/*del1144G*	mature domain/	compound	Chondrodysplasia,	# 200700	(Thomas *et*

	prodomain; no processing/secretion	heterozygous	Grebe type		*al.*, 1997)
mW408R (hW414R)	mature domain; location in type I receptor binding site	heterozygous	Brachypodism		(Masuya *et al.*, 2007)
mW408R (hW414R)	mature domain; location in type I receptor binding site	homozygous	severe Brachypodism, Osteoarthritis		(Masuya *et al.*, 2007)
C429R	mature domain	homozygous	Chondrodysplasia, Grebe type	# 200700	(Faiyaz-Ul-Haque *et al.*, 2008)

Table 1. Table of all known mutations in *GDF5* gene linked to skeletal malformation diseases affecting the limb. Mutations depicted in red represent single nuclear polymorphisms (SNPs) located in 5′ or 3′ regulatory regions of *GDF5* gene. Shown in black are mutations situated in the prodomain, whereas mutations in the mature part are represented in blue. Frameshift mutations are highlighted in italics, non-sense mutations are underlined.

polymorphism is not restricted to cartilage (Egli *et al.*, 2009). In addition, recent analysis showed that expression of GDF-5 could be further modulated epigenetically as both C-alleles of the SNPs rs143383 and rs143384 form CpG sites thereby explaining the intra- and inter-individual variations observed (Reynard *et al.*, 2011). A third SNP influencing GDF-5 expression, 2250ct, is found in the 3′ UTR of *GDF5*. It acts independently from the 5′ SNP rs143383 and can similarly reduce protein expression levels by 20-25% (Egli *et al.*, 2009). The independent reduction in expression by these SNPs can be additive thereby showing that even moderate imbalances in the allelic expression levels of *GDF5* can result in severe disturbances in synovial joint maintenance. This idea is further emphasized by the identification of a duplication in the 3′ UTR of the *BMP2* gene including a distant enhancer of BMP2 expression in BDA2 patients. The phenotype described by Dathe *et al.* resembles those caused by specific mutations in the *GDF5* or the *BMPR1B* gene (Dathe *et al.*, 2009). As BMP-2 is expressed in regions surrounding future joints as well as in the joint interzone during the development of interphalangeal joints in close proximity to GDF-5 expression, one could hypothesize that by either increasing BMP-2 levels due to the duplication of an enhancer or by decreasing the GDF-5 expression due to regulatory SNPs as described above, the fine-tuned balance between signals from different BMPs may be severely disturbed.

3.5. Proper folding and processing of pro-GDF-5 is essential for GDF-5 signaling

Like other ligands of the TGF-β superfamily GDF-5 is expressed and secreted as a dimeric pro-protein consisting of a large (354aa per monomer) pro-part and a smaller (120aa per monomer) mature part at the C-terminus. The C-terminal mature part harbors the characteristic motif present in all TGF-β ligands comprising of seven (BMPs, GDFs) highly conserved cysteine residues (Activins, TGF-βs have two further Cys residues at the N-terminus of the mature part) of which six form the so-called cystine knot. The seventh cysteine residue is involved in an intermolecular disulfide bond thereby stabilizing the (usually homo-)dimeric ligand assembly. The dimeric mature part of TGF-β ligand exhibits a butterfly shaped assembly with the monomeric subunits adopting an architecture resembling a left hand (Sebald *et al.*, 2004). The dimer interface is formed by the palm of the hand, two two-stranded β-sheets resembling two fingers emanate from the cystine knot containing palm. Mutagenesis was used to determine the receptor binding epitopes (Kirsch *et al.*, 2000). The BMP type I receptors bind to the so-called wrist epitope, the type II receptors bind to the so-called knuckle epitope (Kirsch *et al.*, 2000). The location of these receptor binding epitopes were then confirmed by structure analyses of various BMP ligand-receptor complexes (Kirsch *et al.*, 2000, Greenwald *et al.*, 2003, Allendorph *et al.*, 2006, Weber *et al.*, 2007, Kotzsch *et al.*, 2009).

Homozygous non-sense or frame-shift mutations in the pro- or mature part of *GDF5* will result in a complete knockout of *GDF5*. However, also heterozygous non-sense and frame-shift mutations in *GDF5* will severely lower the level of intact protein; assuming equal transcriptional and translational efficiency from both alleles by statistics only 25% of the protein produced will be intact due to its dimeric nature. Hence the complete knockout or partial knockdown of *GDF5* achieved by this type of mutation leads to rather severe skeletal malformation phenotypes such as brachydactyly type C (BDC), symphalangism (SYM1) or multiple synostosis syndrome (SYNS1). One potentially underappreciated possibility is also the formation of nonfunctional heterodimeric ligands if a cell produces more than one TGF-β factor at a time and thus a possible influence of non-sense GDF-5 mutations onto other BMP signals. It is a known fact that in Drosophila the BMP-2 and BMP-7 orthologs Dpp and Screw can form heterodimers with unique functions required for proper development of certain tissues (Shimmi *et al.*, 2005, O'Connor *et al.*, 2006), however in vertebrates existence of such BMP heterodimers has only been postulated or recombinant proteins have been used in the analysis, but existence of such heterodimers has not really been proven *in vivo* (Schmid *et al.*, 2000, Butler & Dodd, 2003) thus a potential "cross"-influence of non-functional GDF-5 mutations on other BMPs can only be hypothesized.

Of the 14 missense mutations known in the *GDF5* gene four are located within the pro-part of the GDF-5 protein. Whereas for the TGF-βs the pro-part fulfills an important regulatory role, termed latency, its role for the BMP and GDF subgroup of the TGF-β superfamily is much less clear. Latency was discovered for TGF-β1 in 1984 showing that TGF-β proteins are secreted as large protein complexes that require activation for TGF-β signaling (Lawrence *et al.*, 1984). It is known today that upon secretion the pro-part of TGF-βs is cleaved in the Golgi apparatus by furin proteases at a site between the pro- and mature part containing a consensus RXXR motif (other proteases might substitute for furin proteases but providing for TGF-β proteins with different N-termini) (Dubois *et al.*, 1995). The pro-part also called latency-associated peptide (LAP) however is still non-covalently attached thereby interfering with TGF-β signaling. Activation corresponding to release of the mature part from this intermediate latent complex is achieved either by physicochemical changes in the environment, e.g. acidification or by further proteolysis. Proteins specifically binding LAP have been identified (Miyazono *et al.*, 1988), these latent TGF-β binding proteins (LTBP) interact with the extracellular matrix and play an important role in the TGF-β activation process (for review see (Annes *et al.*, 2003)). For BMPs a process identical to latency as observed for TGF-βs is not known, but the pro-part of the BMPs possibly enhances the otherwise poor solubility of BMPs under physiolocigal conditions and thus might provide for or enhance their long-range activity (Sengle *et al.*, 2008, Sengle *et al.*, 2011). Recent determination of the structure of the TGF-β1 pro-protein now provides for an insight in the regulatory mechanism of the pro-part at atomic level (Shi *et al.*, 2011). The pro-part embraces the mature part of TGF-β like a straitjacket, a long N-terminal α-helix binds into the type I receptor-binding site (in BMPs and GDFs called wrist epitope) thereby blocking receptor access to this epitope. A proline-rich loop termed latency lasso and a second α-helix encompass the fingertips and the back of the second finger of the mature part of TGF-β hence also blocking the type II receptor epitope. The pro-domain monomers form a dimerization site in the C-terminal region called bowtie, which is located above the butterfly-shaped dimeric TGF-β mature part. Two intermolecular disulfide bonds additionally stabilize the dimerization between the pro-domain subunits. Strikingly, the arrangement of the pro- and mature domain resembles the overall architecture found for the Noggin-BMP7 interaction (Groppe *et al.*, 2002). Both receptor-binding epitopes are tightly blocked from receptor access and the binding of the modulator/pro-domain is strongly enhanced through avidity by forming a covalently linked dimer. The importance of the covalent dimer linkage becomes obvious in the rare bone disorder Camurati-Engelmann disease in which these cysteine residues in the TGF-β1 pro-part are mutated resulting in a disrupted dimerization and leading to increased ligand activation (Janssens *et al.*, 2003, Walton *et al.*, 2010).

Although the sequence homology (as well as differences in the length) between the pro-domains of the various TGF-β members is certainly lower than between their mature parts alignments clearly show that all pro-domains will adopt a similar fold (Shi *et al.*, 2011). A homology model for pro-GDF-5 build on the basis of pro-TGF-β1 structure instantly provides for possible explanations to why the effect of latency is quite different between TGF-βs and members of the BMP subgroup. Particularly for GDF-5 (also true for GDF-6 and -7) many loops in the pro-domain are extended possibly creating further sites for proteolytic activation or degradation, secondly BMPs and GDFs lack the two cysteine residues present in the pro-domain being responsible for covalent linkage (see Fig. 9A). This suggests that the pro-domain association is much less stable for BMPs and GDFs (see mutations of cysteines in the Curati-Engelmann disease) and the release of the mature growth factor domain is facilitated without further need of processing. The four mutations in the GDF-5 pro-domain cluster in three different skeletal malformation phenotypes: M173V – BDC, S204R – BDC, R378Q/P436T (compound heterozygous) – Acromesomelic dysplasia, DuPan syndrome, R380Q – BDA2) indicating a loss-of-GDF-5 function in all cases (Everman *et al.*, 2002, Schwabe *et al.*, 2004, Douzgou *et al.*, 2008, Ploger *et al.*, 2008). On the basis of our own model methionine 173 is placed in close proximity to the first helix element blocking type I receptor binding, whereas serine 204 is placed in the so-called arm domain providing the structural scaffold for the straitjacket architecture. Both missense mutations likely lead to (local) unfolding and thus destabilize the pro-protein complex. This might subsequently lead to lower secretion efficiency and the observed loss-of-function phenotype. The mutation

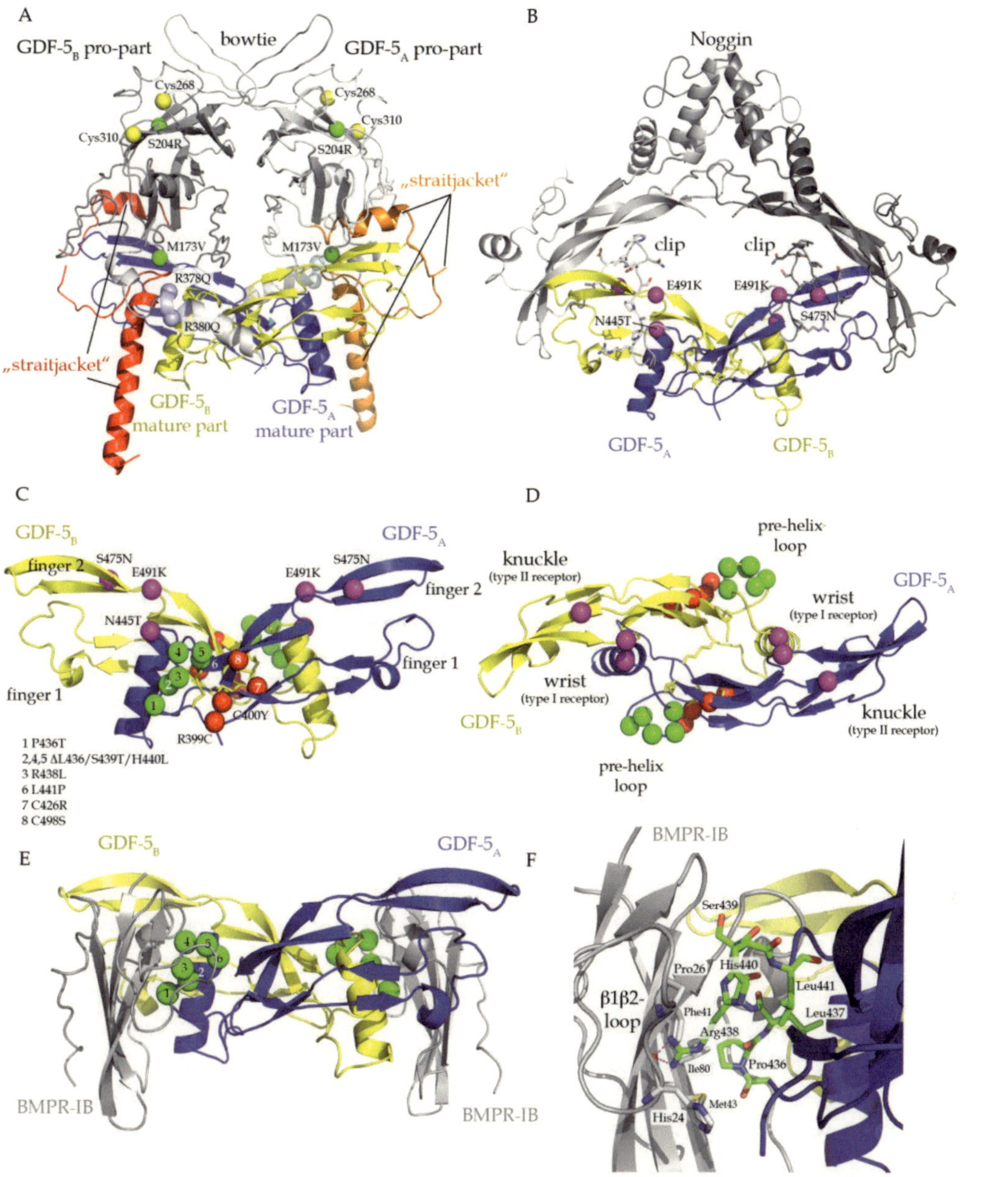

Figure 9. Mutations in GDF-5 and its effect on structure or interactions. A) Homology model of pro-GDF-5 based on the structure of pro-TGF-β1 in ribbon representation (Shi *et al.*, 2011). The mature part of GDF-5 (shown in blue and yellow) is embraced by the pro-part with the N-terminal part resembling a straitjacket (in red and orange). This element comprising of two helices block access to both type I and type II receptor binding epitopes. In contrast to the pro-part of TGF-βs the pro-domains of BMPs and GDFs likely do not have intermolecular disulfides (the potential positions of Cys268 and Cys310 are shown) suggesting that the pro/mature part assembly of BMPs and GDFs might be less stable compared to TGF-βs. Four missense mutations in the pro-part are found to be associated with skeletal malformation diseases: M173V, S204R, R378Q, and R380Q. The first two mutations (marked by green

spheres) possibly cause misfolding of the pro-domain thereby weakening the pro-protein and leading to lower secretion efficiency. The latter two mutations are located in the furin protease site (marked as light-blue spheres) and were shown to lower or abrogate proteolytic processing of the pro-protein. B) Homology model of the Noggin:GDF-5 complex (Schwaerzer *et al.*, 2011) based on the crystal structure of the Noggin:BMP-7 complex (Groppe *et al.*, 2002). Noggin, by a similar mechanism but different structural architecture, embraces GDF-5 thereby blocking receptor binding of either subtype through its clip and finger domains. Three missense mutations in GDF-5 associated with symphalangism were shown to have impaired GDF-5 – Noggin interaction: N445T/K, S475N, and E491K. All three mutations are in close proximity of the Noggin clip region suggesting that through loss of interaction with this element GDF-5 binding to Noggin is attenuated. C) Ribbon representation of the mature part of GDF-5 with the two monomeric subunits shown in blue and yellow. The architecture of a GDF-5 dimer resembles a left hand, the α-helix forming the palm, the two β-sheets depicting two fingers and the N-terminus marking the thumb. Consequentally, the receptor binding epitopes were named wrist (type I receptor), formed by the dorsal side of the fingers and the palm, and knuckle (type II receptor), formed by the ventral side of finger 1 and 2. The location of all known mutations associated with skeletal malformation diseases is depicted by spheres, with color-coding according to their belonging to either cystine knot mutations (red), pre-helix loop mutations (green) or mutations affecting Noggin-binding (magenta). D) As in C but rotated clockwise around the x-axis by 90°. E) Ribbon representation of the complex of GDF-5 (in blue and yellow) bound to the extracellular domain of BMPR-IB (grey). The overview clearly shows that affected residues in the pre-helix loop are in contact with receptor elements suggesting that these mutations alter type I receptor binding. F) Magnification of the interaction between residues in the pre-helix loop of GDF-5 and residues in the binding epitope of BMPR-IB. The complete pre-helix loop is tightly packed to residues in the threestranded β-sheet of BMPR-IB. GDF-5 Arg438 is involved in hydrogen bonds to His24 located in the β1β2-loop of BMPR-IB. The tight turn structures at the N- and C-terminal end of the pre-helix loop also indicate that the mutations involving the exchange of a proline (P436T) or introduction of a proline (L441P) will likely destroy the conformation of the pre-helix loop thereby affecting receptor binding even if these two residues do not form direct contacts with GDF-5.

R380Q targets the pro-domain cleavage site by destroying or attenuating proteolytic processing via furin proteases (Ploger *et al.*, 2008). The now covalent linkage of pro- and mature part of GDF-5 R380Q very likely enhances the competition of the pro-domain with receptor binding and thus leads to loss of or attenuated GDF-5 activity (Ploger *et al.*, 2008). The mechanism by which the double mutation R378Q/P436T causes the skeletal malformation is more complex. As the mutation is compound heterozygous, three GDF-5 variants are potentially produced in the patient. Statistically 50% of the GDF-5 protein would carry both exchanges as a heterodimer and the other 50% would consist of homodimers with either one of the two mutations. Heterozygous carriers of the individual missense mutations R378Q or P436T did not exhibit any skeletal phenotype thus preventing to point towards a particular mutation as disease-causing if found in a homozygous background. For the mutation R378Q it can be assumed that processing of the pro-protein is at least impaired and thus the portion of GDF-5 R378Q homodimer is likely to be inactive as found for R380Q (see Fig. 9) blank (Ploger *et al.*, 2008). The missense mutation P436T is located in the mature part of GDF-5 in the so-called pre-helix loop of the GDF-5 type I receptor-binding epitope (Nickel *et al.*, 2005). Mutation of the equivalent proline residue in BMP-2 strongly decreased binding of this BMP-2 variant to both type I receptors, BMPR-IA and BMPR-IB thus leading to a loss of BMP signaling (Kirsch *et al.*, 2000).

Of the other eight known disease-related amino acid exchanges in the mature part of GDF-5, several mutations involve the exchange of a cysteine residue participating in the formation of the cystine knot, e.g. C400Y, C429R, C498S or introduce additional cysteine residues, e.g. R399C, R438C, which will interfere with proper formation of the cystine knot, thereby leading to a misfolded inactive protein. Several studies show that under conditions mimicking a homozygous background no secretion of the GDF-5 variant is observed (Everman *et al.*, 2002, Dawson *et al.*, 2006). However, mutations involving cysteines can also act dominant-negatively (see Fig. 9). Thomas *et al.* tested the effect of the GDF-5 mutation C400Y, which is found homozygous in chondrodysplasia Grebe type (Thomas *et al.*, 1997). Upon transfection of only the mutated gene into COS-7 cells resembling a homozygous background no GDF-5 protein could be detected in the cell supernatant, however co-transfection of the genes for wildtype GDF-5 and the variant GDF-5 C400Y clearly attenuated GDF-5 protein levels in the supernatant. This effect was dose-dependent indicating that for heterozygous carriers through differential allelic expression a highly variable phenotype could possibly be observed (Thomas *et al.*, 1997). Furthermore, this study also indicated that the mutation might act dominant negative onto other BMPs by selective heterodimerization. By co-transfection of the gene encoding for GDF-5 C400Y together with either BMP-2, BMP-3 or BMP-7, heterodimers could be isolated from the cell supernatant that will most likely be non-functional (Thomas *et al.*, 1997).

3.6. GDF-5 activity is tightly regulated by the BMP antagonist Noggin

All other missense mutations in the *GDF5* gene cluster in two regions of the GDF-5 structure (see Fig. 9C/D). Three missense mutations cluster in close proximity of finger 2 of GDF-5, N445T/K (Seemann *et al.*, 2009), S475N (Akarsu *et al.*, 1999, Schwaerzer *et al.*, 2011) and E491K (Wang *et al.*, 2006). The heterozygous mutations N445T and N445K in GDF-5 were identified in patients suffering from multiple synostosis syndrome (SYNS1) characterized by fusion of carpal bones and proximal symphalangism in fingers II to V (Seemann *et al.*, 2009). Analysis of the recombinant GDF-5 variant in BMPR-IB transfected myoblastic C2C12 cells indicated that the mutation did not lead to a loss of GDF-5 function. In fact analyzing the expression of the osteogenic marker alkaline phosphatase in non-transfected C2C12 cells revealed even a gain of activity exemplified by a small but measureable ALP induction when stimulating with GDF-5 N445T but no induction of ALP expression when using wildtype GDF-5. As this activating mutation is located within the wrist (type I receptor binding) epitope of GDF-5 differences in binding to the BMP type I receptors were assumed. However, competition assays using soluble receptor ectodomains showed that binding of the GDF-5 variant N445T to BMPR-IA as well as BMPR-IB is unaltered (Seemann *et al.*, 2009). Sequence comparison with other BMP factors indicated that one of the mutations found, the exchange of Asn445 to lysine, is native in BMP-9 and BMP-10. As the latter factors are insensitive to Noggin inhibition, Seemann *et al.* assumed that this mutation also renders GDF-5 insensitive to inhibition by Noggin. *In vitro* assays indeed confirmed that GDF-5 N445T is not antagonized by recombinant Noggin protein leading to an increase in GDF-5 signaling activity during early stages of limb and joint development where Noggin and *GDF5* expression patterns overlap (Seemann *et al.*, 2005, Seemann *et al.*, 2009). Another mutation in GDF-5 leading to proximal symphalangism is

E491K discovered in two large Chinese families (Wang *et al.*, 2006). The skeletal malformation phenotype resembles the one seen in aforementioned patients having either the mutation N445T/K (Seemann *et al.*, 2009) or R438L (Seemann *et al.*, 2005) in the *GDF5* gene. Nothing is known about receptor or modulator protein binding of this particular GDF-5 variant, however in the GDF-5 structure Glu491 is in close proximity to Asn445. Moreover, the sidechain carboxamide group of Asn445 is forming a hydrogen bond to the backbone carbonyl of Glu491 possibly suggesting a similar disease-causing molecular mechanism through the loss of inhibition by Noggin as described above by Seemann *et al.* (2009). Modeling of a GDF-5:Noggin complex based on the structure of the BMP-7:Noggin interaction (Groppe *et al.*, 2002) does however not indicate a direct interference of a GDF-5:Noggin interaction by exchanging Glu491 by lysine (see Fig. 9).

The mutation S475N is another mutation in the mature part of GDF-5, which causes multiple synostosis syndrome (SYNS1), a phenotypic description of these heterozygous missense mutations was first reported by Akarsu *et al.* (1999). The phenotype again suggests a gain-of-function in GDF-5 signaling. A detailed analysis of the signaling properties of this GDF-5 variant indeed revealed that GDF-5 S475N is significantly more potent in the chondrogenic differentiation in chicken micromass culture compared to wildtype GDF-5 (Schwaerzer *et al.*, 2011). The mutation is located in the knuckle (type II receptor) epitope of GDF-5 (see Fig. 9C/D). Although no direct structural data is currently available for GDF-5 bound to type I and type II receptors, structure data available on ternary complexes of BMP-2 (Allendorph *et al.*, 2006, Weber *et al.*, 2007) indicated that this highly conserved serine residue is at the center of the BMP/GDF type II receptor interaction. Despite its location exchange of this residue in BMP-2 affected type II receptor binding only marginally (Weber *et al.*, 2007) suggesting that other residues in the BMP-type II receptor interface are more important for the ligand-receptor interaction. However, in GDF-5 Ser475 seems more important for the binding of BMPR-II as indicated by a 7-fold decrease in the binding affinity upon mutation to asparagine, which seems surprising given the fact that this mutant shows an elevated activity compared to wildtype GDF-5 (Schwaerzer *et al.*, 2011). As the BMP type II receptor epitope overlaps heavily with that of Noggin, also the change in binding to Noggin was determined showing that also Noggin binding affinity is similarly decreased by 4-fold. When the effect of Noggin inhibition on BMP factors was investigated by analyzing BMP-induced alkaline phosphatase expression or chondrogenic differentiation in chicken micromass culture in the presence of Noggin, GDF-5 S475N was clearly resistant to antagonizing effects by Noggin, whereas signals from wildtype GDF-5 could be efficiently blocked with Noggin (Schwaerzer *et al.*, 2011). This possibly indicates that the loss in BMP type II receptor binding affinity seen for this variant is overcompensated by the deprivation of Noggin-mediated inhibition (Schwaerzer *et al.*, 2011).

3.7. Type I receptor binding as well as receptor specificity is essential for correct GDF-5 function

A clear hotspot for disease-related mutations is found for the so-called pre-helix loop located in the wrist epitope of GDF-5 (Nickel *et al.*, 2005). This loop is the key interaction element for BMP-type I receptor interaction (Kirsch *et al.*, 2000, Keller *et al.*, 2004, Kotzsch *et al.*, 2008). For BMP-2 and GDF-5 this segment contains the so-called main binding determinant a highly conserved leucine residue, whose polar main chain atoms makes a pair of hydrogen bonds with a conserved glutamine residue present in the BMP type I receptors IA and IB. Mutation of either the leucine to a proline in BMP-2 or GDF-5 or the glutamine residue in BMPR-IA or BMPR-IB leads to a strongly reduced type I receptor affinity (Keller *et al.*, 2004, Kotzsch *et al.*, 2009). In the unbound state this pre-helix loop segment is also rather flexible allowing for geometrical adaptability to different receptor surface geometries. This observation together with the disordered and flexible ligand-binding epitope seen in the BMP type I receptors provides a mechanism for the pronounced ligand-receptor promiscuity seen in the BMP/GDF-subgroup of the TGF-β superfamily (Keller *et al.*, 2004, Allendorph *et al.*, 2007, Klages *et al.*, 2008, Kotzsch *et al.*, 2008, Saremba *et al.*, 2008). Despite structural analyses showed that the pre-helix is flexible before receptor binding, the mutation L441P suggests that in the bound state a geometrically defined conformation is required for (high affinity) binding of BMP type I receptors (Kotzsch *et al.*, 2009). Residue Leu441 is located at the C-terminal end of the pre-helix loop forming a sharp turn together with Ser439 and His440 (see Fig. 9E/F). The sidechain of Leu441 is oriented into the interior of GDF-5 making it implausible that its exchange to proline affects type I receptor binding through altering direct interactions. However, the different backbone torsion angle restraints of a non-proline compared to a proline residue suggest that the L441P mutation alters the conformation of the C-terminal end of the pre-helix loop and that hereby important non-covalent interactions between GDF-5 and its type I receptors are strongly impaired. Although earlier reports claim that the mutation L441P in GDF-5 affects binding to the BMP receptor IB (Faiyaz-Ul-Haque *et al.*, 2002b, Seemann *et al.*, 2005) our own data shows that binding to both BMP type I receptors is strongly attenuated (Kotzsch *et al.*, 2009). A rather complex mutation discovered by Szczaluba *et al.* in patients suffering from DuPan syndrome shows shortening of all toes as well as all fingers but the thumb (Szczaluba *et al.*, 2005). Here in the GDF-5 protein residue Leu437 is deleted and the adjacent residues Ser439 and His440 are mutated to threonine and leucine respectively (see Fig. 9). As these changes grossly alter the sequence as well as conformation of the pre-helix loop, it is not surprising that this GDF-5 compound variant shows no type I receptor binding at all (Kotzsch *et al.*, 2009). Interestingly, although the mutation was found to be heterozygous in the carrier it has a dominant-negative effect (Szczaluba *et al.*, 2005). Misfolding of the mutant protein and hence impaired secretion can be excluded as explanation, as the protein could be recombinantly produced and exhibits wildtype-like affinity to BMP type II receptors. One possible explanation for the quite strong skeletal phenotype might be that this GDF-5 variant is not only inactive but possibly still retains its Noggin-binding capability and therefore can act as a Noggin scavenger similar as to what was described for the BMP-2 variant L51P (Keller *et al.*, 2004).

The probably most interesting mutation in GDF-5 is the exchange of Arg438 to leucine found in patients suffering from proximal symphalangism (Seemann *et al.*, 2005). Based on a structural-function analysis to determine the GDF-5 type I receptor specificity this amino acid position – 438 if the complete pre-pro-protein is considered and position 57 if numbering starts with the mature part of GDF-5 - was shown before to be solely responsible for the BMPR-IB binding preference of GDF-5 (see Fig. 9E/F) (Nickel *et al.,* 2005). The equivalent residue in BMP-2, which binds both BMP type I receptors, BMPR-IA and BMPR-IB, with equally high affinity is alanine. In contrast, in GDF-5 this position is occupied by a large positively charged arginine being also the largest difference in amino acid sequence within the central type I receptor-binding epitope. Upon exchange of Arg438 in GDF-5 to alanine, GDF-5 R438A bound both type I receptors with the same affinity and with binding characteristics indistinguishable from those of BMP-2 (Nickel *et al.,* 2005). Recent structure analysis of GDF-5 bound to its type I receptor BMPR-IB revealed a molecular mechanism by which GDF-5 "discriminates" between both type I receptors (Kotzsch *et al.,* 2009). A loop between the two N-terminal β-strands of the BMP type I receptors can adopt different conformations dependent on the amino acid sequence. As this loop is in contact to the "GDF-5 specificity determining" amino acid Arg438 BMP type I receptors can be selected through the presence or absence of a steric hindrance. BMPs with large bulky sidechains at this position such as GDF-5 of the pre-helix loop can only bind to BMPR-IB, whereas BMPs with small sidechains such as BMP-2 or BMP-4 can bind both BMP type I receptors equally well (Kotzsch *et al.,* 2009).

Analysis of this BMP-2 like GDF-5 variant revealed that in a cell line (ATDC5) having pro-chondrogenic properties and not expressing the BMPR-IB receptor this variant now has the same signaling properties and efficiency as BMP-2 (Nickel *et al.,* 2005). Thus under these conditions GDF-5 can signal via the BMPR-IA receptor and signaling efficiency is only decreased by the lower affinity of wildtype GDF-5 for BMPR-IA. Most interestingly, despite having the same receptor binding properties as BMP-2, GDF-5 R438A still does not induce ALP expression in the myoblastic cell line C2C12 (Klammert *et al.,* 2011). As RT-PCR analysis did not reveal significant differences in BMP receptor expression between both cell lines, ATDC5 and C2C12, other mechanism must exist that determine whether GDF-5 can fully signal through a particular BMP type I receptor. This observation also indicates that GDF-5 by binding to BMPR-IA can activate signaling on some cell types whereas on other cell types it might compete with BMP-2 for BMPR-IA and act as an antagonist (Klammert *et al.,* 2011). The mutation found in SYM1 affected humans, R438L, does not show a complete loss in BMP type I receptor specificity, the larger leucine sidechain in comparison to alanine leads to a 6 to 9-fold higher affinity to BMPR-IB compared to BMPR-IA (Seemann *et al.,* 2005, Kotzsch *et al.,* 2009). However, the result will likely be similar as above in that the mutation R438L renders GDF-5 into a protein that has BMP-2 like receptor binding properties. As BMP-2 is assumed to induce or at least regulate apoptosis in the interdigital mesenchyme (Yokouchi *et al.,* 1996, Merino *et al.,* 1999a), one would first expect increased apoptosis in patients carrying the mutation R438L in GDF-5 due to the presence of an additional BMP-2 like factor (Seemann *et al.,* 2005). However, our latest observation that increased BMPR-IA binding by GDF-5 R438A might not induce full signaling in all cell types possibly indicates that here the gain-of-function mutation in GDF-5 surprisingly leads to a loss of BMP-2 signaling in certain areas of the developing joint by competing for the binding to the same receptor BMPR-IA thereby might impede BMP-2 induced apoptosis which finally results in joint fusion (Klammert *et al.,* 2011).

4. Conclusion

When GDF-5 was discovered, due to its highly defined expression pattern during limb development, which precisely correlates with the location of all future joints throughout the limb, it was assumed immediately that this particular TGF-β factor takes the center stage in the development of all synovial joints. It thus came as a surprise when the *GDF5* knockout mice despite being affected in joint and limb development still showed multiple joints being developed quite normally. Genetic and functional analyses of human skeletal malformation diseases such as brachydactyly or chondroplasia showed that not only a number of other genes can lead to loss of joints or limb deformations similar to those seen in the *GDF5* null mice, but that also different mutations in GDF-5 can result in very distinct malformation phenotypes. Further studies revealed that often these different factors, many of them acting as morphogens themselves, such as Wnts and its (co-)receptors, members of the Sonic Hedgehog family or the FGFs, do not act independently but can be upstream or downstream of the TGF-β signaling cascade or even form positive or negative feedback loops with signaling components of the TGF-β superfamily. This complex regulatory network is further complicated by the fact that components of the TGF-β superfamily - ligands, receptors as well as antagonists – are known to function via highly promiscuous protein-protein interactions. Even if we restrict our focus onto the regulatory signaling network of GDF-5, its highly overlapping receptor binding specificities with other BMPs, such as BMP-2, BMP-6 or BMP-7, all of which are expressed in the direct neighborhood of the developing joint, make immediately clear that mutations altering binding of one particular ligand-receptor pair will ultimately affect the signaling output of other BMP members even when those are not affected by mutations themselves.

One mutation in GDF-5 – R438L – best exemplifies the dilemma. This mutation enables GDF-5 to now efficiently bind to a second BMP type I receptor, BMPR-IA. However this receptor is usually utilized by BMP-2 also present during joint development. As it is not known whether the GDF-5 variant with the altered type I receptor specificity delivers the same signal via this receptor as BMP-2 or whether it can signal at all through this BMP receptor in the present cellular context, developing a molecular disease mechanism explaining the mode of operation for this mutant seems impossible. In addition to this fuzzy BMP ligand-receptor network modulators like Noggin act like hub proteins interacting with multiple BMP ligands with a distinct BMP specificity profile. These interactions are again often linked to feedback loops leading to a precisely defined equilibrium of BMPs, BMP receptors and other modulators, which as a sum deliver a defined biological outcome. Classical morphogens such as the BMPs are considered to function via a concentration gradient, which is then interpreted by the different cells by responding to a particular morphogen threshold. However, the discrepancy of strong *GDF5* expression in all future joint locations and the highly localized effect seen in *GDF5* knockouts suggests that responsiveness to or the differentiation program run by GDF-5 is encoded along the digital ray by the various other morphogens in a temperospatial manner, thus allowing to run the differentiation program for joint formation by GDF-5 only at certain times at very defined places, whereas at other places or at earlier or later developmental stages as defined other factors will take over the GDF-5 function.

Author details

Tina V. Hellmann and Thomas D. Mueller
Dept. Molecular Plant Physiology and Biophysics, Julius-von-Sachs Institute of the University Wuerzburg, Wuerzburg, Germany

Joachim Nickel
Dept. Tissue Engineering and Regenerative Medicine, University Hospital Wuerzburg, Wuerzburg, Germany

Acknowledgement

We thank Markus Peer and Juliane E. Fiebig for helpful discussions and critically reading the manuscript.

5. References

Akarsu, A.N., Rezaie, T., Demirtas, M., Farhud, D.D., and Sarfarazi, M. (1999). Multiple synostosis type 2 (SYNS2) maps to 20q11.2 and caused by a missense mutation in the growth/differentiation factor 5 (GDF5). *Am J Hum Genet,* 65, 4, pp. A281-A281

Allendorph, G.P., Isaacs, M.J., Kawakami, Y., Izpisua Belmonte, J.C., and Choe, S. (2007). BMP-3 and BMP-6 structures illuminate the nature of binding specificity with receptors. *Biochemistry,* 46, 43, pp. 12238-12247

Allendorph, G.P., Vale, W.W., and Choe, S. (2006). Structure of the ternary signaling complex of a TGF-beta superfamily member. *Proc Natl Acad Sci U S A,* 103, 20, pp. 7643-7648

Andl, T., Ahn, K., Kairo, A., Chu, E.Y., Wine-Lee, L., *et al.* (2004). Epithelial Bmpr1a regulates differentiation and proliferation in postnatal hair follicles and is essential for tooth development. *Development,* 131, 10, pp. 2257-2268

Annes, J.P., Munger, J.S., and Rifkin, D.B. (2003). Making sense of latent TGFbeta activation. *J Cell Sci,* 116, Pt 2, pp. 217-224

Babitt, J.L., Zhang, Y., Samad, T.A., Xia, Y., Tang, J., *et al.* (2005). Repulsive guidance molecule (RGMa), a DRAGON homologue, is a bone morphogenetic protein co-receptor. *J Biol Chem,* 280, 33, pp. 29820-29827

Basit, S., Naqvi, S.K., Wasif, N., Ali, G., Ansar, M., *et al.* (2008). A novel insertion mutation in the cartilage-derived morphogenetic protein-1 (CDMP1) gene underlies Grebe-type chondrodysplasia in a consanguineous Pakistani family. *BMC Med Genet,* 9, pp. 102

Bell, J. (1951). On brachydactyly and symphalangism. *The treasury of human inheritance,* 5, 1, pp. 1-31

Bosanac, I., Maun, H.R., Scales, S.J., Wen, X., Lingel, A., *et al.* (2009). The structure of SHH in complex with HHIP reveals a recognition role for the Shh pseudo active site in signaling. *Nat Struct Mol Biol,* 16, 7, pp. 691-697

Brunet, L.J., McMahon, J.A., McMahon, A.P., and Harland, R.M. (1998). Noggin, cartilage morphogenesis, and joint formation in the mammalian skeleton. *Science,* 280, 5368, pp. 1455-1457

Butler, S.J., and Dodd, J. (2003). A role for BMP heterodimers in roof plate-mediated repulsion of commissural axons. *Neuron,* 38, 3, pp. 389-401

Byrnes, A.M., Racacho, L., Nikkel, S.M., Xiao, F., MacDonald, H., *et al.* (2010). Mutations in GDF5 presenting as semidominant brachydactyly A1. *Hum Mutat,* 31, 10, pp. 1155-1162

Carcamo, J., Weis, F.M., Ventura, F., Wieser, R., Wrana, J.L., *et al.* (1994). Type I receptors specify growth-inhibitory and transcriptional responses to transforming growth factor beta and activin. *Mol Cell Biol,* 14, 6, pp. 3810-3821

Caronia, G., Goodman, F.R., McKeown, C.M., Scambler, P.J., and Zappavigna, V. (2003). An I47L substitution in the HOXD13 homeodomain causes a novel human limb malformation by producing a selective loss of function. *Development,* 130, 8, pp. 1701-1712

Chaikuad, A., Sanvitale, C., Mahajan, P., Daga, N., Cooper, C., *et al.* (2010a). Crystal structure of the cytoplasmic domain of the bone morphogenetic protein receptor type-1B (BMPR1B) in complex with FKBP12 and LDN-193189. http://www.rcsb.org Protein Databank (PDB). RCSB

Chaikuad, A., Alfano, I., Shrestha, B., Muniz, J.R.C., Petrie, K., *et al.* (2010b). Crystal structure of the kinase domain of type I activin receptor (ACVR1) in complex with FKBP12 and dorsomorphin. http://www.rcsb.org Protein Databank (PDB). RCSB

Chen, H.B., Shen, J., Ip, Y.T., and Xu, L. (2006). Identification of phosphatases for Smad in the BMP/DPP pathway. *Genes Dev,* 20, 6, pp. 648-653

Craig, F.M., Bentley, G., and Archer, C.W. (1987). The spatial and temporal pattern of collagens I and II and keratan sulphate in the developing chick metatarsophalangeal joint. *Development,* 99, 3, pp. 383-391

Dathe, K., Kjaer, K.W., Brehm, A., Meinecke, P., Nurnberg, P., *et al.* (2009). Duplications involving a conserved regulatory element downstream of BMP2 are associated with brachydactyly type A2. *Am J Hum Genet,* 84, 4, pp. 483-492

Davis, A.P., and Capecchi, M.R. (1996). A mutational analysis of the 5' HoxD genes: dissection of genetic interactions during limb development in the mouse. *Development,* 122, 4, pp. 1175-1185

Dawson, K., Seeman, P., Sebald, E., King, L., Edwards, M., *et al.* (2006). GDF5 is a second locus for multiple-synostosis syndrome. *Am J Hum Genet,* 78, 4, pp. 708-712

Debeer, P., Fryns, J.P., Devriendt, K., Baten, E., Huysmans, C., *et al.* (2004). A novel NOG mutation Pro37Arg in a family with tarsal and carpal synostoses. *Am J Med Genet A,* 128A, 4, pp. 439-440

Derynck, R., Gelbart, W.M., Harland, R.M., Heldin, C.H., Kern, S.E., *et al.* (1996). Nomenclature: vertebrate mediators of TGFbeta family signals. *Cell,* 87, 2, pp. 173

Dixon, M.E., Armstrong, P., Stevens, D.B., and Bamshad, M. (2001). Identical mutations in NOG can cause either tarsal/carpal coalition syndrome or proximal symphalangism. *Genet Med,* 3, 5, pp. 349-353

Douzgou, S., Lehmann, K., Mingarelli, R., Mundlos, S., and Dallapiccola, B. (2008). Compound heterozygosity for GDF5 in Du Pan type chondrodysplasia. *Am J Med Genet A,* 146A, 16, pp. 2116-2121

Dubois, C.M., Laprise, M.H., Blanchette, F., Gentry, L.E., and Leduc, R. (1995). Processing of transforming growth factor beta 1 precursor by human furin convertase. *J Biol Chem,* 270, 18, pp. 10618-10624

Egli, R.J., Southam, L., Wilkins, J.M., Lorenzen, I., Pombo-Suarez, M., *et al.* (2009). Functional analysis of the osteoarthritis susceptibility-associated GDF5 regulatory polymorphism. *Arthritis Rheum,* 60, 7, pp. 2055-2064

Emery, S.B., Meyer, A., Miller, L., and Lesperance, M.M. (2009). Otosclerosis or congenital stapes ankylosis? The diagnostic role of genetic analysis. *Otol Neurotol,* 30, 8, pp. 1204-1208

Everman, D.B., Bartels, C.F., Yang, Y., Yanamandra, N., Goodman, F.R., *et al.* (2002). The mutational spectrum of brachydactyly type C. *Am J Med Genet,* 112, 3, pp. 291-296

Faiyaz-Ul-Haque, M., Ahmad, W., Wahab, A., Haque, S., Azim, A.C., *et al.* (2002a). Frameshift mutation in the cartilage-derived morphogenetic protein 1 (CDMP1) gene and severe acromesomelic chondrodysplasia resembling Grebe-type chondrodysplasia. *Am J Med Genet,* 111, 1, pp. 31-37

Faiyaz-Ul-Haque, M., Ahmad, W., Zaidi, S.H., Haque, S., Teebi, A.S., *et al.* (2002b). Mutation in the cartilage-derived morphogenetic protein-1 (CDMP1) gene in a kindred affected with fibular hypoplasia and complex brachydactyly (DuPan syndrome). *Clin Genet,* 61, 6, pp. 454-458

Faiyaz-Ul-Haque, M., Faqeih, E.A., Al-Zaidan, H., Al-Shammary, A., and Zaidi, S.H. (2008). Grebe-type chondrodysplasia: a novel missense mutation in a conserved cysteine of the growth differentiation factor 5. *J Bone Miner Metab,* 26, 6, pp. 648-652

Francis-West, P.H., Abdelfattah, A., Chen, P., Allen, C., Parish, J., *et al.* (1999). Mechanisms of GDF-5 action during skeletal development. *Development,* 126, 6, pp. 1305-1315

Francois, V., Solloway, M., O'Neill, J.W., Emery, J., and Bier, E. (1994). Dorsal-ventral patterning of the Drosophila embryo depends on a putative negative growth factor encoded by the short gastrulation gene. *Genes Dev,* 8, 21, pp. 2602-2616

Galjaard, R.J., van der Ham, L.I., Posch, N.A., Dijkstra, P.F., Oostra, B.A., *et al.* (2001). Differences in complexity of isolated brachydactyly type C cannot be attributed to locus heterogeneity alone. *Am J Med Genet,* 98, 3, pp. 256-262

Gao, B., Guo, J., She, C., Shu, A., Yang, M., *et al.* (2001). Mutations in IHH, encoding Indian hedgehog, cause brachydactyly type A-1. *Nat Genet,* 28, 4, pp. 386-388

Gao, B., Hu, J., Stricker, S., Cheung, M., Ma, G., *et al.* (2009). A mutation in Ihh that causes digit abnormalities alters its signalling capacity and range. *Nature,* 458, 7242, pp. 1196-1200

Garamszegi, N., Dore, J.J., Jr., Penheiter, S.G., Edens, M., Yao, D., *et al.* (2001). Transforming growth factor beta receptor signaling and endocytosis are linked through a COOH terminal activation motif in the type I receptor. *Mol Biol Cell,* 12, 9, pp. 2881-2893

Gong, Y., Krakow, D., Marcelino, J., Wilkin, D., Chitayat, D., *et al.* (1999). Heterozygous mutations in the gene encoding noggin affect human joint morphogenesis. *Nat Genet,* 21, 3, pp. 302-304

Gray, P.C., Bilezikjian, L.M., and Vale, W. (2002). Antagonism of activin by inhibin and inhibin receptors: a functional role for betaglycan. *Mol Cell Endocrinol,* 188, 1-2, pp. 254-260

Greenwald, J., Groppe, J., Gray, P., Wiater, E., Kwiatkowski, W., *et al.* (2003). The BMP7/ActRII extracellular domain complex provides new insights into the cooperative nature of receptor assembly. *Mol Cell,* 11, 3, pp. 605-617

Groppe, J., Greenwald, J., Wiater, E., Rodriguez-Leon, J., Economides, A.N., *et al.* (2002). Structural basis of BMP signalling inhibition by the cystine knot protein Noggin. *Nature,* 420, 6916, pp. 636-642

Gruneberg, H., and Lee, A.J. (1973). The anatomy and development of brachypodism in the mouse. *J Embryol Exp Morphol,* 30, 1, pp. 119-141

Guo, S., Zhou, J., Gao, B., Hu, J., Wang, H., *et al.* (2010). Missense mutations in IHH impair Indian Hedgehog signaling in C3H10T1/2 cells: Implications for brachydactyly type A1, and new targets for Hedgehog signaling. *Cell Mol Biol Lett,* 15, 1, pp. 153-176

Haines, R.W. (1947). The development of joints. *J Anat,* 81, 1, pp. 33-55

Hatta, T., Konishi, H., Katoh, E., Natsume, T., Ueno, N., *et al.* (2000). Identification of the ligand-binding site of the BMP type IA receptor for BMP-4. *Biopolymers,* 55, 5, pp. 399-406

Hattersley, G., Hewick, R., and Rosen, V. (1995). In-Situ Localization and in-Vitro Activity of Bmp-13. *J Bone Miner Res,* 10, pp. S163-S163

Heinecke, K., Seher, A., Schmitz, W., Mueller, T.D., Sebald, W., *et al.* (2009). Receptor oligomerization and beyond: a case study in bone morphogenetic proteins. *BMC Biol,* 7, pp. 59

Heldin, C.H., Miyazono, K., and ten Dijke, P. (1997). TGF-beta signalling from cell membrane to nucleus through SMAD proteins. *Nature,* 390, 6659, pp. 465-471

Hinchliffe, J.R., and Johnson, D.R. (1980). *The development of the vertebrate limb: an approach through experiment, genetics, and evolution*. Oxford University Press, ISBN 9780198575528

Hirshoren, N., Gross, M., Banin, E., Sosna, J., Bargal, R., *et al.* (2008). P35S mutation in the NOG gene associated with Teunissen-Cremers syndrome and features of multiple NOG joint-fusion syndromes. *Eur J Med Genet,* 51, 4, pp. 351-357

Hogan, B.L. (1996). Bone morphogenetic proteins in development. *Curr Opin Genet Dev,* 6, 4, pp. 432-438

Holley, S.A., Neul, J.L., Attisano, L., Wrana, J.L., Sasai, Y., *et al.* (1996). The Xenopus dorsalizing factor noggin ventralizes Drosophila embryos by preventing DPP from activating its receptor. *Cell,* 86, 4, pp. 607-617

Hoodless, P.A., Haerry, T., Abdollah, S., Stapleton, M., O'Connor, M.B., *et al.* (1996). MADR1, a MAD-related protein that functions in BMP2 signaling pathways. *Cell,* 85, 4, pp. 489-500

Huse, M., Chen, Y.G., Massague, J., and Kuriyan, J. (1999). Crystal structure of the cytoplasmic domain of the type I TGF beta receptor in complex with FKBP12. *Cell,* 96, 3, pp. 425-436

Huse, M., Muir, T.W., Xu, L., Chen, Y.G., Kuriyan, J., *et al.* (2001). The TGF beta receptor activation process: an inhibitor- to substrate-binding switch. *Mol Cell,* 8, 3, pp. 671-682

Janssens, K., ten Dijke, P., Ralston, S.H., Bergmann, C., and Van Hul, W. (2003). Transforming growth factor-beta 1 mutations in Camurati-Engelmann disease lead to increased signaling by altering either activation or secretion of the mutant protein. *J Biol Chem,* 278, 9, pp. 7718-7724

Johnson, D., Kan, S.H., Oldridge, M., Trembath, R.C., Roche, P., *et al.* (2003). Missense mutations in the homeodomain of HOXD13 are associated with brachydactyly types D and E. *Am J Hum Genet,* 72, 4, pp. 984-997

Karp, S.J., Schipani, E., St-Jacques, B., Hunzelman, J., Kronenberg, H., *et al.* (2000). Indian hedgehog coordinates endochondral bone growth and morphogenesis via parathyroid hormone related-protein-dependent and -independent pathways. *Development,* 127, 3, pp. 543-548

Keller, S., Nickel, J., Zhang, J.L., Sebald, W., and Mueller, T.D. (2004). Molecular recognition of BMP-2 and BMP receptor IA. *Nat Struct Mol Biol,* 11, 5, pp. 481-488

Kingsley, D.M. (1994). What do BMPs do in mammals? Clues from the mouse short-ear mutation. *Trends Genet,* 10, 1, pp. 16-21

Kirsch, T., Nickel, J., and Sebald, W. (2000). BMP-2 antagonists emerge from alterations in the low-affinity binding epitope for receptor BMPR-II. *EMBO J* 19, 13, pp. 3314-3324

Klages, J., Kotzsch, A., Coles, M., Sebald, W., Nickel, J., *et al.* (2008). The solution structure of BMPR-IA reveals a local disorder-to-order transition upon BMP-2 binding. *Biochemistry,* 47, 46, pp. 11930-11939

Klammert, U., Kübler, A., Wuerzler, K.K., Sebald, W., Mueller, T.D., *et al.* (2011). Dependent on the Cellular Context GDF-5 can act as potent BMP-2 Inhibitor. *submitted*

Kosaki, K., Sato, S., Hasegawa, T., Matsuo, N., Suzuki, T., *et al.* (2004). Premature ovarian failure in a female with proximal symphalangism and Noggin mutation. *Fertil Steril,* 81, 4, pp. 1137-1139

Kotzsch, A., Nickel, J., Seher, A., Heinecke, K., van Geersdaele, L., *et al.* (2008). Structure analysis of bone morphogenetic protein-2 type I receptor complexes reveals a mechanism of receptor inactivation in juvenile polyposis syndrome. *J Biol Chem,* 283, 9, pp. 5876-5887

Kotzsch, A., Nickel, J., Seher, A., Sebald, W., and Muller, T.D. (2009). Crystal structure analysis reveals a spring-loaded latch as molecular mechanism for GDF-5-type I receptor specificity. *EMBO J* 28, 7, pp. 937-947

Krause, C., Guzman, A., and Knaus, P. (2011). Noggin. *Int J Biochem Cell Biol,* 43, 4, pp. 478-481

Lanske, B., Karaplis, A.C., Lee, K., Luz, A., Vortkamp, A., *et al.* (1996). PTH/PTHrP receptor in early development and Indian hedgehog-regulated bone growth. *Science,* 273, 5275, pp. 663-666

Lawrence, D.A., Pircher, R., Kryceve-Martinerie, C., and Jullien, P. (1984). Normal embryo fibroblasts release transforming growth factors in a latent form. *J Cell Physiol,* 121, 1, pp. 184-188

Lehmann, K., Seemann, P., Boergermann, J., Morin, G., Reif, S., *et al.* (2006). A novel R486Q mutation in BMPR1B resulting in either a brachydactyly type C/symphalangism-like phenotype or brachydactyly type A2. *Eur J Hum Genet,* 14, 12, pp. 1248-1254

Lehmann, K., Seemann, P., Silan, F., Goecke, T.O., Irgang, S., *et al.* (2007). A new subtype of brachydactyly type B caused by point mutations in the bone morphogenetic protein antagonist NOGGIN. *Am J Hum Genet,* 81, 2, pp. 388-396

Lehmann, K., Seemann, P., Stricker, S., Sammar, M., Meyer, B., *et al.* (2003). Mutations in bone morphogenetic protein receptor 1B cause brachydactyly type A2. *Proc Natl Acad Sci U S A,* 100, 21, pp. 12277-12282

Lin, L., Valore, E.V., Nemeth, E., Goodnough, J.B., Gabayan, V., *et al.* (2007). Iron transferrin regulates hepcidin synthesis in primary hepatocyte culture through hemojuvelin and BMP2/4. *Blood,* 110, 6, pp. 2182-2189

Liu, M., Wang, X., Cai, Z., Tang, Z., Cao, K., *et al.* (2006). A novel heterozygous mutation in the Indian hedgehog gene (IHH) is associated with brachydactyly type A1 in a Chinese family. *J Hum Genet,* 51, 8, pp. 727-731

Lopez-Casillas, F., Wrana, J.L., and Massague, J. (1993). Betaglycan presents ligand to the TGF beta signaling receptor. *Cell,* 73, 7, pp. 1435-1444

Lyons, K.M., Pelton, R.W., and Hogan, B.L. (1989). Patterns of expression of murine Vgr-1 and BMP-2a RNA suggest that transforming growth factor-beta-like genes coordinately regulate aspects of embryonic development. *Genes Dev,* 3, 11, pp. 1657-1668

Macias, D., Ganan, Y., Sampath, T.K., Piedra, M.E., Ros, M.A., *et al.* (1997). Role of BMP-2 and OP-1 (BMP-7) in programmed cell death and skeletogenesis during chick limb development. *Development,* 124, 6, pp. 1109-1117

Maloul, A., Rossmeier, K., Mikic, B., Pogue, V., and Battaglia, T. (2006). Geometric and material contributions to whole bone structural behavior in GDF-7-deficient mice. *Connect Tissue Res,* 47, 3, pp. 157-162

Mangino, M., Flex, E., Digilio, M.C., Giannotti, A., and Dallapiccola, B. (2002). Identification of a novel NOG gene mutation (P35S) in an Italian family with symphalangism. *Hum Mutat,* 19, 3, pp. 308

Manjon, C., Sanchez-Herrero, E., and Suzanne, M. (2007). Sharp boundaries of Dpp signalling trigger local cell death required for Drosophila leg morphogenesis. *Nat Cell Biol,* 9, 1, pp. 57-63

Marcelino, J., Sciortino, C.M., Romero, M.F., Ulatowski, L.M., Ballock, R.T., *et al.* (2001). Human disease-causing NOG missense mutations: effects on noggin secretion, dimer formation, and bone morphogenetic protein binding. *Proc Natl Acad Sci U S A,* 98, 20, pp. 11353-11358

Massague, J. (2000). How cells read TGF-beta signals. *Nat Rev Mol Cell Biol,* 1, 3, pp. 169-178

Massague, J., Seoane, J., and Wotton, D. (2005). Smad transcription factors. *Genes Dev,* 19, 23, pp. 2783-2810

Masuya, H., Nishida, K., Furuichi, T., Toki, H., Nishimura, G., *et al.* (2007). A novel dominant-negative mutation in Gdf5 generated by ENU mutagenesis impairs joint formation and causes osteoarthritis in mice. *Hum Mol Genet,* 16, 19, pp. 2366-2375

McLellan, J.S., Yao, S., Zheng, X., Geisbrecht, B.V., Ghirlando, R., *et al.* (2006). Structure of a heparin-dependent complex of Hedgehog and Ihog. *Proc Natl Acad Sci U S A,* 103, 46, pp. 17208-17213

McMahon, J.A., Takada, S., Zimmerman, L.B., Fan, C.M., Harland, R.M., *et al.* (1998). Noggin-mediated antagonism of BMP signaling is required for growth and patterning of the neural tube and somite. *Genes Dev,* 12, 10, pp. 1438-1452

Merino, R., Macias, D., Ganan, Y., Economides, A.N., Wang, X., *et al.* (1999a). Expression and function of Gdf-5 during digit skeletogenesis in the embryonic chick leg bud. *Dev Biol,* 206, 1, pp. 33-45

Merino, R., Rodriguez-Leon, J., Macias, D., Ganan, Y., Economides, A.N., *et al.* (1999b). The BMP antagonist Gremlin regulates outgrowth, chondrogenesis and programmed cell death in the developing limb. *Development,* 126, 23, pp. 5515-5522

Mikic, B., Bierwert, L., and Tsou, D. (2006). Achilles tendon characterization in GDF-7 deficient mice. *J Orthop Res,* 24, 4, pp. 831-841

Minina, E., Schneider, S., Rosowski, M., Lauster, R., and Vortkamp, A. (2005). Expression of Fgf and Tgfbeta signaling related genes during embryonic endochondral ossification. *Gene Expr Patterns,* 6, 1, pp. 102-109

Minina, E., Wenzel, H.M., Kreschel, C., Karp, S., Gaffield, W., *et al.* (2001). BMP and Ihh/PTHrP signaling interact to coordinate chondrocyte proliferation and differentiation. *Development,* 128, 22, pp. 4523-4534

Mishina, Y., Suzuki, A., Ueno, N., and Behringer, R.R. (1995). Bmpr encodes a type I bone morphogenetic protein receptor that is essential for gastrulation during mouse embryogenesis. *Genes Dev,* 9, 24, pp. 3027-3037

Mitrovic, D. (1978). Development of the diarthrodial joints in the rat embryo. *Am J Anat,* 151, 4, pp. 475-485

Miyamoto, Y., Mabuchi, A., Shi, D., Kubo, T., Takatori, Y., *et al.* (2007). A functional polymorphism in the 5' UTR of GDF5 is associated with susceptibility to osteoarthritis. *Nat Genet,* 39, 4, pp. 529-533

Miyazawa, K., Shinozaki, M., Hara, T., Furuya, T., and Miyazono, K. (2002). Two major Smad pathways in TGF-beta superfamily signalling. *Genes Cells,* 7, 12, pp. 1191-1204

Miyazono, K. (2000). TGF-beta signaling by Smad proteins. *Cytokine Growth Factor Rev,* 11, 1-2, pp. 15-22

Miyazono, K., Hellman, U., Wernstedt, C., and Heldin, C.H. (1988). Latent high molecular weight complex of transforming growth factor beta 1. Purification from human platelets and structural characterization. *J Biol Chem,* 263, 13, pp. 6407-6415

Mundlos, S. (2009). The brachydactylies: a molecular disease family. *Clin Genet,* 76, 2, pp. 123-136

Nakao, A., Roijer, E., Imamura, T., Souchelnytskyi, S., Stenman, G., *et al.* (1997). Identification of Smad2, a human Mad-related protein in the transforming growth factor beta signaling pathway. *J Biol Chem,* 272, 5, pp. 2896-2900

Newfeld, S.J., Wisotzkey, R.G., and Kumar, S. (1999). Molecular evolution of a developmental pathway: phylogenetic analyses of transforming growth factor-beta family ligands, receptors and Smad signal transducers. *Genetics,* 152, 2, pp. 783-795

Nickel, J., Kotzsch, A., Sebald, W., and Mueller, T.D. (2005). A single residue of GDF-5 defines binding specificity to BMP receptor IB. *J Mol Biol,* 349, 5, pp. 933-947

Nickel, J., Sebald, W., Groppe, J.C., and Mueller, T.D. (2009). Intricacies of BMP receptor assembly. *Cytokine Growth Factor Rev,* 20, 5-6, pp. 367-377

Nishitoh, H., Ichijo, H., Kimura, M., Matsumoto, T., Makishima, F., *et al.* (1996). Identification of type I and type II serine/threonine kinase receptors for growth/differentiation factor-5. *J Biol Chem,* 271, 35, pp. 21345-21352

O'Connor, M.B., Umulis, D., Othmer, H.G., and Blair, S.S. (2006). Shaping BMP morphogen gradients in the Drosophila embryo and pupal wing. *Development,* 133, 2, pp. 183-193

Oldridge, M., Fortuna, A.M., Maringa, M., Propping, P., Mansour, S., *et al.* (2000). Dominant mutations in ROR2, encoding an orphan receptor tyrosine kinase, cause brachydactyly type B. *Nat Genet,* 24, 3, pp. 275-278

Onichtchouk, D., Chen, Y.G., Dosch, R., Gawantka, V., Delius, H., *et al.* (1999). Silencing of TGF-beta signalling by the pseudoreceptor BAMBI. *Nature,* 401, 6752, pp. 480-485

Owens, E.M., and Solursh, M. (1982). Cell-cell interaction by mouse limb cells during in vitro chondrogenesis: analysis of the brachypod mutation. *Dev Biol,* 91, 2, pp. 376-388

Oxley, C.D., Rashid, R., Goudie, D.R., Stranks, G., Baty, D.U., *et al.* (2008). Growth and skeletal development in families with NOGGIN gene mutations. *Horm Res,* 69, 4, pp. 221-226

Pathi, S., Rutenberg, J.B., Johnson, R.L., and Vortkamp, A. (1999). Interaction of Ihh and BMP/Noggin signaling during cartilage differentiation. *Dev Biol,* 209, 2, pp. 239-253

Perez, W.D., Weller, C.R., Shou, S., and Stadler, H.S. (2010). Survival of Hoxa13 homozygous mutants reveals a novel role in digit patterning and appendicular skeletal development. *Dev Dyn,* 239, 2, pp. 446-457

Ploger, F., Seemann, P., Schmidt-von Kegler, M., Lehmann, K., Seidel, J., *et al.* (2008). Brachydactyly type A2 associated with a defect in proGDF5 processing. *Hum Mol Genet,* 17, 9, pp. 1222-1233

Pogue, R., and Lyons, K. (2006). BMP signaling in the cartilage growth plate. *Curr Top Dev Biol,* 76, pp. 1-48

Polinkovsky, A., Robin, N.H., Thomas, J.T., Irons, M., Lynn, A., *et al.* (1997). Mutations in CDMP1 cause autosomal dominant brachydactyly type C. *Nat Genet,* 17, 1, pp. 18-19

Potti, T.A., Petty, E.M., and Lesperance, M.M. (2011). A comprehensive review of reported heritable noggin-associated syndromes and proposed clinical utility of one broadly inclusive diagnostic term: NOG-related-symphalangism spectrum disorder (NOG-SSD). *Hum Mutat,* 32, 8, pp. 877-886

Reddi, A.H. (1998). Role of morphogenetic proteins in skeletal tissue engineering and regeneration. *Nat Biotechnol,* 16, 3, pp. 247-252

Reynard, L.N., Bui, C., Canty-Laird, E.G., Young, D.A., and Loughlin, J. (2011). Expression of the osteoarthritis-associated gene GDF5 is modulated epigenetically by DNA methylation. *Hum Mol Genet,* 20, 17, pp. 3450-3460

Ricard, N., Bidart, M., Mallet, C., Lesca, G., Giraud, S., *et al.* (2010). Functional analysis of the BMP9 response of ALK1 mutants from HHT2 patients: a diagnostic tool for novel ACVRL1 mutations. *Blood,* 116, 9, pp. 1604-1612

Rosen, V., and Thies, R.S. (1992). The BMP proteins in bone formation and repair. *Trends Genet,* 8, 3, pp. 97-102

Rouault, K., Scotet, V., Autret, S., Gaucher, F., Dubrana, F., *et al.* (2010). Evidence of association between GDF5 polymorphisms and congenital dislocation of the hip in a Caucasian population. *Osteoarthritis Cartilage,* 18, 9, pp. 1144-1149

Rudnik-Schoneborn, S., Takahashi, T., Busse, S., Schmidt, T., Senderek, J., *et al.* (2010). Facioaudiosymphalangism syndrome and growth acceleration associated with a heterozygous NOG mutation. *Am J Med Genet A,* 152A, 6, pp. 1540-1544

Sakou, T., Onishi, T., Yamamoto, T., Nagamine, T., Sampath, T., *et al.* (1999). Localization of Smads, the TGF-beta family intracellular signaling components during endochondral ossification. *J Bone Miner Res,* 14, 7, pp. 1145-1152

Samad, T.A., Rebbapragada, A., Bell, E., Zhang, Y., Sidis, Y., *et al.* (2005). DRAGON, a bone morphogenetic protein co-receptor. *J Biol Chem,* 280, 14, pp. 14122-14129

Saremba, S., Nickel, J., Seher, A., Kotzsch, A., Sebald, W., *et al.* (2008). Type I receptor binding of bone morphogenetic protein 6 is dependent on N-glycosylation of the ligand. *Febs J,* 275, 1, pp. 172-183

Schmid, B., Furthauer, M., Connors, S.A., Trout, J., Thisse, B., *et al.* (2000). Equivalent genetic roles for bmp7/snailhouse and bmp2b/swirl in dorsoventral pattern formation. *Development,* 127, 5, pp. 957-967

Schwabe, G.C., Tinschert, S., Buschow, C., Meinecke, P., Wolff, G., *et al.* (2000). Distinct mutations in the receptor tyrosine kinase gene ROR2 cause brachydactyly type B. *Am J Hum Genet,* 67, 4, pp. 822-831

Schwabe, G.C., Turkmen, S., Leschik, G., Palanduz, S., Stover, B., *et al.* (2004). Brachydactyly type C caused by a homozygous missense mutation in the prodomain of CDMP1. *Am J Med Genet A,* 124A, 4, pp. 356-363

Schwaerzer, G.K., Hiepen, C., Schrewe, H., Nickel, J., Ploeger, F., *et al.* (2011). New insights into the molecular mechanisms of multiple synostoses syndrome: Mutation within the GDF5 knuckle epitope causes noggin-resistance. *J Bone Miner Res,* 27, 2, pp. 429-442

Sebald, W., Nickel, J., Zhang, J.L., and Mueller, T.D. (2004). Molecular recognition in bone morphogenetic protein (BMP)/receptor interaction. *Biol Chem,* 385, 8, pp. 697-710

Seemann, P., Brehm, A., Konig, J., Reissner, C., Stricker, S., *et al.* (2009). Mutations in GDF5 reveal a key residue mediating BMP inhibition by NOGGIN. *PLoS Genet,* 5, 11, pp. e1000747

Seemann, P., Schwappacher, R., Kjaer, K.W., Krakow, D., Lehmann, K., *et al.* (2005). Activating and deactivating mutations in the receptor interaction site of GDF5 cause symphalangism or brachydactyly type A2. *J Clin Invest,* 115, 9, pp. 2373-2381

Seki, K., and Hata, A. (2004). Indian hedgehog gene is a target of the bone morphogenetic protein signaling pathway. *J Biol Chem,* 279, 18, pp. 18544-18549

Sengle, G., Ono, R.N., Lyons, K.M., Bachinger, H.P., and Sakai, L.Y. (2008). A new model for growth factor activation: type II receptors compete with the prodomain for BMP-7. *J Mol Biol,* 381, 4, pp. 1025-1039

Sengle, G., Ono, R.N., Sasaki, T., and Sakai, L.Y. (2011). Prodomains of transforming growth factor beta (TGFbeta) superfamily members specify different functions: extracellular matrix interactions and growth factor bioavailability. *J Biol Chem,* 286, 7, pp. 5087-5099

Settle, S., Marker, P., Gurley, K., Sinha, A., Thacker, A., *et al.* (2001). The BMP family member Gdf7 is required for seminal vesicle growth, branching morphogenesis, and cytodifferentiation. *Dev Biol,* 234, 1, pp. 138-150

Settle, S.H., Jr., Rountree, R.B., Sinha, A., Thacker, A., Higgins, K., *et al.* (2003). Multiple joint and skeletal patterning defects caused by single and double mutations in the mouse Gdf6 and Gdf5 genes. *Dev Biol,* 254, 1, pp. 116-130

Shi, M., Zhu, J., Wang, R., Chen, X., Mi, L., *et al.* (2011). Latent TGF-beta structure and activation. *Nature,* 474, 7351, pp. 343-349

Shi, Y., and Massague, J. (2003). Mechanisms of TGF-beta signaling from cell membrane to the nucleus. *Cell,* 113, 6, pp. 685-700

Shimmi, O., and O'Connor, M.B. (2003). Physical properties of Tld, Sog, Tsg and Dpp protein interactions are predicted to help create a sharp boundary in Bmp signals during dorsoventral patterning of the Drosophila embryo. *Development,* 130, 19, pp. 4673-4682

Shimmi, O., Umulis, D., Othmer, H., and O'Connor, M.B. (2005). Facilitated transport of a Dpp/Scw heterodimer by Sog/Tsg leads to robust patterning of the Drosophila blastoderm embryo. *Cell,* 120, 6, pp. 873-886

Smith, W.C., and Harland, R.M. (1992). Expression cloning of noggin, a new dorsalizing factor localized to the Spemann organizer in Xenopus embryos. *Cell,* 70, 5, pp. 829-840

Song, K., Krause, C., Shi, S., Patterson, M., Suto, R., *et al.* (2010). Identification of a key residue mediating bone morphogenetic protein (BMP)-6 resistance to noggin inhibition allows for engineered BMPs with superior agonist activity. *J Biol Chem,* 285, 16, pp. 12169-12180

Southam, L., Rodriguez-Lopez, J., Wilkins, J.M., Pombo-Suarez, M., Snelling, S., *et al.* (2007). An SNP in the 5'-UTR of GDF5 is associated with osteoarthritis susceptibility in Europeans and with in vivo differences in allelic expression in articular cartilage. *Hum Mol Genet,* 16, 18, pp. 2226-2232

St-Jacques, B., Hammerschmidt, M., and McMahon, A.P. (1999). Indian hedgehog signaling regulates proliferation and differentiation of chondrocytes and is essential for bone formation. *Genes Dev,* 13, 16, pp. 2072-2086

Stelzer, C., Winterpacht, A., Spranger, J., and Zabel, B. (2003). Grebe dysplasia and the spectrum of CDMP1 mutations. *Pediatr Pathol Mol Med,* 22, 1, pp. 77-85

Storm, E.E., Huynh, T.V., Copeland, N.G., Jenkins, N.A., Kingsley, D.M., *et al.* (1994). Limb alterations in brachypodism mice due to mutations in a new member of the TGF beta-superfamily. *Nature,* 368, 6472, pp. 639-643

Storm, E.E., and Kingsley, D.M. (1996). Joint patterning defects caused by single and double mutations in members of the bone morphogenetic protein (BMP) family. *Development*, 122, 12, pp. 3969-3979

Storm, E.E., and Kingsley, D.M. (1999). GDF5 coordinates bone and joint formation during digit development. *Dev Biol*, 209, 1, pp. 11-27

Suzuki, M., Ueno, N., and Kuroiwa, A. (2003). Hox proteins functionally cooperate with the GC box-binding protein system through distinct domains. *J Biol Chem*, 278, 32, pp. 30148-30156

Szczaluba, K., Hilbert, K., Obersztyn, E., Zabel, B., Mazurczak, T., *et al.* (2005). Du Pan syndrome phenotype caused by heterozygous pathogenic mutations in CDMP1 gene. *Am J Med Genet A*, 138, 4, pp. 379-383

Takagi, T., Moribe, H., Kondoh, H., and Higashi, Y. (1998). DeltaEF1, a zinc finger and homeodomain transcription factor, is required for skeleton patterning in multiple lineages. *Development*, 125, 1, pp. 21-31

Takahashi, T., Takahashi, I., Komatsu, M., Sawaishi, Y., Higashi, K., *et al.* (2001). Mutations of the NOG gene in individuals with proximal symphalangism and multiple synostosis syndrome. *Clin Genet*, 60, 6, pp. 447-451

Temtamy, S.A., and Aglan, M.S. (2008). Brachydactyly. *Orphanet J Rare Dis*, 3, pp. 15

ten Dijke, P., Miyazono, K., and Heldin, C.H. (1996). Signaling via hetero-oligomeric complexes of type I and type II serine/threonine kinase receptors. *Curr Opin Cell Biol*, 8, 2, pp. 139-145

Thomas, J.T., Kilpatrick, M.W., Lin, K., Erlacher, L., Lembessis, P., *et al.* (1997). Disruption of human limb morphogenesis by a dominant negative mutation in CDMP1. *Nat Genet*, 17, 1, pp. 58-64

Tylzanowski, P., Mebis, L., and Luyten, F.P. (2006). The Noggin null mouse phenotype is strain dependent and haploinsufficiency leads to skeletal defects. *Dev Dyn*, 235, 6, pp. 1599-1607

Ueno, N., Ling, N., Ying, S.Y., Esch, F., Shimasaki, S., *et al.* (1987). Isolation and partial characterization of follistatin: a single-chain Mr 35,000 monomeric protein that inhibits the release of follicle-stimulating hormone. *Proc Natl Acad Sci U S A*, 84, 23, pp. 8282-8286

van den Ende, J.J., Mattelaer, P., Declau, F., Vanhoenacker, F., Claes, J., *et al.* (2005). The facio-audio-symphalangism syndrome in a four generation family with a nonsense mutation in the NOG-gene. *Clin Dysmorphol*, 14, 2, pp. 73-80

Villavicencio-Lorini, P., Kuss, P., Friedrich, J., Haupt, J., Farooq, M., *et al.* (2010). Homeobox genes d11-d13 and a13 control mouse autopod cortical bone and joint formation. *J Clin Invest*, 120, 6, pp. 1994-2004

Vortkamp, A., Lee, K., Lanske, B., Segre, G.V., Kronenberg, H.M., *et al.* (1996). Regulation of rate of cartilage differentiation by Indian hedgehog and PTH-related protein. *Science*, 273, 5275, pp. 613-622

Walton, K.L., Makanji, Y., Chen, J., Wilce, M.C., Chan, K.L., *et al.* (2010). Two distinct regions of latency-associated peptide coordinate stability of the latent transforming growth factor-beta1 complex. *J Biol Chem*, 285, 22, pp. 17029-17037

Wanek, N., Muneoka, K., Holler-Dinsmore, G., Burton, R., and Bryant, S.V. (1989). A staging system for mouse limb development. *J Exp Zool,* 249, 1, pp. 41-49

Wang, X., Xiao, F., Yang, Q., Liang, B., Tang, Z., *et al.* (2006). A novel mutation in GDF5 causes autosomal dominant symphalangism in two Chinese families. *Am J Med Genet A,* 140A, 17, pp. 1846-1853

Weber, D., Kotzsch, A., Nickel, J., Harth, S., Seher, A., *et al.* (2007). A silent H-bond can be mutationally activated for high-affinity interaction of BMP-2 and activin type IIB receptor. *BMC Struct Biol,* 7, pp. 6

Weekamp, H.H., Kremer, H., Hoefsloot, L.H., Kuijpers-Jagtman, A.M., Cruysberg, J.R., *et al.* (2005). Teunissen-Cremers syndrome: a clinical, surgical, and genetic report. *Otol Neurotol,* 26, 1, pp. 38-51

Wiater, E., and Vale, W. (2003). Inhibin is an antagonist of bone morphogenetic protein signaling. *J Biol Chem,* 278, 10, pp. 7934-7941

Wieser, R., Wrana, J.L., and Massague, J. (1995). GS domain mutations that constitutively activate T beta R-I, the downstream signaling component in the TGF-beta receptor complex. *EMBO J,* 14, 10, pp. 2199-2208

Wolfman, N.M., Celeste, A.J., Cox, K., Hattersley, G., Nelson, R., *et al.* (1995). Preliminary Characterization of the Biological-Activities Rhbmp-12. *J Bone Miner Res,* 10, pp. S148-S148

Wolfman, N.M., Hattersley, G., Cox, K., Celeste, A.J., Nelson, R., *et al.* (1997). Ectopic induction of tendon and ligament in rats by growth and differentiation factors 5, 6, and 7, members of the TGF-beta gene family. *J Clin Invest,* 100, 2, pp. 321-330

Wotton, D., and Massague, J. (2001). Smad transcriptional corepressors in TGF beta family signaling. *Curr Top Microbiol Immunol,* 254, pp. 145-164

Wu, M.Y., and Hill, C.S. (2009). Tgf-beta superfamily signaling in embryonic development and homeostasis. *Dev Cell,* 16, 3, pp. 329-343

Yi, S.E., LaPolt, P.S., Yoon, B.S., Chen, J.Y., Lu, J.K., *et al.* (2001). The type I BMP receptor BmprIB is essential for female reproductive function. *Proc Natl Acad Sci U S A,* 98, 14, pp. 7994-7999

Yokouchi, Y., Sakiyama, J., Kameda, T., Iba, H., Suzuki, A., *et al.* (1996). BMP-2/-4 mediate programmed cell death in chicken limb buds. *Development,* 122, 12, pp. 3725-3734

Zhao, G.Q. (2003). Consequences of knocking out BMP signaling in the mouse. *Genesis,* 35, 1, pp. 43-56

Zhao, X., Sun, M., Zhao, J., Leyva, J.A., Zhu, H., *et al.* (2007). Mutations in HOXD13 underlie syndactyly type V and a novel brachydactyly-syndactyly syndrome. *Am J Hum Genet,* 80, 2, pp. 361-371

Zhu, H., Kavsak, P., Abdollah, S., Wrana, J.L., and Thomsen, G.H. (1999). A SMAD ubiquitin ligase targets the BMP pathway and affects embryonic pattern formation. *Nature,* 400, 6745, pp. 687-693

Zimmerman, L.B., De Jesus-Escobar, J.M., and Harland, R.M. (1996). The Spemann organizer signal noggin binds and inactivates bone morphogenetic protein 4. *Cell,* 86, 4, pp. 599-606

Zou, H., Wieser, R., Massague, J., and Niswander, L. (1997). Distinct roles of type I bone morphogenetic protein receptors in the formation and differentiation of cartilage. *Genes Dev*, 11, 17, pp. 2191-2203

Missense Mutation in the *LDLR* Gene: A Wide Spectrum in the Severity of Familial Hypercholesterolemia

Mathilde Varret and Jean-Pierre Rabès

Additional information is available at the end of the chapter

http://dx.doi.org/10.5772/36432

1. Introduction

Hypercholesterolemia is a major risk factor for atherosclerosis and its premature cardiovascular complications. Hypercholesterolemia can be multifactorial (diet, genetic background...) or - less frequently - monogenic, leading to Autosomal Dominant Hypercholesterolemia (ADH, OMIM #143890). ADH is characterised by a selective elevation of plasmatic Low Density Lipoprotein (LDL) levels, tendinous xanthoma and premature coronary heart disease. ADH has proven to be genetically heterogeneous and associated with defects in at least 3 different genes: *LDLR* (LDL receptor), *APOB* (apolipoprotein B) and *PCSK9* (proprotein convertase subtilisin-kexin type 9).

Familial hypercholesterolemia (FH, OMIM #606945) is the most frequent form of ADH and is due to mutations within the gene encoding the LDL specific receptor. FH is an autosomal co-dominant trait, with homozygotes being more severely affected than heterozygotes (Goldstein and Brown, 1989). FH is also one of the most common inherited disorders with a frequency of heterozygotes estimated to be 1:500 and a frequency of homozygotes being ≈ $1:10^6$ in most populations. In certain communities, such as French Canadians (Moorjani et al. 1989), Finns (Koivisto et al. 1992), Afrikaners (Kotze et al. 1989; Leitersdorf et al. 1989), Druze (Landsberger et al. 1992) and Lebanese (Lehrman et al. 1987), FH frequency can be as high as 1/67 because of founder effects.

2. The LDL receptor

The human low-density lipoprotein receptor mediates the transport of LDL into cells via endocytosis, and thus plays a major role in the clearance of lipoproteins from the blood. In 1973, by studying homozygous patient fibroblasts, Michael S. Brown and Joseph L.

Goldstein showed that the deficient protein in Familial Hypercholesterolemia was the LDL receptor (Goldstein and Brown, 1985).

The *LDLR* gene is localised at 19p13.1-p13.3, spans 45 kb and includes 18 exons (Lindgren et al. 1985; Yamamoto et al. 1984). It is ubiquitously expressed and encodes a glycoprotein of 839 amino acids that is pivotal in cholesterol homeostasis. The correspondence between the 6 functional domains of the protein and the exons of the *LDLR* gene is now well-established (Figure 1) (See Jeon and Blacklow 2005 for a review).

1. The signal peptide (21 amino acids) encoded by exon 1 is necessary for transport to the cell membrane and is cleaved during translocation into the endoplasmic reticulum (ER).
2. The ligand binding domain, encoded by exons 2 to 6 mediates the interaction with lipoproteins. This domain is made of seven modules named LDL receptor type A repeat (LR) and homologous to sequences of the protein C9 of the complement cascade (Südolf et al. 1985). Each LR module is about 40 residues long, has six conserved cysteine residues, and contains a conserved acidic region near the C-terminus which serves as a calcium-binding site (Yamamoto et al. 1984, Fass et al. 1997). Mutational studies of the seven LR modules of the LDL receptor indicate that modules 3-7 all contribute significantly to the binding of LDL particles (Russel et al. 1989). Each of the LR5 and LR6 modules is essentially structurally independent of the other (North et al. 1999).
3. The EGF precursor homology domain (400 amino acids encoded by exons 7 to 14) is made of three 40 amino acids repeats homologous to the EGF precursor, and is involved in the dissociation of the receptor and the lipoprotein in the endocytosis machinery. The two first repeats are contiguous and separated from the third by a 280 amino acid sequence that contains five copies of a conserved motif (YWTD) repeated once for each of 40-60 amino acids. The first epidermal growth factor-like repeat (EGF-A) in the EGF homology domain interacts in a sequence-specific manner with proprotein convertase subtilisin/kexin type 9 (PCSK9) (Zhang et al. 2007, Kwon et al. 2008). PCSK9 post-translationally regulates hepatic LDL receptors by binding to them on the cell surface and by leading to their degradation. Gain-of-function mutations that increase the affinity of PCSK9 toward the receptor and increase plasma LDL-cholesterol levels in humans, have been reported in the *PCSK9* gene associated with Autosomal Dominant Hypercholesterolemia (Abifadel et al. 2003, 2009). Loss-of-function mutations that decrease the affinity of PCSK9 toward the receptor have also been reported in the *PCSK9* gene associated with low plasma levels of LDL (Cohen et al. 2005).
4. Exon 15 encodes a 58 amino acid sequence that is enriched in serines and threonines, which serve as attachment sites for O-linked sugar chains. The absence of this exon has no significant functional consequence in cultured hamster fibroblasts (Davis et al. 1986).
5. The 22 amino acids membrane-anchoring domain, encoded by exon 16 and the 5′ end of exon 17, is essential to the attachment of the receptor to the cell membrane.
6. The 50 amino acid cytoplasmic tails, encoded by the remainder of exon 17 and the 5′ end of exon 18, are involved in the endocytosis of the protein. The NPXY motif was shown to interact with the AP-2 clathrin adaptor and thus is important in the localisation of the receptor in coated pits on the cell surface. The NPXY motif was also

shown to interact with the phosphotyrosine binding (PTB) domain of a specific clathrin adaptor protein encoded by the *LDLRAP1* gene. Mutations in the *LDLRAP1* gene have been reported in Autosomal Recessive Hypercholesterolemia (Garcia et al. 2001, Soutar 2010).

The reminder of exon 18 specifies the 2,6 kb 3' untranslated region of the mRNA.

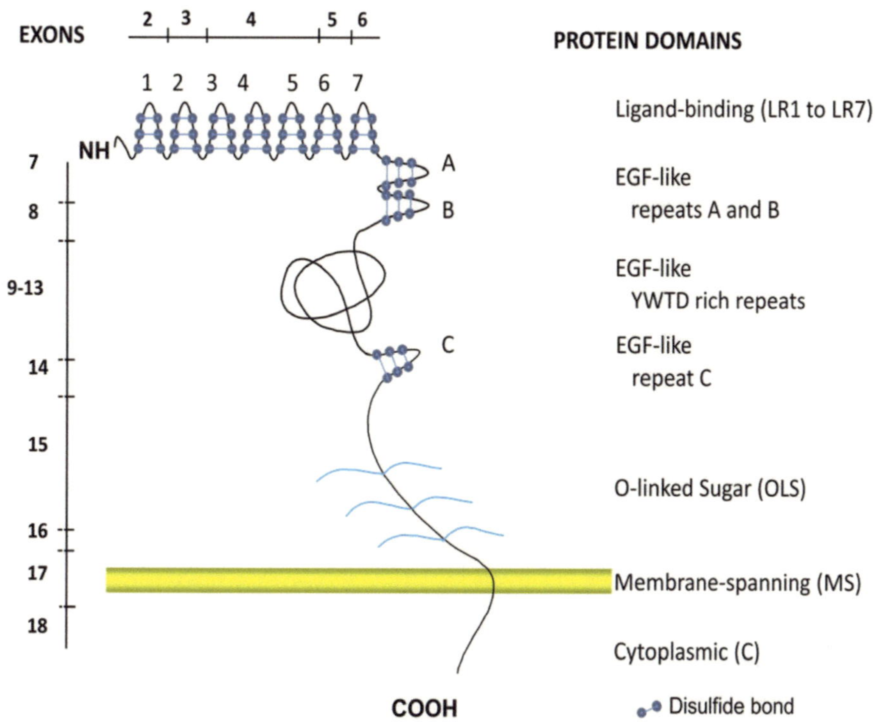

Figure 1. Correspondence between functional domains of the protein and exons of the *LDLR* gene.

In normal fibroblasts, the precursor protein is modified in the ER: the 21 amino acid signal peptide is cleaved and the precursor of 120 kDa is O-glycosylated to give rise to the 160 kDa protein. The resultant mature protein is transported from the Golgi apparatus to the cell surface within 30 minutes. The transmembrane receptor is present at the surface of most cell types and mediates the transport of LDL into cells, via receptor-mediated endocytosis, thus playing a pivotal role in cholesterol homeostasis (Goldstein and Brown, 2009). By endosome acidification, the lipoparticle is dissociated from the receptor, degraded and the receptor recycles back into the membrane.

3. Mutations in the *LDLR* gene

Mutations involving a small number of nucleotides, from point mutations to small deletions or insertions, account for 90% of all mutations in the *LDLR* gene, while the remaining are major rearrangements due to unequal recombination between the 30 *Alu* sequences identified throughout the gene (Hobbs et al. 1990). To date, more than 1400 point mutations and small deletions or insertions associated with FH have been reported in the *LDLR* gene (http://www.ucl.ac.uk/fh and www.umd.be/LDLR/).

The UMD-LDLR database (www.umd.be/LDLR/) actually includes 1404 point mutations, small deletions or insertions and mutations affecting splicing (intronic mutations) in the *LDLR* gene reported in the literature. It cannot accommodate mutations from the UTR and promoter regions, and large deletions or insertions or indels. In addition, two mutations that affect the same allele are entered as two different records linked by the same sample ID. If the same mutation has been reported in apparently unrelated patients (for example, the c.1A>C (p.Met1Leu) identified in Spanish (Chaves et al. 2001), British (Day et al. 1997) and Dutch patients (Fouchier et al. 2005), separate entries were made for each patient as recurrent mutations, in the absence of haplotypes demonstrating a common ancestor.

Among these 1404 small DNA variations of the *LDLR* gene, 58.5% are missense mutations, 21.7% are small deletions or insertions, 10.4 % are nonsense and 9.4% are splice site mutations. A large majority of these small DNA variations are single nucleotide substitutions (76.6%, 1076/1404), including 75.1% missense, 13.6% nonsense and 11.3% splice site mutations.

3.1. Missense mutations

Missense mutations are the most numerous of the small DNA variations (58.5%, 821/1404) reported in the *LDLR* gene in association with Familial Hypercholesterolemia (FH). Like the other small DNA variations in the *LDLR* gene, missense mutations are widely distributed throughout the whole sequence of the gene (Figure 2). Therefore, no real mutation hot spot can be defined which sustains the need to scan the whole gene sequence to identify FH-causing mutations in the diagnostic procedures.

The CpG dinucleotide has been shown to be a hot spot for mutations in humans because it can undergo oxidative deamination of 5-methyl cytosine (Krawczak et al. 1998). The *LDLR* gene sequence includes 123 CpG dinucleotides, accounting for 4.8% of the coding sequence. This ratio is similar to the mean percentage of CpG (3.7%) in the coding sequence of a large number of genes involved in human diseases and localised on autosomes (Cooper and Krawczak 1990). Missense mutations are the only substitutions in the *LDLR* gene occurring at the CpG dinucleotide for 4.8% (46/954) of all the single nucleotide variations. Interestingly, in the *LDLR* gene, the percentage of substitution occurring at the CpG (4.8%) is significantly lower than the mean observed for disease-causing mutations in other genes (37%) (Cooper and Krawczak 1990). There is no explanation, to date, for this observation.

In the LDL receptor protein, the most numerous amino acids are aspartate (8.7%), serine (8.1%), leucine (7.7%), cysteine (7.3%), glycine (7.2%) and valine (6.7%). The less represented amino acids are methionine (1.3%), tyrosine (2.0%), histidine (2.2%), tryptophane (2.3%) and phenylalanine (3.0%). This distribution of amino acids is consistent with the one reported for human proteins in general, with an exception for cysteine that is less abundant (3%) (Lewin

1990). The LDL receptor is known to be a cysteine-rich protein in which disulphide bonds between two cysteines are essential for ensuring the correct folding of 10 major modules necessary for protein activity (Russell et al. 1989, Kurniawan et al. 2001).

The number of mutations affecting an amino acid is not always related to its frequency in the protein. Cysteine, tryptophane and aspartate are more frequently affected than others residues, indicating that they are essential actors of protein activity. Substitutions affect 57 (90%) of the 63 cysteines of the LDL receptor, 43 (57%) of the 75 aspartates and 12 (60%) of the 20 tryptophanes. Cysteines are involved in the folding of the ligand binding and EGF-like domains. Aspartates are also highly conserved residues of the repeated modules of the LDL binding domain. Their negative charges are involved in bonds with positively charged residues of the apo B and apo E ligands. Apart from its hydrophobicity, tryptophane does not have a structural or functional role as manifest as those of a cysteine or a charged residue. However, along with methionine, tryptophane is the only amino acid encoded by a single codon, probably explaining its "more mutable" trait observed here.

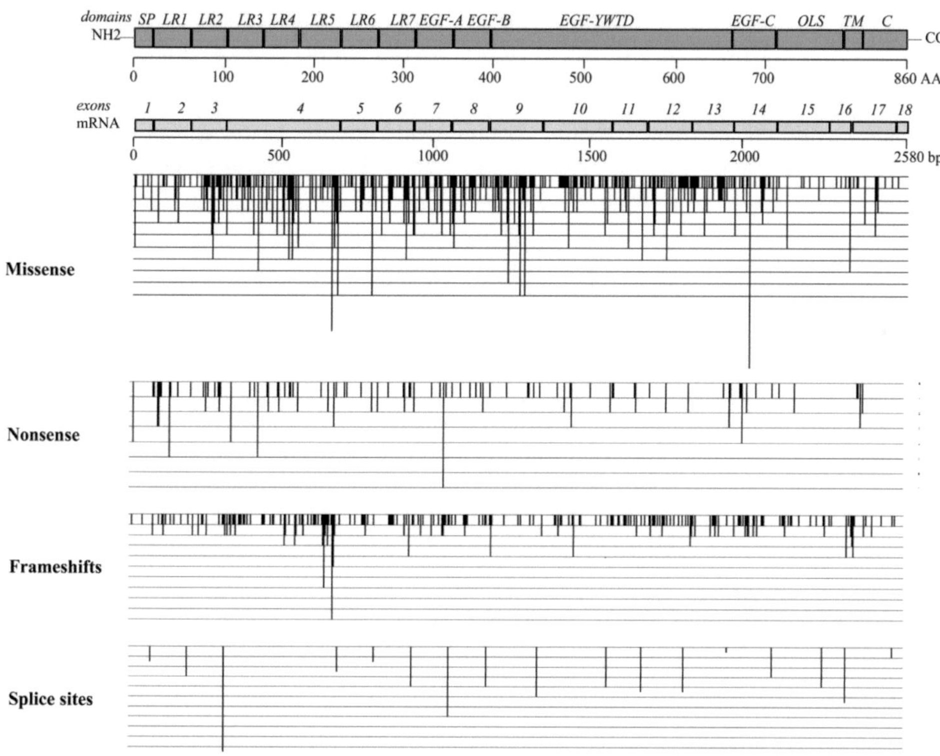

Figure 2. Distribution of point mutations within the LDL receptor gene (*LDLR*).

A certain proportion of the disease-causing substitutions (missense and nonsense mutations), ~25%, have been shown to alter functional splicing signals within exons, such as exonic splicing enhancers (ESE), to create an alternative splice site within exons that is used preferentially, or induce the loss of the consensus exonic splice site (Cartegni et al. 2002,

Sterne-Weiler et al. 2011). Within the *LDLR* gene, 28.4% of the reported missense mutations are predicted to alter functional splicing signals. The missense mutation c.2140G>C (p.Glu714Gln) that was predicted to be benign with four prediction tools for substitutions (Polyphen*, SIFT*, Pmut* and SNPs3D*) was predicted to create the loss of the intron 14 donor splice site with either NetGene2* and NNSPLICE* prediction tools for splice site mutations (Marduel et al. 2010). It is clear, however, that mRNA analyses are necessary to support these predictions, as performed for a small number of exonic substitutions. The conservative amino acid substitution c.2389 G>T (p.V776L) that would be unlikely to affect LDL receptor function, concerns the last nucleotide of exon 16 and causes exon 16 skipping (Bourbon et al. 2009). These missense mutations would therefore be likely to exert their major pathological effects on splicing rather than through an alteration in the amino acid sequence of the LDL receptor. This is reinforced by the observation of several silent substitutions associated with the clinical phenotype of familial hypercholesterolemia. The silent mutation p.Leu605Leu (c.1813C>T) was predicted to create a new donor splice site AGGT at position 1813 in exon 12. The use of this new donor site would lead to the substitution of leucine 605 by a threonine, the deletion of 11 amino acids (from Alanine 606 to Aspartate 616), a frameshift and the appearance of a premature termination 49 codons further on (Marduel et al. 2010). The variant, c.621C>T (p.Gly207Gly), was found to be associated with altered splicing. The nucleotide change leading to p.Gly207Gly resulted in the generation of new 3'-splice donor site in exon 4 of the LDL receptor gene. Splicing of this alternate splice site leads to an in-frame 75-base pair deletion in a stable mRNA of exon 4 and nonsense-mediated mRNA decay (Defesche et al. 2008). The silent mutation, p.Arg406Arg, that also introduces a new splice site, causes a deletion of 31 bp in the *LDLR* mRNA sequence, and introduces a premature termination 4 codons further on (Bourbon et al. 2007).

NetGene2	http://www.cbs.dtu.dk/services/NetGene2/
NNSPLICE	http://www.fruitfly.org/seq_tools/splice.html
Polyphen	http://genetics.bwh.harvard.edu/pph/
SIFT	http://sift.jcvi.org/
Pmut	http://mmb2.pcb.ub.es:8080/PMut/
SNP3D	http://www.snps3d.org/

Tools for *in silico* prediction of protein function.

3.2. Frameshift mutations

Among the 1404 small DNA variations of the *LDLR* gene, a total of 305 (21.7%) are small deletions or insertions, including 261 (85.6%) independent mutations leading to a frameshift and 55 (14.4%) in-frame deletions or insertions. This proportion of in-frame small deletions or insertions is consistent with observations made for other disease-causing genes (Cooper, Antonarakis and Krawczak 1995). The frameshift mutations are due to either a small deletion (176/261, 12.5%) or insertion/duplication (85/261, 6.0%) of a few nucleotides (from 1 to 49 for deletions, from 1 to 23 for insertions). The sequence context analysis provides evidence that a repeated motif flanking the frameshift event could be involved in the aetiology of the mutation in 48.0% of the deletional events and in 29.2% of the insertional events.

Half of the frameshift mutations involved a single nucleotide: 58.5% (103/176) among deletions and 56.5% (48/85) among insertions. In half of the deletion cases and in half the insertion cases, the single nucleotide deletion/insertion occurs within runs of 2 to 7 identical bases. Runs of identical bases are known to cause deletions/insertions according to the slipped mispairing mechanism occurring at DNA replication (Ball et al. 2005).

Deletions involving larger sequences (from 2 to 49 bp) can be divided into three different types: (1) One of the repeated flanking sequences is included in the deletion, which is also explained by the slipped mispairing mechanism occurring at DNA replication (Ball et al. 2005); (2) The repeated sequences flanking the deletion are not included in the frameshift mutation, which is explained by homologous recombination between palindromic or symmetric repeated sequences (Cooper 1995); (3) Parts of the flanking repeated sequences are included in the deletion. To date, no molecular mechanism has been identified to explain such deletional events.

Insertions involving larger sequences (from 2 to 23 bp) can be explained by the same mechanisms as described for deletions, and can be divided into two different types: (1) The inserted sequence is a duplication; (2) The inserted sequence is new within the *LDLR* gene sequence. This latter observation raises the hypothesis that very probably insertions do not occur at random but rather in order to create repeated sequences that were not present in the original gene sequence. A consensus sequence, GTAAGT, was frequently identified flanking small deletions or insertions (Ball et al. 2005). In the *LDLR* gene sequence, this consensus is present at the 3′ end of exon 4 at position c.681-687. Among the 96 deletions (in frame and frameshift) in the *LDLR* gene, 11 (11.5%) are at this position pointing to a discrete hot spot for insertions, as observed in Figure 2 and in accordance with previous reports (Kotze et al. 1996).

3.3. Nonsense mutations

Nonsense mutations represent 10.4% (146/1404) of the small DNA variations in the *LDLR* gene, and 13.6% (146/1076) of the FH-causing substitutions.

Among the 860 codons of the *LDLR* gene sequence, 253 potential stop codons (codons that can be turned into a stop codon with only one substitution) were identified (29.4%) and were not equally distributed throughout the whole gene. In exons 2 to 8, more than 33% of the protein codons are potential stop codons, while less than 21% of the protein codons are potential stop codons in exons 9, 10, 13, 15 and 16. Among these 253 potential stop codons, 93 of them (36.8%) are affected by a mutational event.

The number of mutations affecting potential stop codons is not always related to their frequency in each exon. Potential stop codons are more frequently affected by mutation in exons 3, 9, 10 and 14, with 57.1%, 50.0%, 46.2% and 53.3% respectively of potential stop codons in each exon carrying a mutational event. Conversely, in exons 1, 12, 13 and 17,

16.7%, 18.2%, 20.0% and 26.7% respectively of the potential stop codons are affected by a mutational event.

3.4. Splice site mutations

Among the 1404 small DNA variations of the *LDLR* gene, a total of 132 (9.4%) are splice site mutations and, among the 1076 single nucleotide FH-causing substitutions, 122 (11.4%) are intronic. From the analysis of a large number of genes, a mean proportion of 15% for splice site mutations among disease-causing DNA substitutions was evaluated (Krawczak et al. 2007). The expected frequency of splice site substitutions within the *LDLR* gene is 9% (Cooper and Krawczak 1990). The number of FH-causing splice site substitutions observed in this wide review of the literature (9.5%) is thus consistent with the expected value for the *LDLR* gene.

Among the 132 splice site mutations of the *LDLR* gene, 14 (10.6%) are mid-intronic mutations situated at more than 10 bp of intron/exon junctions. Half of the intronic mutational events in the *LDLR* gene (55.3%, 73/132) affect the two canonical "AG" and "GT" highly conserved dinucleotides of the acceptor and donor splice sites respectively. Accordingly to the analysis of a large number of disease-causing mutations in different genes (Krawckak et al. 1992), within the *LDLR* gene intronic mutations affecting a donor splice site are more frequent (65.1%, 86/132) than mutations affecting an acceptor splice site (36.4%, 48/132).

4. Comparative analysis of mutations in the *LDLR* gene

To facilitate the mutational analysis of the *LDLR* gene and promote the analysis of the relationship between genotype and phenotype, in 1997 we created a software package along with a computerised database: UMD-LDLR. For each mutation, information is provided at several levels: at the gene level (exon and codon number, wild type and mutant codon, mutational event, mutation name), at the mRNA level (size, processing), at the protein level (wild type and mutant amino acid, affected domain, activity, mutation class), and at the personal level (ethnic background, age, sex, body mass index and familial history of coronary heart disease). The software package contains routines for the analysis of the LDLR database that were developed with the 4th dimensionR (4D) package from ACI. The use of the 4D SGDB gives access to optimised multi-criteria research and sorting tools to select records from any field. Moreover, 13 routines were specifically developed (Varret et al. 1997, 1998, Villèger et al. 2002, Béroud et al. 2005, www.umd.be/LDLR/).

The aim of this study was to analyse these four mutation groups at the molecular, biological and clinical level.

4.1. Analysis of *LDLR* mutations at the molecular level

4.1.1. Frequency of mutational events

DNA substitutions are of two types: transitions are interchanges of two-ring purines (A>G and G>A) or of one-ring pyrimidines (C>T and T>C) and, therefore, involve bases of similar shape; transversions are interchanges of purine for pyrimidine bases, which involve exchange of one-ring and two-ring structures. Therefore, there are twice as many possible transversions as there are transitions. However, among human diseases-causing substitutions, transitions (63%) are observed more frequently than transversions (37%) (Cooper and Krawczak 1990).

Accordingly, in the *LDLR* gene, missense mutations due to transitions (55.9%, 459/821) are more frequent than substitutions due to transversions (42.5%, 349/821) (Figure 3). Like exonic mutational events, small DNA variations at the splice site are substitutions (92.4%, 122/132) or small deletions/insertions (9.1%, 12/132). Again, among the intronic substitutions, transitions (59.8%, 73/122) are observed more frequently than transversions (40.1%, 49/122) (Figure 3). Interestingly, in the *LDLR* gene, the ratio of transversion/transition is different for nonsense mutations. The transversions are the more frequent mutational event leading to a stop codon (52.7%, 77/146) compared to transitions (47.3%, 69/146) (Figure 3).

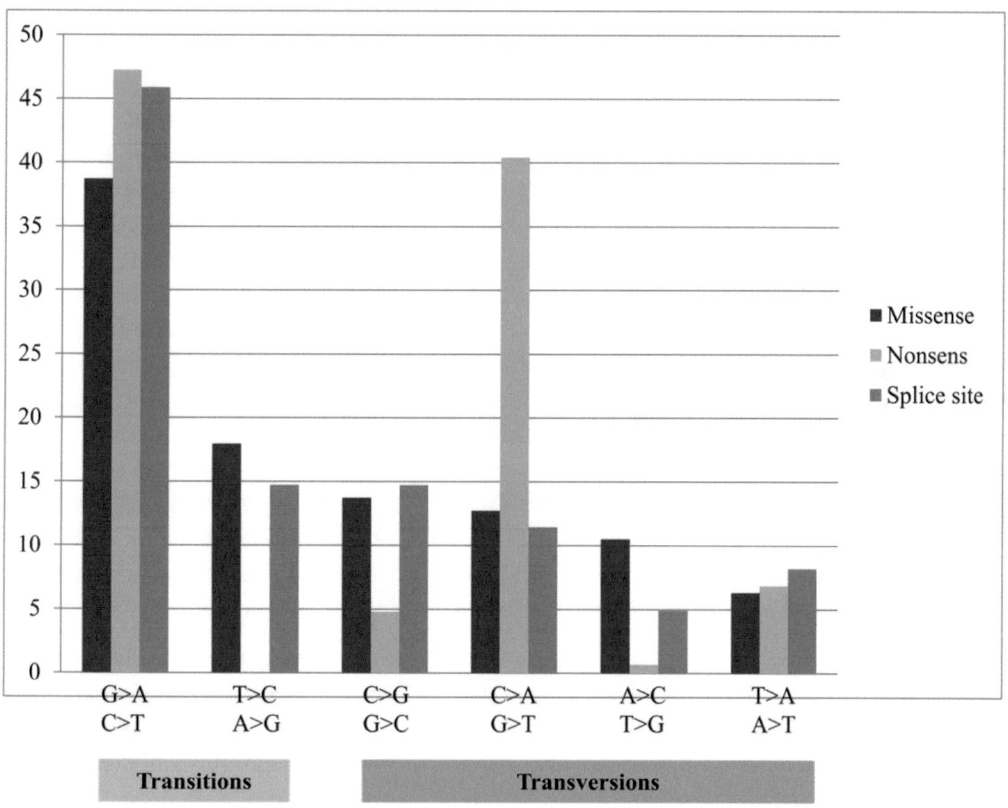

Figure 3. Molecular events frequency of the different groups of mutations. Values are given in % of each event within each group of mutation.

Because of the constraints mediated by the genetic code, transition A>G and transversion A>C, G>C cannot be at the origin of a stop codon. Thus, only two transitional events (G>A and C>T) and 6 transversional events (A>T, C>A, C>G, G>T, T>A and T>G) lead to a stop codon, which means that half of the transitional events and a quarter of the transversional events are not involved in nonsense mutations. These constraints can explain the observed difference in the ratio of transversion/transition between missense and nonsense mutations.

However, the ratio of transversion/transition is consistent with the one observed for human diseases-causing substitutions (Cooper and Krawczak 1990) when the three groups of mutations are taken together (missense, nonsense and splice). Altogether, transitions (55.9%, 601/1076) are observed more frequently than transversions (44.1%, 475/1076).

4.1.2. Distribution of the substitutions in the 18 exons of the LDLR gene

The expected number of mutations in each exon is estimated by the 'Stat exons' tool of the UMD software according to the size and the composition (mutability of each codon) of each exon (Béroud et al. 2000 and 2005). This analysis enables the detection of a statistically significant difference between observed and expected mutations.

For exons 1, 5, 8 and 10 to 14, all types of substitutions are distributed as expected. There is a significant excess of all substitutions (missense and nonsense) within exons 3 and 4 (Table 1), indicating discrete mutational hot-spots and underlining the essential role played by the encoded domains in protein function. Exon 3 encodes the second LR motif of the ligand binding domain in the LDL receptor. To date, there is no data revealing a more essential function of this LR motif when compared to the six others. Exon 4 encodes the three central LR motifs (LR3, LR4 and LR5) of the ligand binding domain in the LDL receptor. The LR5 motif have been shown to be the only one of the seven LR motifs to be able to bind the two ligands of the receptor, apo B and apo E, while the 6 other motifs only bind apo B (Russel et al. 1989). Thus, the mutations affecting this motif are associated with a more severe alteration of lipoprotein catabolism and, therefore, have a higher tendency to be selected by FH definition criteria. There is a significant deficit of all substitutions (missense and nonsense) within exons 15 and 16 (Table 1) indicating discrete mutational cold-spots. Exon 15 encodes the O-linked sugar domain of the LDL receptor that has been shown to have no significant functional activity (Davis et al. 1986). To date, there is no explanation as to the observed deficit of substitutions within exon 16 which encodes the membrane-anchoring domain that is essential to the attachment of the receptor to the cell membrane.

The two types of exonic substitutions (missense and nonsense) are differently distributed in exons 2, 6, 7, 9, 17 and 18 of the *LDLR* gene (Table 1). Missense mutations are the only ones presenting a significant excess in exons 6 and 9 and a significant deficit in exons 17 and 18 (Table 1), maybe reflecting a bias in this analysis due to the different number of mutations of each type. Nonsense mutations are less numerous than missense mutations, a significant difference is thus less probably obtained for nonsenses than for missenses. Nevertheless, these observations indicate discrete mutational hot-spots within exons 6 and 9 and discrete mutational cold-spots within exons 17 and 18. Exon 6 encodes the last LR motif of the ligand binding domain in the LDL receptor. To date, there is no data revealing a more essential function of this LR motif when compared with the six others. Exon 9 encodes the NH2-

terminal part of the EGF-like domain which is rich in YWTD repeats which are essential for the correct folding of the receptor at the cell surface. To date, there is no explanation as to the observed deficit of substitutions within exons 17 and 18 encoding the COOH-terminal part of the membrane-anchoring domain and the cytoplasmic tail, which are essential for the attachment of the receptor to the cell membrane and in the endocytosis of the protein.

In exon 2, we observed a significant deficit of missenses and a significant excess of nonsenses (Table 1). Exon 2 encodes the first LR motif of the ligand binding domain in the LDL receptor. To date, there is no data revealing a more or less essential function of this LR motif when compared with the six others.

Interestingly, nonsense mutations are the only ones that present a significant excess in exon 7 of the *LDLR* gene (Table 1). This excess relies upon the high frequency of the c.1048C>T, p.Arg350X mutation, formerly called FH-Fossum. Indeed, this mutation is reported in 9 apparently unrelated patients from different geographic origins: Norway (Solberg et al. 1994), the Netherlands (Lombardi et al. 1995), the U.K. (Day et al. 1997), Poland (Gorski et al. 1998), Germany (Thiart et al. 1998), Canada (Gaudet et al. 1999), Japan (Yu et al. 2002), Denmark (Damgaard et al. 2005) and Spain (Brusgaard et al. 2006). In the absence of haplotypes demonstrating a common ancestor, these mutational events are supposed to be recurrent and to correspond to a mutational hot-spot in the *LDLR* gene.

Exon	**Expected mutations (%)**	**Observed missenses**		**Observed nonsenses**		**Observed exonic substitutions**	
		%	**significance**	%	**significance**	%	**significance**
1	**2,6**	1,7	ns	2,7	ns	1,9	ns
2	**5,0**	2,5	< 0.01	11,6	< 0.001	3,9	ns
3	**4,8**	6,4	< 0.05	6,8	< 0.05	6,5	< 0.02
4	**14,9**	20,5	< 0.001	20,5	< 0.001	20,5	< 0.001
5	**4,8**	4,4	ns	3,4	ns	4,3	ns
6	**4,9**	7,0	< 0.01	5,5	ns	6,8	< 0.01
7	**4,7**	5,2	ns	8,9	< 0.02	5,7	ns
8	**5,0**	5,3	ns	4,8	ns	5,2	ns
9	**6,6**	11,2	< 0.001	4,1	ns	10,1	< 0.001
10	**8,7**	7,3	ns	6,2	ns	7,1	ns
11	**4,7**	4,9	ns	4,8	ns	4,9	ns
12	**5,2**	6,4	ns	2,1	ns	5,7	ns
13	**5,6**	5,3	ns	2,1	ns	4,8	ns
14	**5,9**	6,4	ns	9,6	ns	6,9	ns
15	**6,4**	1,6	< 0.001	2,1	< 0.05	1,7	< 0.001
16	**2,8**	1,5	< 0.05	0,0	< 0.05	1,3	< 0.01
17	**6,1**	2,3	< 0.001	4,8	ns	2,7	< 0.001
18	**1,3**	0,1	< 0.01	0,0	ns	0,1	< 0.001

Table 1. Distribution of the different exonic substitutions throughout the 18 exons of the *LDLR* gene.

4.2. Analysis of *LDLR* mutations at the biological level

4.2.1. Functional classes of LDLR gene's mutations

Mutations in the *LDLR* gene have been classified into 5 functional groups based on the characteristics of the mutant protein produced and analysed in patients' fibroblasts (Hobbs et al 1992):

Class 1 mutations disrupt the synthesis of the LDL receptor and no precursor is produced (null alleles).

Class 2 mutations block transport to the Golgi apparatus: mutations are reported in class 2A when a complete defect in transport to the cell membrane is observed and in class 2B when receptors are transported at a detectable - but markedly reduced - rate.

Class 3 mutations produce proteins that reach the membrane but fail to bind the LDL.

Class 4 mutations produce a receptor that binds the lipoprotein but which cannot be internalised. The mutations affecting the cytoplasmic domain alone are classed 4A, while those also affecting the membrane-spanning region are classed 4B.

Class 5 mutations block the acid-dependant dissociation of the receptor and the ligand in the endosome, an essential event for receptor recycling.

The link between the functional class type of the mutation and the severity of the disease has been established, and patients carrying a class 1 mutation are more severely affected than those with a mutation from another functional group (Hobbs et al 1992). In the UMD-LDLR database, among the 288 single nucleotide mutations with available data concerning the functional group, 42.0% (121/288) are class 2B, 31.9% (92/288) are class 1, 13.5% (39/288) are class 5, 7.6% (22/288) are class 2A, 3.8% (11/288) are class 4A and 1.0% (3/288) are class 3. Class 1 mutations are mainly nonsense and frameshift mutations (66.3% nonsenses, 30.4% frameshifts and 3.3% missenses) and 62% of them are localised in exons 2 to 6, encoding the ligand binding domain for one half and in exons 7 to 14 encoding the EGF-like domain for the other half (Figure 4). Class 2B mutations are mainly missense mutations (92.6% missenses and 7.4% frameshifts) and 71% of them are localised in exons 2 to 6, encoding the ligand binding domain (Figure 4). Class 5 mutations are mainly missense mutations (95% missenses and 5% splice site mutations) and 95% of them are localised in exons 7 to 14, encoding the EGF-like domain (Figure 4). Class 2A, 3 and 4A mutations are mainly missense mutations (59% missenses, 22% nonsenses and 19% frameshifts) and 67% of them are localised in exons 7 to 14, encoding the EGF-like domain. As expected, the localisation of these different classes of mutations is consistent with the functional definition of each class. The higher prevalence of mutations at the origin of truncated proteins (nonsenses and frameshifts) within the class 1 functional group is consistent with the expected null allele effect of these kinds of mutations. Altogether, these observations are globally in agreement with the admitted dogma according to which mutations leading to a protein of abnormal size (nonsense, frameshift and splice) are at the origin of a more severe phenotype than missense mutations.

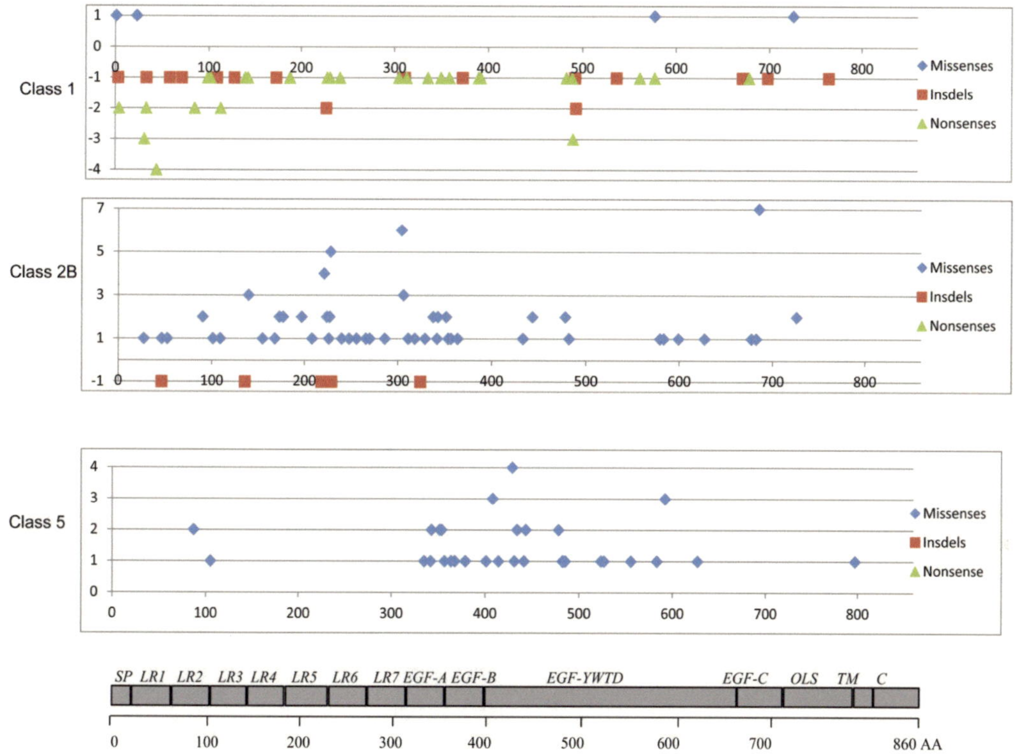

Figure 4. Distribution of the different mutations according to the three main functional classes.

4.2.2. LDL receptor activity

In the UMD-LDLR database, the LDL receptor activity measured in patients' fibroblasts is available for 91 single nucleotide mutations: assays were performed for 24 heterozygote carriers, 22 homozygote carriers and 45 compound heterozygotes.. For homozygote carriers of a missense mutation, the mean LDL receptor activity is 8.7% rather than 2.7% for carriers of a mutation leading to a protein of abnormal size (nonsense, frameshift and splice) (Figure 5). For heterozygote carriers of a missense mutation, the mean LDL receptor activity is 33.2% rather than 19.8% for carriers of an abnormal-protein mutation. Moreover, a gradient can be drawn for compound heterozygotes with a mean LDL receptor activity of 13.3%, 7.3% and 3.6% for carriers of two missense mutations, one missense and one abnormal-protein mutation and two abnormal-protein mutations respectively (Figure 5). Once again, these observations are globally in agreement with an admittedly more severe phenotype for mutations leading to a protein of abnormal size when compared with missense mutations. However, missense mutations in the *LDLR* gene are associated with a larger spectrum of LDL receptor activity in fibroblasts (from 2% to 67% for heterozygotes and from 2% to 22.5% for homozygotes) when compared with mutations leading to a protein of abnormal size (from 2% to 47% for heterozygotes and from 2% to 11% for homozygotes).

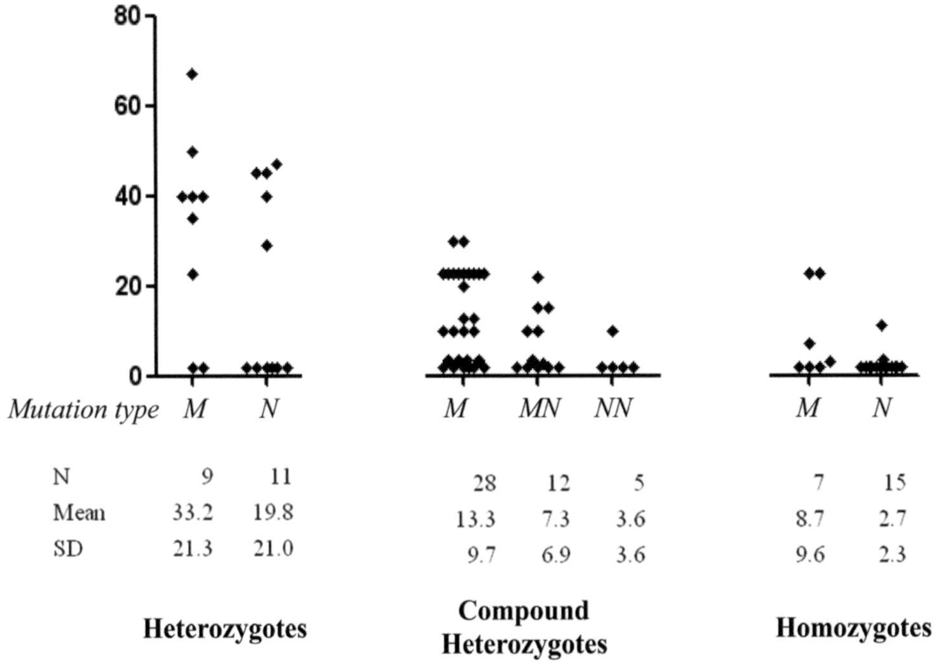

Figure 5. LDL receptor activity in fibroblast from mutation carriers. The values are expressed as % of LDL binding compared with the values obtained for normocholesterolemic subjects. M: missense. N: null allele (frameshift, splice, nonsense).

4.3. Analysis of *LDLR* mutations at the biochemical/clinical level

4.3.1. Plasmatic lipid levels among LDLR gene mutations carriers

Among the 1061 unique events included in the UMD-LDLR database, lipid values are available for only 307 of them (29%), corresponding with 25 homozygote carriers and 282 heterozygote carriers of different molecular events within the *LDLR* gene (Table 2). According to the biochemical definition of familial hypercholesterolemia, triglycerides and HDL-cholesterol levels were within the normal range while the total- and LDL-cholesterol levels were elevated. As expected for a co-dominant disease, the total- and LDL-cholesterol levels were higher for homozygote mutation carriers than for molecular heterozygotes. No differences were observed between the four groups of mutations (missenses, frameshifts, splice sites and nonsenses), suggesting a similar effect of missense and mutations leading to a protein of abnormal size (nonsense, frameshift and splice) on the biochemical expression of the disease. Furthermore, no differences were observed among the distribution of total- and LDL-cholesterol levels among the four groups of mutations (Figure 6).

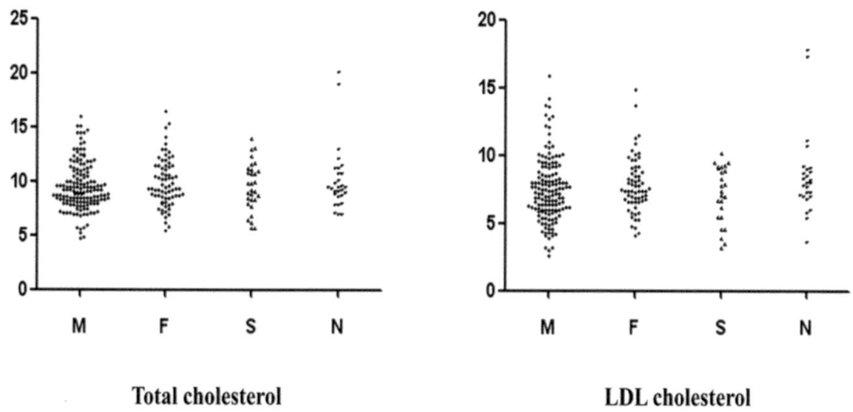

Figure 6. Distribution of total- and LDL-cholesterol plasmatic levels for heterozygotes carriers of a missense (M), a frameshift (F), a splice site (S) or a nonsense (N) mutation in the LDLR gene.

		HDL-Cholesterol	LDL-Cholesterol	Total Cholesterol	Triglycerides
Heterozygotes					
Missense	N	133	144	152	137
	Mean (SD)	1.31 (0.51)	7.50 (2.38)	9.50 (2.18)	1.66 (0.94)
Frameshift	N	60	63	73	64
	Mean (SD)	1.21 (0.34)	7.84 (2.05)	9.89 (2.22)	1.39 (0.89)
Splice	N	22	25	30	24
	Mean (SD)	1.28 (0.41)	7.17 (2.08)	9.56 (2.20)	1.49 (0.54)
Nonsenses	N	24	24	27	27
	Mean (SD)	1.17 (0.40)	7.74 (1.64)	9.43 (1.53)	1.46 (0.73)
Homozygotes					
Missense	N	13	15	14	12
	Mean (SD)	1.04 (0.41)	15.55 (4.96)	17.39 (4.49)	1.42 (0.72)
Frameshift	N	3	3	3	2
	Mean (SD)	0.66 (0.21)	16.01 (1.17)	17.43 (0.93)	1.23 (0.04)
Splice	N	3	3	5	4
	Mean (SD)	0.67 (0.16)	15.25 (1.79)	18.06 (4.74)	1.34 (0.17)
Nonsenses	N	2	2	2	2
	Mean (SD)	0.87 (0.52)	17.54 (0.37)	19.56 (0.76)	2.00 (1.27)

Table 2. Mean plasmatic lipid levels for heterozygotes and homozygote carriers of missense, frameshift, splice site or nonsense mutations in the *LDLR* gene. Values are in mmol/L.

4.3.2. Clinical expression of familial hypercholesterolemia among LDLR gene mutation carriers

Of the 1061 unique events reported in the UMD-LDLR database, clinical data is available for only 230 of them (22%) including 25 homozygote carriers and 215 heterozygote carriers of different molecular events within the *LDLR* gene (Table 3). This clinical data concerns tendinous cholesterol deposits - such as xanthomas - and the diagnosis of premature coronary artery disease (CAD). Tendinous xanthomas are more frequently observed for the carriers of a mutation leading to a protein of abnormal size rather than for the heterozygotes for a missense mutation (Table 3). Once more, this observation is in agreement with the admitted dogma according to which mutations leading to a protein of abnormal size (nonsense, frameshift and splice) are at the origin of a more severe phenotype than are missense mutations. However, no differences were observed for the occurrence of CAD between missenses and those mutations leading to a protein of abnormal size (Table 3). This latter observation suggests a similar effect with regard to missense and mutation leading to a protein of abnormal size (nonsense, frameshift and splice) in the clinical expression of the disease.

	Missenses			Frameshifts, Splice sites, Nonsenses		
Sex ratio (M/F)	1.06 (83/78)			1.09 (60/55)		
Age (mean years ± SD)	39.6 ± 17.5			36.8 ± 14.9		
	N	Yes (%)	No (%)	N	Yes (%)	No (%)
CAD	100	58	42	99	52	48
Tendinous xanthomas	106	50	50	109	65	35

Table 3. Clinical expression of familial hypercholesterolemia for heterozygotes carriers of different mutations in the *LDLR* gene.

5. Conclusion

To date, it seems logical that mutations leading to a protein of abnormal size (nonsense, frameshift and splice) are at the origin of a more severe phenotype than missense mutations. The genotype/phenotype correlations performed with the UMD-LDLR database provide molecular, biological and clinical evidence that underlies this dogma. Moreover, missense mutations in the *LDLR* gene are the source of a wider spectrum in the severity of FH, than are mutations leading to a protein of abnormal size, from an almost normal phenotype to very severe forms of the disease.

Mutations in the *LDLR* gene are numerous and frequently recurrent but, conversely, rarely sporadic. These observations reveal not only the high mutability at one time of this gene, but also that these mutations were probably selected through time. It can be postulated that a hypercholesterolemic mutation could have given a selective advantage to carriers and may be a member of the pool of alleles that constitute the «"thrifty genotype" (Neel at al. 1998). The thrifty genotype hypothesis suggested that, in the early years of life, the hypercholesterolemic genotype was thrifty in the sense of being exceptionally efficient in the utilisation of food. It would thereby confer a survival advantage during times of food shortage. However, in contemporary societies, as food is usually available in unlimited amounts, the thrifty genotype no longer provides a survival advantage but instead renders its owners more susceptible to hypercholesterolemia.

Author details

Mathilde Varret
INSERM U698, Paris, France
Université Paris Denis Diderot, France

Jean-Pierre Rabès
INSERM U698, Paris, France
AP-HP, Hôpital A. Paré, Laboratoire de Biochimie et Génétique Moléculaire, Boulogne-Billancourt, France
Université Versailles Saint-Quentin-en-Yvelines, UFR de Médecine Paris Ile-de-France Ouest, Guyancourt, France

6. References

Abifadel M, Varret M, Rabès JP, Allard D, Ouguerram K, Devillers M, Cruaud C, Benjannet S, Wickham L, Erlich D, Derré A, Villéger L, Farnier M, Beucler I, Bruckert E, Chambaz J, Chanu B, Lecerf JM, Luc G, Moulin P, Weissenbach J, Prat A, Krempf M, Junien C, Seidah NG, Boileau C. Mutations in PCSK9 cause autosomal dominant hypercholesterolemia. Nat Genet. 2003: 34(2): 154-6.

Abifadel M, Rabès JP, Devillers M, Munnich A, Erlich D, Junien C, Varret M, Boileau C. Mutations and polymorphisms in the proprotein convertase subtilisin kexin 9 (PCSK9) gene in cholesterol metabolism and disease. Hum Mutat. 2009: 30(4): 520-9.

Ball EV, Stenson PD, Abeysinghe SS, Krawczak M, Cooper DN, Chuzhanova NA. Microdeletions and microinsertions causing human genetic disease: common mechanisms of mutagenesis and the role of local DNA sequence complexity. Hum Mutat. 2005: 26(3): 205-13.

Béroud C, Collod-Beroud G, Boileau C et al. UMD (Universal Mutation Database): a generic software to build and analyze locus-specific databases. Human Mutation 2000: 15: 86-94.

Béroud C, Hamroun D, Collod-Beroud G et al. UMD (Universal Mutation Database): 2005 update. Hum Mut 2005: 26(3): 184-191.

Bourbon M, Sun XM, Soutar AK. A rare polymorphism in the low density lipoprotein (LDL) gene that affects mRNA splicing. Atherosclerosis. 2007: 195(1): e17-20

Bourbon M, Duarte MA, Alves AC, Medeiros AM, Marques L, Soutar AK. Genetic diagnosis of familial hypercholesterolaemia: the importance of functional analysis of potential splice-site mutations. J Med Genet. 2009: 46(5): 352-7.

Brown MS, Goldstein JL. A receptor-mediated pathway for cholesterol homeostasis. Science 1986: 232(4746): 34–47.

Brusgaard K, Jordan P, Hansen H, Hansen AB, Hørder M.

Molecular genetic analysis of 1053 Danish individuals with clinical signs of familial hypercholesterolemia. Clin Genet. 2006: 69(3): 277-83.

Cartegni L, Chew SL, Krainer AR. Listening to silence and understanding nonsense: exonic mutations that affect splicing. Nat Rev Genet. 2002: 3(4): 285-98.

Chaves FJ, Real JT, García-García AB, Civera M, Armengod ME, Ascaso JF, Carmena R. Genetic diagnosis of familial hypercholesterolemia in a South European outbreed population: influence of low-density lipoprotein (LDL) receptor gene mutations on treatment response to simvastatin in total, LDL, and high-density lipoprotein cholesterol. J Clin Endocrinol Metab. 2001: 86(10): 4926-32.

Cohen J, Pertsemlidis A, Kotowski IK, Graham R, Garcia CK, Hobbs HH. Low LDL cholesterol in individuals of African descent resulting from frequent nonsense mutations in PCSK9. Nat Genet. 2005: 37(2):161-5.

Cooper DN, Krawczak M. The mutational spectrum of single base-pair substitutions causing human genetic disease: patterns and predictions. Hum Genet 1990: 85(1): 55-74.

Cooper DN, Antonarakis SE and Krawczak M. The nature and mechanisms of human gene mutation. In: Scriver CR, Beaudet AL, Sly WS and Valle D eds. The metabolic basis of inherited diseases. New York: Mc Graw-Hill, 1995.

Crick FHC. Codon – anticodon pairing: the wobble hypothesis. J. Mol. Biol., 19(1966), pp. 548–555.

Damgaard D, Nissen PH, Jensen LG, Nielsen GG, Stenderup A, Larsen ML, Faergeman O. Detection of large deletions in the LDL receptor gene with quantitative PCR methods. BMC Med Genet. 2005: 6: 15.

Davis CG, Elhammer A, Russell DW, et al. Deletion of clustered O-linked carbohydrates does not impair function of low density lipoprotein receptor in transfected fibroblasts. J Biol Chem. 1986: 261(6): 2828-38.

Day IN, Haddad L, O'Dell SD, Day LB, Whittall RA, Humphries SE. Identification of a common low density lipoprotein receptor mutation (R329X) in the south of England: complete linkage disequilibrium with an allele of microsatellite D19S394. J Med Genet. 1997: 34(2): 111-6.

Defesche JC, Schuurman EJ, Klaaijsen LN, Khoo KL, Wiegman A, Stalenhoef AF. Silent exonic mutations in the low-density lipoprotein receptor gene that cause familial hypercholesterolemia by affecting mRNA splicing. Clin Genet. 2008: 73(6): 573-8.

Fass D, Blacklow S, Kim PS, Berger JM. Molecular basis of familial hypercholesterolaemia from structure of LDL receptor module. Nature 1997: 388(6643): 691-3.

Fouchier SW, Kastelein JJ, Defesche JC. Update of the molecular basis of familial hypercholesterolemia in The Netherlands. Hum Mutat. 2005: 26(6): 550-6.

Garcia CK, Wilund K, Arca M, et al. Autosomal recessive hypercholesterolemia caused by mutations in a putative LDL receptor adaptor protein. Science 2001: 292(5520): 1394-8.

Gaudet D, Vohl MC, Couture P, Moorjani S, Tremblay G, Perron P, Gagné C, Després JP. Contribution of receptor negative versus receptor defective mutations in the LDL-receptor gene to angiographically assessed coronary artery disease among young (25-49 years) versus middle-aged (50-64 years) men. Atherosclerosis. 1999 : 143(1): 153-61.

Goldstein JL, Schrott HG, Hazzard WR et al. Hyperlipidemia in coronary heart disease. II. Genetic analysis of lipid levels in 176 families and delineation of a new inherited disorder, combined hyperlipidemia. J Clin Invest 1973: 52(7): 1544–1568.

Goldstein J, Brown M. Familial hypercholesterlemia. In: Scriver C, Beaudet A, Sly W, eds. The metabolic basis of inherited diseases. New York: Mc Graw-Hill, 1989: 1215–1250.

Goldstein JL, Brown MS. History of Discovery: The LDL receptor. Arterioscler Thromb Vasc Biol 2009: 29(4): 431-8.

Górski B, Kubalska J, Naruszewicz M, Lubiński J. LDL-R and Apo-B-100 gene mutations in Polish familial hypercholesterolemias. Hum Genet 1998: 102(5): 562-5.

Hobbs HH, Russell DW, Brown MS, Goldstein JL. The LDL receptor locus in familial hypercholesterolemia: mutational analysis of a membrane protein. Annu Rev Genet 1990: 24: 133-170.

Hobbs HH, Brown MS, Goldstein JL. Molecular genetics of the LDL receptor gene in familial hypercholesterolemia. Hum Mutat 1992: 1: 445-66.

Jeon H, Blacklow SC. Structure and physiologic function of the low-density lipoprotein receptor. Annu Rev Biochem. 2005: 74: 535-62.

Koivisto UM, Turtola H, Aalto-Setala K, et al. The familial hypercholesterolemia (FH)-North Karelia mutation of the low density lipoprotein receptor gene deletes seven nucleotides of exon 6 and is a common cause of FH in Finland. J Clin Invest 1992: 90: 219-28.

Kotze MJ, Langenhoven E, Warnich L, et al. The identification of two low-density lipoprotein receptor gene mutations in South African familial hypercholesterolaemia. S Afr Med J 1989: 76: 399-401.

Kotze MJ, Thiart R, Loubser O, de Villiers JN, Santos M, Vargas MA, Peeters AV. Mutation analysis reveals an insertional hotspot in exon 4 of the LDL receptor gene. Hum Genet. 1996: 98(4): 476-8.

Krawczak M, Cooper DN. Single base-pair substitutions in pathology and evolution: two sides to the same coin. Hum Mutat. 1996: 8(1): 23-31.

Krawczak M, Ball EV, Cooper DN. Neighboring-nucleotide effects on the rates of germ-line single-base-pair substitution in human genes. Am J Hum Genet 1998: 63(2): 474-88.

Krawczak M, Thomas NS, Hundrieser B, Mort M, Wittig M, Hampe J, Cooper DN. Single base-pair substitutions in exon-intron junctions of human genes: nature, distribution, and consequences for mRNA splicing. Hum Mutat. 2007: 28(2): 150-8.

Kurniawan ND, Aliabadizadeh K, Brereton IM, Kroon PA, Smith R. NMR structure and backbone dynamics of a concatemer of epidermal growth factor homology modules of the human low-density lipoprotein receptor. J Mol Biol. 2001: 311(2): 341-56.

Kwon HJ, Lagace TA, McNutt MC, Horton JD, Deisenhofer J. Molecular basis for LDL receptor recognition by PCSK9. Proc Natl Acad Sci U S A. 2008: 105(6): 1820-5.

Landsberger D, Meiner V, Reshef A, et al. A nonsense mutation in the LDL receptor gene leads to familial hypercholesterolemia in the Druze sect. Am J Hum Genet 1992: 50: 427-33.

Lehrman MA, Schneider WJ, Brown MS, et al. The Lebanese allele at the low density lipoprotein receptor locus. Nonsense mutation produces truncated receptor that is retained in endoplasmic reticulum. J Biol Chem 1987: 262: 401-10.

Leitersdorf E, Van der Westhuyzen DR, Coetzee GA, Hobbs HH. Two common low density lipoprotein receptor gene mutations cause familial hypercholesterolemia in Afrikaners. J Clin Invest 1989: 84: 954-61.

Lewin B, in "Genes IV" (Oxford Cell Press, New-York, 1990).

Lindgren V, Luskey KL, Russell DW, Francke U. Human genes involved in cholesterol metabolism: chromosomal mapping of the loci for the low density lipoprotein receptor and 3-hydroxy-3- methylglutaryl-coenzyme A reductase with cDNA probes. Proc Natl Acad Sci USA 1985: 82: 8567-71.

Lombardi P, Sijbrands EJ, van de Giessen K, Smelt AH, Kastelein JJ, Frants RR, Havekes LM. Mutations in the low density lipoprotein receptor gene of familial hypercholesterolemic patients detected by denaturing gradient gel electrophoresis and direct sequencing. J Lipid Res. 1995: 36(4): 860-7.

Marduel M, Carrie A, Sassolas A et al. Molecular spectrum of autosomal dominant hypercholesterolemia in France. Human Mutation 2010: 31: E1811-1824.

Moorjani S, Roy M, Gagne C, et al. Homozygous familial hypercholesterolemia among French Canadians in Quebec Province. Arteriosclerosis 1989: 9: 211-6.

Neel JV, Weder AB, Julius S. Type II diabetes, essential hypertension, and obesity as 'syndromes of impaired genetic homeostasis': the 'thrifty genotype' hypothesis enters the 21st century. Perspect Biol Med 1998: 42: 44–74.

North CL, Blacklow SC. Structural independence of ligand-binding modules five and six of the LDL receptor. Biochemistry 1999: 38(13): 3926-35.

Russell DW, Brown MS, Goldstein JL. Different combinations of cysteine-rich repeats mediate binding of low density lipoprotein receptor to two different proteins. J Biol Chem 1989: 264(36): 21682-8.

Solberg K, Rødningen OK, Tonstad S, Ose L, Leren TP. Familial hypercholesterolaemia caused by a non-sense mutation in codon 329 of the LDL receptor gene. Scand J Clin Lab Invest. 1994: 54(8): 605-9.

Soutar AK. Rare genetic causes of autosomal dominant or recessive hypercholesterolaemia. IUBMB Life. 2010: 62(2): 125-31.

Sterne-Weiler T, Howard J, Mort M, Cooper DN, Sanford JR. Loss of exon identity is a common mechanism of human inherited disease. Genome Res. 2011: 21(10): 1563-71.

Sudhof TC, Russell DW, Goldstein JL, et al. Cassette of eight exons shared by genes for LDL receptor and EGF precursor. Science 1985: 228: 893-5.

Thiart R, Loubser O, de Villiers JN, Marx MP, Zaire R, Raal FJ, Kotze MJ. Two novel and two known low-density lipoprotein receptor gene mutations in German patients with familial hypercholesterolemia. Hum Mutat. 1998: Suppl 1: S232-3.

Varret M, Rabes JP, Collod-Beroud G et al. Software and database for the analysis of mutations in the human LDL receptor gene. Nucleic Acids Research 1997: 25(1): 172-180.

Varret M, Rabes JP, Thiart R et al. LDLR Database (second edition): new additions to the database and the software, and results of the first molecular analysis. Nucleic Acids Research 1998: 26(1): 248-252.

Villèger L, Abifadel M, Allard D et al. The UMD-LDLR database: additions to the software and 490 new entries to the database. Human Mutation 2002: 20(2): 81-87.

Yamamoto T, Davis CG, Brown MS, et al. The human LDL receptor: a cysteine-rich protein with multiple Alu sequences in its mRNA. Cell 1984: 39: 27-38.

Yu W, Nohara A, Higashikata T, Lu H, Inazu A, Mabuchi H. Molecular genetic analysis of familial hypercholesterolemia: spectrum and regional difference of LDL receptor gene mutations in Japanese population. Atherosclerosis. 2002: 165(2): 335-42.

Zhang DW, Lagace TA, Garuti R, Zhao Z, McDonald M, Horton JD, Cohen JC, Hobbs HH. Binding of proprotein convertase subtilisin/kexin type 9 to epidermal growth factor-like repeat A of low density lipoprotein receptor decreases receptor recycling and increases degradation. J Biol Chem. 2007: 282(25): 18602-12.

Chapter 4

Missense Mutation in Cancer in Correlation to Its Phenotype – VHL as a Model

Suad AlFadhli

Additional information is available at the end of the chapter

http://dx.doi.org/10.5772/36727

1. Introduction

Cancer is a complex genetic disease caused by abnormal alteration (mutations) in DNA sequences that leads to dyregulation of normal cellular processes thereby driving tumor growth. The study of such causal mutations is a central focus of cancer biology for two reasons; first is to reveal the molecular mechanisms of tumorigenesis, second is to provide insight in the development of novel therapeutic and diagnostic approaches. Although hundreds of genes are known to be mutated in cancers our understanding of mutational events in cancer cells remains incomplete (Futreal PA et al, 2004). This however has widely opened the field of cancer genomics studies which aims to provide new insights into the molecular mechanisms that lead to tumorigenesis.

As we are in the era of evidence-based molecular diagnosis, predictive testing, genetic counseling, gene-informed cancer risk assessment, and preventative and personalized medicine, therefore, studying the Mendelian genetics of the familial forms of cancer is one approach that can set up the basis for gene-informed risk assessment and management for the patient and family. Herein we selected a Mendelian genetics form of familial cancer such as hereditary tumor syndromic endocrine neoplasias caused by highly penetrant germline mutations leading to pheochromocytoma-paraganglioma syndromes. An example of such syndromes are autosomal dominant disorders; von Hippel-Lindau (VHL); Multiple endocrine neoplasia syndrome type 1 (MEN-1), loss-of-function germline mutations in the tumor suppressor gene MEN1 increase the risk of developing pituitary, parathyroid and pancreatic islet tumors, and less commonly thymic carcinoids, lipomas and benign adrenocortical tumors. In the case of multiple endocrine neoplasia type 2 (MEN 2), gain-of-function germline mutations clustered in specific codons of the RET proto-oncogene increase the risk of developing medullary thyroid carcinoma (MTC), phaeochromocytoma and parathyroid tumors. PTEN mutations in Cowden syndrome (CS), associated with breast, thyroid, and endometrial neoplasias. Identification and characterization of germline mutations in the predisposition genes of the great majority of these syndromes has empowered the clinical practice by the retrieved genetic information which guides medical management.

This review focuses specifically on the analysis of missense mutations in oncogenes and the tumor suppressor genes, though these genes can also be mutated through a variety of other mechanisms such as DNA amplification, translocation, and deletion. Unlike synonymous or silent mutations, which do not cause amino acid changes, missense mutations are non-synonymous amino acid substitutions that are typically caused by single-base nucleotide point mutations. However, many random missense mutations are not expected to alter protein function due to plasticity built into many amino acid residues.

2. Cancer and the "two hits" of Knudson's hypothesis

Before proceeding into missense mutation in tumor suppressor gene we ought to introduce the "two hits" of Knudson's hypothesis. Alfred Knudson Jr in 1971 published his inspiring statistical analysis of the childhood cancer retinoblastoma where he found that retinoblastoma tend to be multifocal in familial cases and unifocal in sporadic presentation (Knudson A. G. Jr, 1971). Knudson postulated that patients with the familial form of the cancer would be born with one mutant allele and that all cells in that organ or tissue would be at risk, accounting for early onset and the multifocal nature of the disease. In contrast, sporadic tumors would develop only if a mutation occurred in both alleles within the same cell, and, as each event would be expected to occur with low frequency, most tumors would develop late in life and in a unifocal manner. His observations led him to propose a two-hit theory of carcinogenesis. The "two hits" of Knudson's hypothesis, which has proved true for many tumors, recognized that familial forms of cancer might hold the key to the identification of important regulatory elements known as tumor-suppressor genes (Ayerbes et al, 2008;.

3. Missense mutations in oncogenes and the tumor suppressor genes

Using the second generation sequencing approaches provided detailed information on the frequency and position of single point mutations as well as structural aberrations of cancer genomes such as small insertions and deletions, focal copy number alterations, and genomic rearrangementsm (Wood LD et al, 2007;. Jones S et al, 2008; Greenman C et al, 2007; Sjoblom T et al, 2006; Pleasance ED et al 2010a,b; Cancer Genome Atlas Research Network, 2008). The findings show that the complexity of each cancer genome is far greater than expected and that extensive variations exist between different cancer types as well as between different tumor samples of the same cancer type. Several recent studies have used the Catalogue Of Somatic Mutations In Cancer (COSMIC) database to discriminate oncogenes and the tumor suppressor genes by using the difference in their mutation patterns in order to understand oncogenesis and diagnose cancers (Forbes SA et al, 2008; Stehr H et al, 2011; Liu H, 2011). Such investigations at the systems level are currently being performed for many of oncogenes and the tumor suppressor genes as part of the Mutanom project (http://www.mutanom.org).

Stehr H *et al* study describes in a quantitative way, the opposing structural effects of cancer-associated missense mutations in oncogenes and tumor suppressors. Using COSMIC database (Forbes SA, 2008). Stehr H *et al* has assessed the effects of 1992 mutations cancer-associated mutations representing two common mechanisms through which tumorigenesis is initiated: via gain-of-function of oncogenes and loss-of-function of tumor suppressors (Vogelstein B et al, 1993). Then compared them to the effects of natural variants and randomized mutations. They focused on mechanisms of cancer mutations that have a consequence at the structural level. Another significant body of work has been published on consequences of mutations in a structural context (Ng PC, 2003, 2006; Ramensky V, et al, 2002; Wang Z et al, 2001; Karchin R et al, 2009). These studies differ in that either they focus on estimating the effects of individual mutations or they use different sets of disease mutations.

Studies of structural effects of mutations have found that disease mutations primarily occur in the protein core (Ramensky V, et al, 2002; Wang Z et al, 2001). This trend was confirmed only for the set of tumor suppressors. In contrast, core residues in oncogenes are significantly less often mutated than expected by chance. This is in agreement with Stehr H *et al* results for protein stability. Mutations located in the protein core are often destabilizing and result in loss-of-function. Thus, Stehr H *et al* data suggests that the loss-of-function of tumor suppressors is often caused by destabilization of the protein. They also suggested that specific mutations of functional sites that can either disable enzymatic activity and regulatory mechanisms or increase protein activity are often responsible for oncogene activation. Stehr H *et al* results show that the most frequently mutated types of functional sites in oncogenes are ATP and GTP binding sites and that the frequency of mutation is significantly higher than expected. This suggests that mutations of ATP and GTP binding sites are specific and common mechanisms of oncogene activation. Examples for such activating mutations near ATP binding sites have been described in the literature (Davies H et al, 2002; Shu HK et al, 1990, Jeffers M, et al, 1997).

Liu H *et al* investigated >120,000 mutation samples in 66 well-known tumor suppressor genes and oncogenes of the COSMIC database, and found a set of significant differences in mutation patterns (e.g., non-3n-indel, non-sense SNP and mutation hotspot) between them. They also developed indices to readily distinguish one from another and predict clearly the unknown oncogenesis genes as tumor suppressors (e.g., ASXL1, HNF1A and KDM6A) or oncogenes (e.g., FOXL2, MYD88 and TSHR). Based on their results, a third gene group was classified, which has a mutational pattern between tumor suppressors and oncogenes. The concept of the third gene group was thought to help in understanding gene function in different cancers or individual patients and to know the exact function of genes in oncogenesis.

4. The clinical of VHL disease

von Hippel-Lindau (VHL) disease (MIM 193300) is a dominantly inherited familial cancer syndrome. It is caused by mutations in the VHL tumor suppressor gene with an incidence of

1:31-36000 live births worldwide across all ethnic backgrounds, with similar prevalence in both genders (Maher *et al.*, 1991; Maher, *et al.*2004). The prevalence however was shown to be higher in some population withtin the same ethnicity such as 1:39 000 in South-West Germany and 1:53 000 in Eastern England (Maher ER et al, 1991; Neumann H et al, 1991). VHL is characterized by marked age-dependent penetrance and phenotypic variability. The factors that affect the actual clinical expression and tumor formation, including age of onset, tissue and organ-specific lesions, severity of lesions, and recurrence, are unknown. VHL main clinical manifestations are:

4.1. Hemangioplastoms

Hemangioplastoms of the central nervous system (CNS) which are typically located in the cerebellum, but can also occur at the brainstem, spinal cord, and rarely, at the lumbosacral nerve roots and supratentorial (Neumann et al., 1995). Retinal or CNS hemangioblastomas are often the earliest manifestations of VHL disease and the most common, occurring in up to 80% of patients (Maher et al., 1990b; Melmon and Rosen, 1964; Weil et al., 2003). VHL-associated cerebellar hemangioblastomas are diagnosed at a mean age of 29–33 years, much earlier than sporadic cerebellar hemangioblastomas (Hes et al., 2000a, 2000b; Wanebo et al., 2003). These lesions are rarely malignant, but enlargement or bleeding within the CNS can result in neurological damage and death (Pavesi et al., 2008). A lower incidence of CNS hemangioblastomas has been documented in specific ethnic populations (12% Finland (Niemela M et al., 1999); 5% German (Zbar B et al., 1999). Patients with cerebellar haemangioblastomas typically present with symptoms of increased intracranial pressure and limb or truncal ataxia (depending on the precise location of the tumor). Wanebo et al. (2003) showed most CNS hemangioblastomas were associated with cysts that were often larger than other hemangioblastomas.

4.2. Pheochromocytoma

Pheochromocytomas are endocrine neoplasias with intra- or extra-adrenal gland lesions that appear histologically as an expansion of large chromaffin positive cells, derived from neural crest cells (Lee et al., 2005). Seven to 18% of VHL patients are afflicted with pheochromocytomas (Crossey et al., 1994a; Garcia et al., 1997). The absence or present of this phenotype will type the VHL into type 1or 2 (A,B,C), respectively (Woodward ER et al., 1997; Hofstra RMW et al., 1996). Untreated pheochromocytomas can result in hypertension and subsequent acute heart disease, brain edema, and stroke.

4.3. Clear cell renal cell carcinoma (RCC)

Clear cell renal cell carcinoma (RCC) occurs in up to 70% of patients with VHL and is a frequent cause of death. 70% of VHL patients have the risk of developing RCC by 60 years old (Maher et al., 1990b, 1991; Whaley et al., 1994), at an average age of 44 years versus the average age of 62 years, at which sporadic RCC develops in the general population (http://www.umd.be/VHL/W_VHL /clinic.shtml). Renal cysts are common in VHL patients as well; however, unlike the completely benign cysts in the general population, renal cysts in VHL patients might degenerate into RCC (Kaelin et al., 2004). However, it is unlikely that RCC in all VHL patients originates from cysts, or that all cysts will eventually become malignant. RCC often overproduces VEGF, and thus can be very vascular (Berse et al., 1992; Sato et al., 1994; Takahashi et al., 1994).

4.4. Others clinical manifestations

VHL patient can also have low-grade adenocarcinomas of the temporal bone, also known as endolymphatic sac tumors (ELST), pancreatic tumor, and epididymal or board ligament cystadenomas (Gruber et al., 1980; Neumann and Wiestler, 1991; Maher et al., 2004; Kaelin et al., 2007). ELST in VHL cases can be detected by MRI or CT imaging in up to 11% of patients (Manski TJ, et al., 1997). Although often asymptomatic, the most frequent clinical presentation is hearing loss (mean age 22 years), but tinnitus and vertigo also occur in many cases. In addition to the inherited risk for developing cancer, VHL patients develop cystic disease in various organs including the kidney, pancreas, and liver (Hough et al., 1994; Lubensky et al., 1998; Maher et al., 1990b; Maher, 2004).

Tumor growth commonly cycled between growth and quiescent phases. Patients with numerous tumors experienced growth and quiescent phases simultaneously, suggesting that a combination of acquired genetic lesions and hormonal activity influence tumor growth.

5. VHL clinical classification:

Molecular genetic mutation and phenotypic clustering has allowed development of a clinical classification, although intra-familial variability is well recognized.

As mentioned previously VHL disease can be classified into VHL Type 1 or Type 2 depending on the phenotype. Type 1 describes those with typical VHL manifestations such as emangioblastomas and RCC, but does not include pheochromocytomas. Once a pheochromocytoma occurs the classification becomes Type 2. Type 2, accounting for 7–20% of VHL kindreds, is further subdivided into: (2A) pheochromocytomas and other typical VHL manifestations except RCC, (2B) the full spectrum of VHL disease including pheochromocytomas, RCC, and other typical VHL manifestation, and Type (2C) identifies those with familial risk of isolated pheochromocytoma (Gross D et al, 1996; Martin R, et al., 1998), although there are some kindreds without identified VHL mutation raising the possibility of another genetic locus (Woodward ER et al, 1997; Crossey et al., 1994b; Garcia et al., 1997; Mulvihill et al., 1997).

6. Morbidity and Mortality of VHL

The morbidity of VHL disease depends on the organ system involved. For example, retinal hemangioblastomas can result in retinal detachment and/or blindness (Webster et al., 1999). Mortality is often due to either metastasis of RCC or complications of CNS hemangioblastomas (Filling-Katz et al., 1991; Maher et al., 1990b; Neumann et al., 1992); however, due to improved screening guidelines, life expectancy of VHL patients has improved.

7. VHL gene and pVHL function

The human VHL gene is a 10-kb region located on the short arm of chromosome 3 (3p25.3) (Richards et al., 1993) and consists of 3 exons (Kuzmin et al., 1995; Latif et al., 1993a, 1993b): Exon1 spans codons 1–113, exon 2 spans codons 114–154, and exon 3 spans codons 155–213. Two protein products are encoded by VHL: a 30-kDa full-length protein (p30, 213 amino acids, NM_000551.2 [variant 1 mRNA]) and a shorter protein product of 19-kDa (p19, 160 amino acids NM_198156.1 [variant 2 mRNA]), which is generated by alternative translation initiation at an internal methionine at position 54 (Blankenship et al., 1999). Although evolutionary conservation of VHL sequence is very strong over most of the pVHL19 sequence, the first 53 amino acids included in pVHL30 are less well conserved and functional studies suggest that the two pVHL isoforms have equivalent effects (Woodward ER et al, 2000; Iliopoulos O et al, 1998). The VHL mRNA and protein is widely expressed in both fetal and adult tissues (Richards FM et al., 1996; Corless CL et al., 1997) and can be found in all multicellular organisms examined to date without known similarity to other proteins (van M et al., 2001). Remarkable progress has been made in elaborating the function of pVHL and the role its inactivation plays in the pathophysiology of this disorder, including dysregulation of angiogenesis and tumor formation.

Given the lack of primary sequence homology to other proteins, the function of pVHL has been derived from studying pVHL interactors and associated proteins. Roles in oxygen-dependent angiogenesis, tumorigenesis, fibronectin matrix assembly and cytoskeleton organization, cell cycle control and cellular differentiation have been proposed. The N-terminal acidic domain of VHLp30 contains eight repetitions of a five-residue acidic repeat, which are absent in VHLp19. Phosphorylation of this acidic domain participates in tumor suppression and this domain binds the Kinesin-2 adaptor KAP3, thus mediating microtubule-binding (Lolkema et al., 2005, 2007). This domain is also responsible for binding metastasis suppressor Nm23H2, a protein known to regulate dynamin-dependent endocystosis (Hsu et al., 2006). Further downstream, the β-sheet domain (residues 63–154) binds HIF0a subunits at residues 65–117 and the α-helical domain (residues 155–192) binds the Elongin B and Elongin C (Elongin BC) complex at residues 158–184 (Feldman et al., 1999). Binding of pVHL to the Elongin BC is mediated by the chaperonin TRiC/ CCT. Elongin BC binding to pVHL requires TRiC, and VHL mutations causing defects in binding to Elongin BC are associated with VHL disease (Feldman et al., 1999). pVHL inactivation leads to an overexpression of hypoxia-inducible factor (HIF) and upregulation of its targets (vascular endothelial growth factor (VEGF), erythropoietin, transforming growth factor (TGF)-beta, alpha). Whether this is the sole etiologic factor causing characteristic VHL hemangioblastoma formation remains to be clarified. Evidence also suggests that pVHL inactivation alters fibronectin extracellular matrix formation, and that pVHL may participate in cellular differentiation and cell cycle control. Ongoing studies are directed at elaborating the biologic consequences that these pathways play in the angiogenesis and tumor formation central to VHL. Additionally, VHL protein has functions that are independent of HIF-1alpha and HIF-2alpha and are thought to be important for its tumor-suppressor action, assembly of the extracellular matrix, control of microtubule dynamics, regulation of apoptosis, and possibly stabilization of TP53 proteins (Frew IJ and Krek W. 2007).

8. Molecular genetics of VHL disease

Germline mutations, including large deletions/rearrangements, in the *VHL* gene, linked to 3p25-p26, are etiologic for virtually all VHL disease (Latif, F. et al., 1993; Stolle, C. et al., 1998; Zbar, B. et al., 1996). These VHL germline mutations may be also detected in patients with autosomal dominant familial non-syndromic phaeochromocytoma (Woodward ER et al., 1997; Neumann HP et al., 2002). Specific VHL missense mutations can cause an autosomal recessive form of polycythaemia without any evidence of VHL disease (AngSO et al., 2002; Gordeuk VR et al., 2004). Germ-line mutation confers genetic risk of tumor formation in concert with somatic second VHL allele loss or DNA methylation inactivation. However, somatic loss or inactivation of the wild-type vhl allele has been demonstrated in central nervous system (CNS) sporadic hemangioblastomas (Gnarra JR et al., 1994; Kanno H et al., 2000; Foster K et al., 1994; Herman JG et al 1994; Oberstrass J, et al., 1996; Tse J et al., 1997; Lee J-Y et al., 1998), in sporadic and VHL-associated renal cell carcinomas (RCCs) (Latif F et al, 1993; Shuin T et al., 1994; Phillips JL et al., 2001), pheochromocytoma (Bender BU et al., 2000; Linehan WM et al., 2001) and in endolymphatic sac tumors (ELSTs) (Vortmeyer AO et al., 2000).

More than 300 germline mutations have been identified in familial VHL. These occur throughout the coding region with only a few mutations appearing in multiple families (Zbar B et al., 1996; Beroud C et al., 1996). The new mutation rate has been estimated at between 3 and 20% (Latif F et al., 1993; Richard S et al., 1994; Schimke RN et al., 2000). Although decreased penetrance has been described (Maddock IF et al., 1994), comprehensive familial molecular data have not yet been reported to clarify this rate.

There has been limited correlation between specific mutation and phenotype, although some data on genotype-phenotype correlations have been reported (Neumann H et al., 1998; Hes F et al., 2000). Such correlations have revealed that certain missense mutations confer a high risk of pheochromocytoma (VHL type 1) whereas loss of pVHL through large deletions or nonsense-mediated decay appears to be incompatible with pheochromocytoma development (VHL type 2). [Chen et al., 1995; Cybulski et al., 2002; Glavac et al., 1996; Hes et al., 2000a, 2000b; Maher et al., 1996; Neumann and Bender, 1998; Ong et al., 2007; Zbar et al., 1996].

Interestingly, missense mutations causing amino acid changes on the surface of pVHL appear to have a higher risk for pheochromocytomas than missense mutations occurring deep within the protein; surface missense mutations also appear to have a higher risk for pheochromocytomas than deletions, nonsense, and frameshift mutations [Ong et al., 2007]. Thus, pheochromocytoma development appears to be related to an intact, but altered pVHL, which has seeded the hypothesis that these mutations may induce gain-of-function possibly through a dominant negative effect [Hoffman et al., 2001; Lee et al., 2005; Maher and Kaelin, 1997; Stebbins et al., 1999]. Nordstrom-O'Brien et al., 2010, analyzed 1548 VHL families and provided a wealth of data for genotype–phenotype correlations. They found 52% had missense mutations most frequently occurred at codons 65, 76, 78, 98, splice mutations at codon 155, 158, 161, 162, and 167. 13% had frameshift, 11% had nonsense, 6% had in-frame deletions/ insertions, 11% had large/complete deletions, and 7% had splice mutations. Mutations that predict absence of functional protein (deletion, frame-shift, nonsense, and splice) are associated in 96-97% of cases with type 1 phenotype and show an increased risk of RCC (including type 2b cases). This suggests that expressed dysfunctional protein may be required for pheochromocytoma formation. Missense mutations are associated with type 2 phenotype (hemangioblastoma and pheochromocytoma +/- RCC) in 69-98% of cases (Stolle C et al., 1998; Chen F et al., 1995; Zbar B et al., 1996). While Nordstrom-O'Brien et al., found 83.5% of VHL Type 2 families mainly had missense mutations. However, this is not as high as some studies, reporting up to 96% of those with pheochromocytomas to have missense mutations (Zbar et al., 1996). Nordstrom-O'Brien et al., found low percentage of VHL Type 2 families (0.5-7%) had other types of mutation such as nonsense, frameshift, splice, in-frame deletion/insertions, and partial deletions. The small percentage of nonsense and partial deletions along with the absence of complete deletions supports theories that an intact though altered pVHL is associated with pheochromocytomas. Stratifying missense mutations into those that resulted in substitution of a surface amino acid and those that disrupted structural integrity demonstrated that surface amino acid substitutions conferred a higher pheochromocytoma risk (Ong KR et al., 2007). Although loss of heterozygosity has been reported in endolymphatic sac tumors (ELST) tumors (Kawahara N et al., 1999; Vortmeyer AO et al., 1997) no predominant mutation has been identified.

It may be difficult, however, to predict functional biologic consequences from specific point mutations without direct functional assays as reported in recent RCC *in-vitro* mutation panel studies.

The recent characterization of the VHL protein crystal structure might suggests possible functional consequences of specific mutations. If we focus on the structure of the pVHL we can predict the effect of the mutation on the functionality of the pVHL and therefore the phenotype resulted. Mutation-specific dysfunction may depend on protein destabilization, altered interactor binding at the various pVHP binding domains or potential alteration in binding to other factors involved in tumor suppressor/activator activity. pVHL has two domains: an amino-terminal domain rich in β-sheet (the β-domain) and a smaller carboxyterminal α-helical domain (the α-domain). A large portion of the α-domain surface interacts with Elongin C, which binds to other members (e.g., Elongin B, Cul2, and Rbx1) of an SCF-like E3 ubiquitin-protein ligase complex as mentioned earlier. Obviously, loss of function VHL mutations prevents Elongin C binding and target ubiquitylation (Clifford et al., 2001). The β-domain on the other side has a macromolecular binding site targets the HIF-1α and HIF-2α regulatory subunits for proteasomal degradation. Whereas Type 1 and Type 2B mutations impair pVHL binding to Elongin C, Type 2A mutations map to the β-domain

HIF-binding site and do not affect the ability of pVHL to bind Elongin C (Clifford et al., 2001). Therefore, classifying missense substitutions according to their predicted effect on pVHL structure enhances the ability to predict pheochromocytoma risk (Ong KR et al., 2007)

Nordstrom-O'Brien et al 2010 suggested that increased identification of new mutations and new patients with previously described mutations gives momentum to the search for the exact role of pVHL in its normal and mutated form. Understanding such functions and its association with specific mutations allows for identification of disease risks in individual patients. Such insight will offer improved diagnostics, surveillance, and treatment of VHL patients (Nordstrom-O'Brien et al., 2010).

Ongoing delineation of clinical subtypes may allow for better genotype-phenotype correlations, prediction of clinical progression and molecular mutation-directed clinical management. There is significant intra-familial difference in clinical expressivity and as of yet limited knowledge about modifiers of this phenotypic variation (Webster AR, et al, 1998). Prediction of the clinical course in any one patient based on molecular data is therefore difficult.

Author details

Suad AlFadhli
Molecular Genetics, Kuwait University, Kuwait

9. References

Ang SO, Chen H, HirotaK et al: Disruption of oxygen homeostasis underlies congenital Chuvash polycythemia. Nat Genet 2002; 32: 614–621.

Ayerbes VM, Gallego AG, Prado DS, Fonseca JP, Campelo G R, Aparicio ALM. Origin of renal cell carcinomas. Clin Transl Oncol. 2008 Nov;10(11):697-712.

Bender BU, Gutsche M, Glasker S, et al. Differential genetic alterations in von Hippel-Lindau syndrome-associated and sporadic pheochromocytomas. J Clin Endocrinol Metab 2000; 85:4568-4574.

Beroud C, Joly D, Gallou C, et al. Software and database for the analysis of mutation in VHL gene [www.umd.necker.fr:2005]. Nucleic Acids Res 1998; 26:256-258.

Berse B, Brown LF, Van de Water L, Dvorak HF, Senger DR. Vascular permeability factor (vascular endothelial growth factor) gene is expressed differentially in normal tissues, macrophages, and tumors. Mol Biol Cell 1992; 3:211–220.

Blankenship C, Naglich JG, Whaley JM, Seizinger B, Kley N. Alternate choice of initiation codon produces a biologically active product of the von Hippel Lindau gene with tumor suppressor activity. Oncogene 1999;18:1529–1535.

Cancer Genome Atlas Research Network: Comprehensive genomic characterization defines human glioblastoma genes and core pathways. Nature 2008; 455:1061-1068.

Chen F, Kishida T, Yao M, et al. Germline mutations in the von Hippel-Lindau disease tumor suppressor gene: correlations with phenotype. Hum Mutat 1995; 5:66-75.

Clifford SC, Cockman ME, Smallwood AC, Mole DR, Woodward ER, Maxwell PH, Ratcliffe PJ, Maher ER. Contrasting effects on HIF-1alpha regulation by disease-causing pVHL mutations correlate with patterns of tumourigenesis in von Hippel-Lindau disease. Hum Mol Genet 2001;10:1029–1038.

Corless CL, Kibel AS, Iliopoulos O et al: Immunostaining of the von Hippel-Lindau gene product in normal and neoplastic human tissues. Hum Path 1997; 28: 459–464.

Crossey PA, Foster K, Richards FM, Phipps ME, Latif F, Tory K, Jones MH, Bentley E, Kumar R, Lerman MI, Zbar B, Affara NA, Ferguson-Smith MA, Maher ER. Molecular genetic investigations of the mechanism of tumourigenesis in von Hippel-Lindau disease: analysis of allele loss in VHL tumours. Hum Genet 1994a; 93:53–58.

Crossey PA, Richards FM, Foster K, Green JS, Prowse A, Latif F, Lerman MI, Zbar B Affara NA, Ferguson-Smith MA, Maher ER. Identification of intragenic mutations in the von Hippel-Lindau disease tumour suppressor gene and correlation with disease phenotype. Hum Mol Genet 1994b;3:1303–1308.

Cybulski C, Krzystolik K, Murgia A, Gorski B, et al. Germline mutations in the von Hippel-Lindau (VHL) gene in patients from Poland: disease presentation in patients with deletions of the entire VHL gene. J Med Genet 2002;39:E38.

Davies H, Bignell GR, Cox C, Stephens P, Edkins S, Clegg S, Teague J, Woffendin H, Garnett MJ, Bottomley W, et al: Mutations of the BRAF gene in human cancer. Nature 2002; 417:949-954.

Feldman DE, Thulasiraman V, Ferreyra RG, Frydman J. Formation of the VHLelongin BC tumor suppressor complex is mediated by the chaperonin TRiC. Mol Cell 1999;4:1051–1061.

Filling-Katz MR, Choyke PL, Oldfield E, Charnas L, Patronas NJ, Glenn GM, GorinMB, Morgan JK, Linehan WM, Seizinger BR, Zbar B. Central nervous system involvement in Von Hippel-Lindau disease. Neurology 1991;41:41–46.

Forbes SA, Bhamra G, Bamford S, Dawson E, Kok C, Clements J, Menzies A, Teague JW, Futreal PA, Stratton MR: The Catalogue of Somatic Mutations in Cancer (COSMIC). Curr Protoc Hum Genet 2008; Chapter 10, Unit 10 11.

Foster K, Prowse A, van den Berg A, et al. Somatic mutations of the von Hippel-Lindau disease tumour suppressor gene in non-familial clear cell renal carcinoma. Hum Mol Genet 1994; 3:2169-2173.

Frew IJ and Krek W. Multitasking by pVHL in tumour suppression. *Curr Opin Cell Biol* 2007;19:685-690.

Futreal PA, Coin L, Marshall M, Down T, Hubbard T, Wooster R, Rahman N, Stratton MR. A census of human cancer genes. Nat Rev Cancer. 2004;4(3):177-83.

Greenman C, Stephens P, Smith R, Dalgliesh GL, Hunter C, Bignell G, Davies H, Teague J, Butler A, Stevens C, et al: Patterns of somatic mutation in human cancer genomes. Nature 2007; 446:153-158.

Garcia A, Matias-Guiu X, Cabezas R, Chico A, Prat J, Baiget M, De Leiva A. Molecular diagnosis of von Hippel-Lindau disease in a kindred with a predominance of familial phaeochromocytoma. Clin Endocrinol (Oxf) 1997; 46:359–363

Glavac D, Neumann HP, Wittke C, Jaenig H, Masek O, Streicher T, Pausch F, Engelhardt D, Plate KH, Hofler H, Chen F, Zbar B, Brauch H. Mutations in the VHL tumor suppressor gene and associated lesions in families with von Hippel-Lindau disease from central Europe. Hum Genet 1996; 98:271–280.

Gnarra JR, Tory K, Weng Y, et al. Mutations of the VHL tumour suppressor gene in renal carcinoma. Nat Genet 1994; 7:85-90.

Gordeuk VR, Sergueeva AI, Miasnikova GY et al: Congenital disorder of oxygen-sensing: association of the homozygous Chuvash polycythemia VHL mutation with thrombosis and vascular abnormalities but not tumors. Blood 2004; 103: 3924–3932.

Gross D, Avishai N, Meiner V, et al. Familial pheochromocytoma associated with a novel mutation in the von Hippel-Lindau gene. J Clin Endocrinol Metab 1996; 81:147-149.

Gruber MB, Healey GB, Toguri AG, Warren MM. Papillary cystadenoma of epididymis: component of von Hippel-Lindau syndrome. Urology 1980; 16:305–306.

Herman JG, Latif F, Weng Y, et al. Silencing of the VHL tumor-suppressor gene by DNA methylation in renal carcinoma. Proc Natl Acad Sci USA 1994; 91:9700-9704.

Hes F, Zewald R, Peeters T, Sijmons R, Links T, Verheij J, Matthijs G, Leguis E, Mortier G, van der Torren K, Rosman M, Lips C, Pearson P, van der Luijt R. Genotype–phenotype correlations in families with deletions in the von Hippel-Lindau (VHL) gene. Hum Genet 2000a;106:425–431.

Hes FJ, McKee S, Taphoorn MJ, Rehal P, van Der Luijt RB, McMahon R, van Der Smagt JJ, Dow D, Zewald RA, Whittaker J, Lips CJ, MacDonald F, Pearson PL, Maher ER. Cryptic von Hippel-Lindau disease: germline mutations in patients with haemangioblastoma only. J Med Genet 2000b; 37:939–943.

Hoffman MA, Ohh M, Yang H, Klco JM, Ivan M, Kaelin Jr WG. von Hippel-Lindau protein mutants linked to type 2C VHL disease preserve the ability to downregulate HIF. Hum Mol Genet 2001; 10:1019–1027.

Hofstra RMW, Stelwagen T, Stulp RP, et al. Extensive mutation screening of RET in sporadic medullary thyroid carcinoma and of RET and VHL in sporadic pheochromocytoma reveals involvement of these genes in only a minority of cases. J Clin Endocrinol Metab 1996; 81:2881

Hough DM, Stephens DH, Johnson CD, Binkovitz LA. Pancreatic lesions in von Hippel-Lindau disease: prevalence, clinical significance, and CT findings. AJR Am J Roentgenol 1994;162:1091–1094.

Hsu T, Adereth Y, Kose N, Dammai V. Endocytic function of von Hippel-Lindau tumor suppressor protein regulates surface localization of fibroblast growth factor receptor 1 and cell motility. J Biol Chem 2006; 281:12069–12080.

Iliopoulos O, Ohh M, Kaelin Jr WG: pVHL19 is a biologically active product of the von Hippel-Lindau gene arising from internal translation initiation. Proc Natl Acad Sci USA 1998; 95: 11661–1166.

Ivan M, KaelinWG.The vonHippel-Lindau tumor suppressor protein. Curr Opin Genet Dev 2001; 11:27-34.

Jeffers M, Schmidt L, Nakaigawa N, Webb CP, Weirich G, Kishida T, Zbar B, VandeWoude GF: Activating mutations for the met tyrosine kinase receptor in human cancer. Proc Natl Acad Sci USA 1997; 94:11445-11450.

Jones S, Zhang X, Parsons DW, Lin JC, Leary RJ, Angenendt P, Mankoo P, Carter H, Kamiyama H, Jimeno A, et al: Core signaling pathways in human pancreatic cancers revealed by global genomic analyses. Science (New York, NY) 2008; 321:1801-1806.

Kaelin Jr WG. The von Hippel-Lindau tumor suppressor gene and kidney cancer. Clin Cancer Res 2004; 10(18 Pt 2):6290S–6295S.

Kaelin WG. Von Hippel-Lindau disease. Annu Rev Pathol 2007; 2:145–173.

Kanno H, Saljooque F, Yamamoto I, et al. Role of the von Hippel-Lindau tumor suppressor protein during neuronal differentiation. Cancer Res 2000; 60:2820-2824.

Karchin R: Next generation tools for the annotation of human SNPs. Brief Bioinform 2009; 10:35-52.

Kawahara N, Kume H, Ueki K, et al. VHL gene inactivation in an endolymphatic sac tumor associated with von Hippel-Lindau disease. Neurology 1999; 53:208-210.

Knudson A. G. Jr Mutation and cancer: statistical study of retinoblastoma. Proc. Natl. Acad. Sci. USA 1971;68:820–823

Kuzmin I, Duh FM, Latif F, Geil L, Zbar B, Lerman MI. 1995. Identification of the promoter of the human von Hippel-Lindau disease tumor suppressor gene. Oncogene. 1995;10(11):2185-94.

Latif F, Duh FM, Gnarra J, Tory K, Kuzmin I, Yao M, Stackhouse T, Modi W, Geil L, Schmidt L, Li H, Orcutt ML, Maher E, Richards F, Phipps M, Ferguson-Smith M, Le Paslier D, Linehan WM, Zbar B, Lerman MI. von Hippel-Lindau syndrome: cloning and identification of the plasma membrane Ca(11)-transporting ATPase isoform 2 gene that resides in the von Hippel-Lindau gene region. Cancer Res 1993a;53:861–867.

Latif F, Tory K, Gnarra J, Yao M, Duh FM, Orcutt ML, Stackhouse T, Kuzmin I, Modi W, Geil L, and many others. Identification of the von Hippel-Lindau disease tumor suppressor gene. Science 1993b; 260:1317–1320.

Lee J-Y, Dong S-M, Park W-S, et al. Loss of heterozygosity and somatic mutations of the VHL tumor suppressor gene in sporadic cerebellar hemangioblastomas. Cancer Res 1998; 58:504-508.

Lee S, Nakamura E, Yang H, Wei W, Linggi MS, Sajan MP, Farese RV, Freeman RS, Carter BD, Kaelin Jr WG, Schlisio S. Neuronal apoptosis linked to EglN3 prolyl hydroxylase and familial pheochromocytoma genes: developmental culling and cancer. Cancer Cell 8: 2005; 155–167.

Linehan WM, Eisenhofer G, Walther MM, Goldstein DS. Recent advances in genetics, diagnosis, localization and treatment of pheochromocytoma. Ann Intern Med 2001; 134:315-329.

Liu H, Xing Y, Yang S, Tian D. Remarkable difference of somatic mutation patterns between oncogenes and tumor suppressor genes. Oncol Rep. 2011;26(6):1539-46.

Lolkema MP, Gervais ML, Snijckers CM, Hill RP, Giles RH, Voest EE, Ohh M. Tumor suppression by the von Hippel-Lindau protein requires phosphorylation of the acidic domain. J Biol Chem 2005; 80:22205–22211.

Lolkema MP, Mans DA, Snijckers CM, van Noort M, van Beest M, Voest EE, Giles RH. The von Hippel-Lindau tumour suppressor interacts with microtubules through kinesin-2. FEBS Lett 2007; 581:4571–4576.

Lubensky IA, Pack S, Ault D, Vortmeyer AO, Libutti SK, Choyke PL, Walther MM, Linehan WM, Zhuang Z. Multiple neuroendocrine tumors of the pancreas in von Hippel-Lindau disease patients: histopathological and molecular genetic analysis. Am J Pathol 1998; 153:223–231.

Maddock IF, Moran A, Maher ER, et al. A genetic register for von Hippel-Lindau disease. J Med Genet 1996; 33:120-127.

Maher ER. Von Hippel-Lindau disease. Curr Mol Med 2004; 4:833–842.

Maher ER, Iselius L, Yates JR, Littler M, Benjamin C, Harris R, Sampson J,Williams A, Ferguson-Smith MA, Morton N. Von Hippel-Lindau disease: a genetic study. J Med Genet 1991; 28:443–447

Maher ER, Kaelin Jr WG. von Hippel-Lindau disease. Medicine (Baltimore) 1997; 76:381–391.

Maher ER, Webster AR, Richards FM, Green JS, Crossey PA, Payne SJ, Moore AT. Phenotypic expression in von Hippel-Lindau disease: correlations with germline VHL gene mutations. J Med Genet 1996; 33:328–332.

Maher ER, Yates JR, Harries R, Benjamin C, Harris R, Moore AT, Ferguson-Smith MA. Clinical features and natural history of von Hippel-Lindau disease. Q J Med 1990b; 77:1151–1163.

Manski TJ, Heffner DK, Glenn GM et al: Endolymphatic sac tumors—A source of morbid hearing loss in von Hippel-Lindau disease. Jama-Journal of the American Medical Association 1997; 277: 1461–1466.

Martin R, Hockey A, Walpole I, et al. Variable penetrance of familial pheochromocytoma associated with the von Hippel-Lindau gene mutation, S68W. Mutations in brief no 150. Online Hum Mutat 1998; 12:71.

Melmon KL, Rosen SW. Lindau's disease. Review of the literature and study of a large kindred. Am J Med 1964; 36:595–617.

Mulvihill JJ, Ferrell RE, Carty SE, Tisherman SE, Zbar B. Familial pheochromocytoma due to mutant von Hippel-Lindau disease gene. Arch Intern Med 1997; 157:1390–1391.

Neumann H, Bender B. Genotype-phenotype correlations in von Hippel-Lindau disease. J Intern Med 1998; 243:541±545..

Neumann HP, Wiestler OD. Clustering of features of von Hippel-Lindau syndrome: evidence for a complex genetic locus. Lancet 1991; 337:1052–1054.

Neumann HP, Bausch B, McWhinney SR et al: Germ-line mutations in nonsyndromic Phaeochromocytoma. N Engl J Med 2002; 346: 1459–6621.

Neumann HP, Eng C, Mulligan LM, Glavac D, Zauner I, Ponder BA, Crossey PA, Maher ER, Brauch H. Consequences of direct genetic testing for germline mutations in the clinical management of families with multiple endocrine neoplasia, type II. JAMA 1995; 274:1149–1151.

Neumann HP, Eggert HR, Scheremet R, Schumacher M, Mohadjer M, Wakhloo AK, Volk B, Hettmannsperger U, Riegler P, Schollmeyer P. Central nervous system lesions in von Hippel-Lindau syndrome. J Neurol Neurosurg Psychiatry 1992; 55:898–901.

Neumann HP, Wiestler OD. Clustering of features and genetics of von Hippel-Lindau syndrome. Lancet 1991; 338: 258.

Ng PC, Henikoff S. Predicting the effects of amino acid substitutions on protein function. Annu Rev Genomics Hum Genet 2006;7:61-80.

Ng PC, Henikoff S: SIFT: Predicting amino acid changes that affect protein function. Nucleic acids research 2003; 31:3812-3814.

Niemela M, Lemeta S, Summanen P, et al. Long-term prognosis of haemangioblastoma of the CNS: impact of von Hippel-Lindau disease. Acta Neurochir 1999; 141:1147±1156.

Nordstrom-O'Brien M, van der Luijt RB, van Rooijen E, van den Ouweland AM, Majoor-Krakauer DF, Lolkema MP, van Brussel A, Voest EE, Giles RH.Genetic analysis of von Hippel-Lindau disease. Hum Mutat. 2010; 31(5):521-37.

Oberstrass J, Reifenberger G, Reifenberger J, et al. Mutations of the von Hippel-Lindau tumour suppressor gene in capillary haemangioblastomas of the central nervous system. J Pathol 1996; 179:151-156.

Ong KR, Woodward ER, Killick P, Lim C, Macdonald F, Maher ER. Genotype–phenotype correlations in von Hippel-Lindau disease. Hum Mutat 2007; 28:143–149

Pavesi G, Feletti A, Berlucchi S, Opocher G, Martella M, Murgia A, Scienza R. Neurosurgical treatment of von Hippel-Lindau-associated hemangioblastomas: benefits, risks and outcome. J Neurosurg Sci 2008; 52:29–36.

Phillips JL, Ghadimi BM, Wangsa D, et al. Molecular cytogenetic characterization of early and late renal cell carcinomas in von Hippel-Lindau disease. Genes Chromosomes Cancer 2001; 31:1-9.

Pleasance ED, Cheetham RK, Stephens PJ, McBride DJ, Humphray SJ, Greenman CD, Varela I, Lin ML, Ordonez GR, Bignell GR, et al: A comprehensive catalogue of somatic mutations from a human cancer genome. Nature 2010a; 463:191-196.

Pleasance ED, Stephens PJ, O'Meara S, McBride DJ, Meynert A, Jones D, Lin ML, Beare D, Lau KW, Greenman C, et al: A small-cell lung cancer genome with complex signatures of tobacco exposure. Nature 2010b; 463:184-190.

Ramensky V, Bork P, Sunyaev S: Human non-synonymous SNPs: server and survey. Nucleic acids research 2002; 30:3894-3900.

Richards FM, Maher ER, Latif F, Phipps ME, Tory K, Lush M, Crossey PA, Oostra B, Enblad P, Gustavson KH, Green J, Turner G, Yates JRW, Linehan WM, Affara NA, Lerman M, Zbar B, Ferguson-Smith MA. Detailed genetic mapping of the von Hippel-Lindau disease tumour suppressor gene. J Med Genet 1993; 30:104–107.

Richards FM, Payne SJ, Zbar B et al: Molecular Analysis of De-Novo Germline Mutations in the von Hippel-Lindau Disease Gene. Hum Mol Gen 1995; 4:2139–2143.

Richards FM, Schofield PN, Fleming S: Expression of the von Hippel-Lindau disease tumour suppressor gene during human embryogenesis. Hum Mol Gen 1996; 5: 639–644.

Richard S, Chauveau D, Chretien Y, et al. Renal lesions and pheochromocytoma in von Hippel-Lindau disease. Adv Nephrol 1994; 23:1-27.

Sato K, Terada K, Sugiyama T, Takahashi S, Saito M, Moriyama M, Kakinuma H, Suzuki Y, Kato M, Kato T. Frequent overexpression of vascular endothelial growth factor gene in human renal cell carcinoma. Tohoku J Exp Med 1994; 173:355–360.

Schimke RN, Collins D, Stolle CA. Von Hippel-Lindau syndrome. In: GeneClinics: clinical genetic information resource; www.geneclinics.org/profiles/vhl.

Shu HK, Pelley RJ, Kung HJ: Tissue-specific transformation by epidermal growth factor receptor: a single point mutation within the ATP-binding pocket of the erbB product increases its intrinsic kinase activity and activates its sarcomagenic potential. Proc Natl Acad Sci USA 1990; 87:9103-9107.

Shuin T, Kondo K, Torigoe S, et al. Frequent somatic mutations and loss of heterozygosity of the von Hippel-Lindau tumor suppressor gene in primary human renal cell carcinomas. Cancer Res 1994; 54:2852-2855.

Sjoblom T, Jones S, Wood LD, Parsons DW, Lin J, Barber TD, Mandelker D, Leary RJ, Ptak J, Silliman N, et al: The consensus coding sequences of human breast and colorectal cancers. Science 2006; 314:268-274.

Stebbins CE, Kaelin Jr WG, Pavletich NP. Structure of the VHL–ElonginC–ElonginB complex: implications for VHL tumor suppressor function. Science 1999; 284:455–461.

Stehr H, Jang SH, Duarte JM, Wierling C, Lehrach H, Lappe M, Lange BM. The structural impact of cancer-associated missense mutations in oncogenes and tumor suppressors. Mol Cancer. 2011;10:54.

Stolle C, Glenn G, Zbar B, et al. Improved detection of germline mutations in the von Hippel-Lindau disease tumor suppressor gene. Hum Mutat 1998; 12:417-423.

Takahashi A, Sasaki H, Kim SJ, Tobisu K, Kakizoe T, Tsukamoto T, Kumamoto Y, Sugimura T, Terada M. Markedly increased amounts of messenger RNAs for vascular endothelial growth factor and placenta growth factor in renal cell carcinoma associated with angiogenesis. Cancer Res 1994; 54: 4233–4237.

Tse J, Wong J, Lo K-W, et al. Molecular genetic analysis of the von Hippel-Lindau disease tumor suppressor gene in familial and sporadic cerebellar hemangioblastomas. Am J Clin Pathol 1997; 107:459-466.

Vogelstein B, Kinzler KW: The multistep nature of cancer. Trends Genet 1993; 9:138-141.

Vortmeyer AO, Huang SC, Koch CA, et al. Somatic von Hippel-Lindau gene mutations detected in sporadic endolymphatic sac tumors. Cancer Res 2000; 60:5963-5965.

Vortmeyer AO, Choo D, Pack SD, et al. Von Hippel-Lindau disease gene alterations associated with endolymphatic sac tumor. J Natl Cancer Inst 1997; 89:970-972.

Wanebo JE, Lonser RR, Glenn GM, Oldfield EH. The natural history of hemangioblastomas of the central nervous system in patients with von Hippel-Lindau disease. J Neurosurg 2003.; 98:82–94.

Wang Z, Moult J: SNPs, protein structure, and disease. Human Mutation 2001, 17:263-270.

Webster AR, Maher ER, Moore AT. Clinical characteristics of ocular angiomatosis in von Hippel-Lindau disease and correlation with germline mutation. Arch Ophthalmol 1999; 117:371–378.

Webster AR, Richards FM, MacRonald FE, et al. An analysis of phenotypic variation in the familial cancer syndrome von Hippel-Lindau disease: evidence for modifier effects. Am J Hum Genet 1998; 63:1025-1035.

Weil RJ, Lonser RR, DeVroom HL, Wanebo JE, Oldfield EH. Surgical management of brainstem hemangioblastomas in patients with von Hippel-Lindau disease. J Neurosurg 2003; 98:95–105

Whaley JM, Naglich J, Gelbert L, Hsia YE, Lamiell JM, Green JS, Collins D, Neumann HP, Laidlaw J, Li FP, Klein-Szanto AJP, Seizinger BR, Kley N. Germ-line mutations in the von Hippel-Lindau tumor-suppressor gene are similar to somatic von Hippel-Lindau aberrations in sporadic renal cell carcinoma. Am J Hum Genet 1994; 55:1092–1102.

Wood LD, Parsons DW, Jones S, Lin J, Sjoblom T, Leary RJ, Shen D, Boca SM, Barber T, Ptak J, et al: The genomic landscapes of human breast and colorectal cancers. Science 2007; 318:1108-1113.

Woodward ER, Buchberger A, Clifford SC et al: Comparative sequence analysis of the VHL tumor suppressor gene. Genomics 2000; 65: 253–265.

Woodward ER, Eng C, McMaon R, et al. Genetic predisposition to phaeochromocytoma: analysis of candidate genes GDNF, RET and VHL. Hum Mol Genet 1997; 6:1051-1056.

Woodward ER, Eng C, McMaon R, et al. Genetic predisposition to phaeochromocytoma: analysis of candidate genes GDNF, RET and VHL Hum Mol Genet 1997; 6:1051-1056.

Woodward ER, Eng C, McMahon R et al: Genetic predisposition to phaeochromocytoma: Analysis of candidate genes GDNF, RET and VHL. Hum Mol Genet 1997; 6: 1051–1056.

Zbar B, Kaelin W, Maher E, et al. Third International Meeting on von Hippel-Lindau disease. Cancer Res 1999; 59:2251-2253.

Zbar, B., Kishida, F. Chen, *et al*. Germlinemutations in the von Hippel-Lindau disease (VHL) gene in families from North American, Europe and Japan. Hum. Mutat. 1996; 8:348–357.

Zbar B, Kishida T, Chen F, et al. Germline mutations in the von Hippel-Lindau disease (VHL) gene in families from North America, Europe, and Japan. Hum Mutat 1996; 284:455461.

Zbar B, Kishida T, Chen F, Schmidt L, Maher ER, Richards FM, Crossey PA,Webster AR, Affara NA, Ferguson-Smith MA, Brauch H, Glavac D,

Neumann HP, Tisherman S, Mulvihill JJ, Gross DJ, Shuin T, Whaley J,Seizinger B, Kley N, Olschwang S, Boisson C, Richard S, Lips CH,Lerman M, Linehan WM. Germline mutations in the Von Hippel-Lindaudisease (VHL) gene in families from North America, Europe, and Japan. Hum Mutat 1996; 8:348–357.

Chapter 5

Genotype-Phenotype Disturbances of Some Biomarkers in Colorectal Cancer

Mihaela Tica, Valeria Tica, Alexandru Naumescu,
Mihaela Uta, Ovidiu Vlaicu and Elena Ionica

Additional information is available at the end of the chapter

http://dx.doi.org/10.5772/48366

1. Introduction

Colorectal carcinoma (CRC) is one of the most common human cancers. In 2008, 1.233.000 new CRC patients were diagnosed worldwide and about 608.000 deaths caused by colorectal cancer were estimated making it the fourth most common cause of death from cancer in the world. Five-year survival for CRC patients indicates a percent of 54.0% in Europe. Additionally, from the five-year survival, it was observed 74.0% of survival for patients with stage I, 66.5% for patients with stage IIA, 73.1% for patients with stage IIIA and only 5.7% for patients with stage IV disease (Stanczak, 2011). The success of colorectal cancer screening programs has resulted in an increasing number of biopsies of early neoplastic lesions with subtle histological features, making development of ancillary diagnostic testing for CRC essential. The incorporation of ancillary techniques, such as immunohistochemistry, cytochemical staining, electron microscopy, cytogenetic and, more recently, molecular testing, has made a significant impact in the diagnosis and management of solid tumors. Interpretation of hematoxylin-eosin stained slides by light microscopy remains the basic of anatomic pathology. However, an expanding menu of molecular assays continues to be implemented owing to their clinical utility in diagnosis, prognosis and risk assessment, therapy selection, as well as cancer screening and minimal residual disease detection. Carcinomas tend to carry multiple, complex, non-recurrent chromosomal and molecular aberrations, and they were not traditionally considered ideal candidates for molecular testing. However, this is changing with the discovery and implementation of new diagnostic, prognostic, and therapeutic molecular markers. Although single molecular biomarkers have proved useful, technical advances allowed performing the global genomic, epigenomic, or proteomic profiling of solid tumor malignancies. The research continues for more definitive molecular indicators that correlate with histological features and patient response to therapy and/ or survival.

Increasing understanding of cancer biology is beginning to explain the reasons for therapeutic failures. Signal transduction research have revealed that the receptors, enzymes and transcription factors that regulate cell fate are virtually all connected into an complex network of cross-regulatory interactions. The cell fate control system is not only interconnected but also highly redundant, such that if a gene or protein is disabled, another can perform a similar function (Rizzo, P, 2008). Key molecular mechanisms implicated in the genesis of CRC include chromosomal instability, DNA repair defects, and aberrant methylation. Chromosomal instability causes structural chromosomal anomalies, usually during DNA replication, with subsequent loss of tumor suppressor genes. DNA repair defects are caused by mutations in genes responsible for the repair of base-base DNA mismatches. These can be found as germline mutations or somatic methylation anomalies in acquired cases of CRC. A significant proportion of cases of CRC associated with mismatch repair anomalies occur on the right side of the colon and have a characteristic histological appearance. DNA repair defects can be detected indirectly by the associated epiphenomenon of microsatellite instability or unrepaired strand slippage within microsatellite regions.

Taking all these into account, we can conclude that study of colorectal carcinogenesis provides fundamental insights into the general mechanisms of cancer evolution. Now, it is believed that there are two patho-genetically distinct pathways for the development of colon cancer involving stepwise accumulation of multiple mutations. However, the genes involved and the mechanisms by which the mutations arisen are different.

The pathway, sometimes called the APC/ β-caterin pathway, is characterized by chromosomal instability that results in stepwise accumulation of mutations in a series of oncogenes and tumor suppressor genes. The molecular evolution of colon cancer along this pathway occurs through a series of morphologically identifiable stages. Initially, there is localized colon epithelial proliferation. This is followed by the formation of small adenomas that progressively enlarge, become more dysplastic, and ultimately develop into invasive cancers. This is referred to as the adenoma-carcinoma sequence. The genes that are correlated with this pathway are as follows:

Adenomatous Polyposis Coli (APC) - *APC* gene is located on chromosome 5 in 5q21 locus, and the mutations appearing at its level are responsible for the progression of CRC. Reported mutations in the *APC* gene include missense mutations and deletions, resulting in synthesis of truncated APC proteins. While "inherited" mutations are not clustered in a certain region of the gene but appear at the 5′-end or in nearby it, somatic mutations are clustered in the central region. The *APC* gene mutation is the genetic basis for FAP (Familial Adenomatous Polyposis) syndrome and fulfills the "first hit" concept advanced by Knudson in the 1970s. FAP patients have hundreds to thousands of colorectal adenomas and early onset carcinoma and allelic mutation of the *APC* gene followed by a loss of heterozygosity (LOH) is a common feature. Loss of this gene is believed to be the earliest event in the formation of adenomas. APC is involved in cell migration and adhesion and regulates levels of β-catenin (Senda T, 2005), an important mediator of the Wnt/ β-catenin signaling pathway. More than 80% of CRC have inactivated *APC*, and 50% of cancers without *APC* mutations have β-catenin mutations (Muhammad WS, 2010). *APC* gene product, a 310kDa protein located both in the cytoplasm and in the nucleus, interacting with β-catenin on the signaling pathway of Wnt-1. At the N-terminus site, the APC protein contains Armadillo-repeat binding domains and oligomerization domain and at the C-terminus site there are EB1 and tumor suppressor protein DLG binding domains. The APC protein also contains three 15-amino acids and seven 20-amino acids repeat regions from which the second one was show to be involved in the negative regulation of β-catenin protein expression in cells. At the 5'-end *APC* gene we can found the mutation cluster region (MCR) which is responsible for most of the mutations in *APC* gene which create truncated proteins. The truncated proteins contain ASEF (APC-stimulated guanine nucleotide exchange factor) and β-catenin binding sites in the armadillo-repeat domain but loose the β-catenin regulatory activity which is located in the 20-amino acids repeat domain (Narayan S, 2003). The diverse effects of mutations in *APC* gene indicates that this molecule plays a key role in the regulation of cell growth in a number of colonic and extracolonic tissues.

β-Catenin is a member of the cadherin-based cell adhesive complex, which also acts as a transcription factor if the protein is translocated to the nucleus. When it is not bound to E-cadherin and participating in cell-to-cell adhesion, a cytoplasmic degradation complex (consisting of APC, Axin, GSK-3β, and β-catenin) leads to β-catenin phosphorylation and degradation. When *APC* gene loss the normal function, β-catenin is not efficiently degraded and accumulates in the cytoplasm and is translocated to the nucleus where bind to a family of transcription factors called T-cell factor (TCF) or lymphoid enhancer factor (LEF) proteins and lead to transcriptional activation of certain target genes like c-Myc and Cyclin D. β-Catenine gene (*CTNNB1*) is located on the 3p chromosome and modifications in expression are associated with both early and tardive genetic events (Stanczak A, 2011). Most human cancers that involve *CTNNB1*mutations possess changes in exon 3 (amino acid residues in the N-terminus region), which provides loses binding affinity to GSK-3β, the kinase that phosphorylates and degrades β-catenin, in normal cells (Samowitz W.S., 1999). *APC* mutations are present in 80% of sporadic carcinomas (Knudson AG, 2001). Mutations in the *CTNNB1* gene at various key phosphorylation sites have been identified in CRC and several other solid tumors and it seem to prevent destruction of β-catenin by the proteasome pathway, which then leads to constitutive activation of Wnt signaling.

The **E-cadherin** gene (*CDH1*) is located on chromosome 16q22.1 and it contains 2.6 kb of coding sequences with 16 exons. There are overwhelming genetic data to support the role of E-cadherin as a tumor/ invasion suppressor in epithelial cells, and loss of expression, as well as mutations, has been described in a number of epithelial cancers. The implication of the *CDH1* gene in the process of carcinogenesis was initially associated with the gastric cancer because at this gene level somatic mutations which were associated with different types of diffuse gastric cancer (Becker KF, 1994) were observed. Subsequent research showed the existence of some germline mutations of *CDH1* in the families with dominant autosomal susceptibility for the hereditary diffuse gastric cancer (Suriano G, 2005). The genetic studies up to the present are sustaining the suppressor invasive/tumoral role of E-cadenin in the epithelial cells, and the expression loss along with mutations were described in some types of epithelial cancers (breast, colorectal, thyroid, endometrium, ovary cancer). Allelic imbalances of the LOH type were frequently observed in metastasizing malignancies derived from liver, prostate and breast. It is presumed that the loss of function contributes to the cancer progression by increasing the level of proliferation, invasion and/or metastasis. The E-caderin phenotypic expression in carcinomas is very well known, but the studies on the appearance of allelic imbalances at the *CDH1* level are rare. E-cadenin expression modifications are frequently associated with a high tumoral level, like the disease of prostate, breast, bladder, pancreas, stomach and colon. The mature protein product belongs to the family of cell–cell adhesion molecules and it plays a fundamental role in the maintenance of cell differentiation and the normal architecture of epithelial tissues (Stanczak A., 2011, Handschuh G, 1999). As an epithelial cell adhesion molecule E-cadherin mediates the contact between neighboring epithelial cells, including the colorectal epithelial cells, and helps to establish the defined membrane domains and cell polarity (Goodwin and Yap 2004). The extracellular domain of E-cadherin is responsible for homotypic binding of adjacent cells, and the cytoplasmic domain of E-cadherin facilitates adhesion through interaction with catenin proteins (Bryant and Stow 2004). The ectodomain of this protein mediates bacterial adhesion to mammalian cells and the cytoplasmic domain is required for internalization. Identified transcript variants arise from mutation at consensus splice sites. E-cadherin expression in epithelial cells is crucial for the establishment and maintenance of epithelial cell polarity.

BRCA1 gene mapped on the long arm of chromosome 17 (17q12-21) was identified by positional cloning methods. Mutations at the level of this gene are responsible in part for inherited predisposition to ovary, breast, prostate and colon cancers. However, whether these mutations are a factor in sporadic forms of these tumours remains unclear. Loss of *BRCA1* heterozygosity represents a molecular alteration presented in colorectal cancer, with unfavorable consequence in survival rates and that can be considered an independent prognosis factor in steps I and II of colorectal cancer stages (Roukos D., 2010). *BRCA1* is a large gene with many functional domains, each with different biological features. The C terminal region is related to the transactivation region of the protein and residues 758–1064 to the domain binding to Rad51, thus working as a complex to repair double stranded DNA breaks. In relation to its repair role, *BRCA1* is also related to co-activation of p53. The relationship of truncating germline mutations in the *BRCA1* gene and breast and ovarian cancers is established. Mutations in this gene are responsible in part for the inherited predisposition to breast and ovarian cancers, and probably for one third of all site specific inherited breast cancer. In previous studies, researchers found a high percentage of LOH in the 17q21 region in sporadic CRC cases. BRCA proteins have a significant role in multiple pathways, signaling cell cycle delays for DNA lesions or leading to apoptosis for severe damage. BRCA proteins function in transcriptional regulation and chromatin remodeling, and they are required to repair double-strand breaks. Double-strand breaks in mammalian chromosomes stimulate the activity of recombination repair enzymes by more than 100-fold. In transformed colon cells of *BRCA1* mutation carriers, BRCA1 functions are probably lost. In almost all colorectal cancers, the mutated *APC* gene, lead to MYC over-expression and as consequence involve BRCA1 over-expression. BRCA1 directly link MYC at double-strand break repair and participate to the preserving genome integrity. When *BRCA1* is mutated and have only one normal allele, MYC-associated loss of homology - directed recombination repair should occur earlier than in individuals with two normal *BRCA1* alleles. BRCA1 expression is reduced in at least some sporadic colon adenocarcinomas and somatic loss of one normal *BRCA1* allele is common not only in hereditary but also in sporadic CRC tumors (Friedenson B, 2004).

Group IIA PLA$_2$ is a 14-kDa enzyme found in a number of tissues and secretory products (Nevaleine TJ, 1993). The plasma concentration of the enzyme increases dramatically in severe infections and other diseases involving generalized inflammation and cancer (Ogawa M, 1991). In the gastrointestinal tract, expression of group IIA PLA$_2$ has been localized in Paneth cells of the small intestine (Nevaleine TJ, 1995), metaplastic Paneth cells of gastric (Nevaleine TJ, 1995) and colonic mucosa (Haapamaki MM, 1999) as well as columnar epithelial cells of inflammeted colonic mucosa. Functional defects in PLA$_2$ in tumor cells may interfere with the regulatory mechanisms of tumor growth. The *PLA2G2A* gene function is relevant in tumorigenesis, and is a good candidate gene modifying the *Apc* gene in the Min (multiple intestinal neoplasias) mice. On the one hand, it has been suggested that a mutation resulting in splice variants of the *Pla2g2a* gene and in different truncated forms of its protein accounts for the increased number of polyps in mice carrying the Min mutation. Numerous studies suggested that *Pla2g2a* is a candidate gene for *Mom-1*. The analysis of a mouse/ human hybrid panel showed that the *PLA2G2A* gene, located on the human chromosome 1p, is a candidate gene for the MOM-1 locus, (Spirio LN, 1996; Ishiguro Y, 1999; Mounier CM, 2008). It was also observed that the *PLA2G2A* gene is intact, but an allelic imbalance (AI), or an allelic loss, was found at one of the alleles and a loss of heterozygosity (LOH) was identified on *PLA2G2A* regions (Mihalcea, A, 2009).

The **EGFR** is a member of the HER (human epidermal growth factor receptor) family, and includes HER1 (EGFR, ErbB-1), HER2 (ErbB-2), HER3 (ErbB-3), and HER4 (ErbB-4) (Boss JL, 1989). The natural ligands for EGFR include EGF, transforming growth factor (TGF), amphiregulin, heregulin, heparin-binding EGF, and cellulin. Ligand binding induces receptor dimerisation and subsequent auto-phosphorylation that activates critical pathways for cellular survival and proliferation such as PI3K/Akt, Stat, Src and MAPK. EGFR mediates signaling by activating the MAPK and PI3K signaling cascades (Jhawer M, 2008). EGFR modifications have been described in many cancers as a consequence of mutations or gene amplifications that induce protein over-expression, structural rearrangements and autocrine loops. EGFR abnormalities may have a relevant role in both carcinogenesis and clinical progression of CRC. EGFR is differentially expressed in normal, premalignant, and malignant tissues, and over-expression of EGFR has been documented in up to nearly 90% of cases of metastatic CRC (Boss JL, 1989; Arteaga CL, 2001). In addition, EGFR is over-expressed in a wide range of solid tumors and is involved in their growth and proliferation through various mechanisms. Given the documented role of EGFR in the development and progression of cancers, this receptor signaling pathway represents a rational target for drug development (Vokes EE, 2006; Lee JJ, 2007). Recent clinical data have shown that advanced colorectal cancer with tumor-promoting mutations of these pathways -- including activating mutations in KRAS, BRAF, and the p110 subunit of PI3K-- do not respond to anti-EGFR therapy.

The variability in clinical presentation, aggressiveness, and patterns of treatment failure suggests distinct genotypes and phenotypes identification, which can help future treatment strategies. A new concept called "personalized medicine" may be another beginning of a new era and it has been designed to offer every patient a suitable therapy. By this new approach, "Personalized medicine" can be defined as the tailoring of medical treatment to a specific subset of patients who are usually identified by genetic markers or other molecular profiling strategies. There is an increasing interest in this therapeutic strategy on the part of pharmaceutical and bio-pharmaceutical companies, consumers, and third party payers. Consequently, the level of clinical trial activity surrounding personalized medicines is intensifying as sponsors seek ways to target their therapies to patient populations that would most benefit from them. The aim of the present chapter is to elaborate an experimental model in order to improve the "personalized" therapeutically strategy, by evaluating some key gene expression involved into a crosstalk signaling, in colorectal cancer.

By our study design we have evaluated the comparative expression at proteic and genetic level of several key point proteins (*APC, PLA2G2A, CDH1, BRCA1,* and *EGFR*). Our *in vivo* experiment involved diagnosis testing of CRC patients and molecular biology testing on biological samples in order to clarify the cross-talk of interested genes and to better understand the CRC typology among Romanian patients.

The idea of applying such a model to our studies was generated during the research that we conducted in our projects. We have noticed that between different proteins and genes is a very close relationship, which depends on the tumor type, cell grade and staging. Following a study of a large number of articles published in the international databases we observed that other researchers have drawn the same conclusion.

2. Results and discussion

2.1. Tissue samples and blood

Samples were obtained with the consent of 93 patients, consisting of histopatologically confirmed colorectal adenomas. Samples were obtained during colonoscopy with biopsy forceps, by harvesting at least four fragments from all the quadrants of the pathological tissue. The surgical intervention for CRC treatment included radical and palliative techniques (right or left hemicolectomy, segmentary colectomy, low anterior rectal resection–Dixon, Milles operation, Hartmann operation). All tumors were histologically (HP) examined by pathologist in order to: (a) confirm the diagnosis of adenocarcinoma, (b) confirm the presence of tumor and evaluate the percentage of tumor cells in these samples, and (c) carry out pathological staging. The complete HP diagnosis included: degree of differentiation (well/ moderate/ poor), vascular, neural and lymphatic invasion, status of the margins of resection (invaded/ noninvaded) and also TNM stadialisation. After surgical resection, tumor tissues were cut in small pieces, frozen immediately in liquid nitrogen and stored at - 80^{0}C until they were analyzed.

For the initial patients group, only 75 patients who had at least 75% tumor cells were taken in consideration for molecular biology analyses. To perform immunohistochemistry by immunofluorescence (IHF) analyses, five micrometers thick tissue serial sections were incubated with primary antibodies diluted in BSA (bovine serum albumin) in PBS (phosphate buffered saline). After washing with PBS, FITC-conjugated secondary antibodies (Invitrogen) were applied and then the samples were washed again. The protein expression was evaluated by fluorescent microscopy. In order to analyze the mutational status, DNA was extracted from patients' venous blood (as control) and from tumours. DNA preparation was performed using the *Wizard® Genomic DNA Purification kit* (Promega) according to the manufacturer's recommendations. The extracted DNA was stored at -80^{0}C until molecular biology analyses.

2.2. Clinicopathological characteristics

The medical records of all 93 patients provided their birth date and sex, and the following parameters: tumor location, tumor size, lymph node metastases, pathological stage, vascular and neural invasion and tumoral differentiation grading.

Out of 93 cases, there were 40 womens and 53 mens. The mean age was 50 years. The majority had T3 tumors (31.8%); T2 tumors (25.80%) according to tumor stage of the TNM classification of colon and rectum neoplasm and 53 patients (57%) had lymph node involvement (N+). In the study lot, 17 cases (18.27%) presented metastasis at the time at CRC diagnosis. These were predominantly localized in the liver (12 cases, 70.58%) and rarely in the lungs (4 cases, 23.52%).

Regarding the histopathological type of colorectal tumors, the vast majority was adenocarcinomas (ADK) with different grades of differentiation. Most of the tumors (42 cases: 45.16%) were well differentiated (G1) while 33 cases (35.48 %) were moderately differentiated (G2) and 18 cases (19.35%) poor differentiated (G3) tumors. Beside typical adenocarcinoma another histopathological type of tumors was rare and was localized: i) to the right colon - especially mucinous ADK (5 cases from a total of 9 cases in the all study lot) and 1 adenosquamous carcinoma; ii) to the left colon - 2 cases of mucinous ADK and 1 case of "signet-ring" cell carcinoma; iii) to the rectum - 2 mucinous ADK, 1 squamocellular carcinoma and 1 case of anaplazic carcinoma. Patients characteristic is summarized in Table 1.

Our study has not taken into consideration the diet, because most of the patients do not know the food properties or they use food with pro-carcinogen potential. Regarding the diet, we consider that the patient instruction is extremely useful and has to be done by the surgeon doctor after the surgical treatment and then by the family doctor. This approach allows both secondary prophylaxis and control of possible relapses/ recidivists. A monitoring of the patients included in the study will shows the efficiency of medical control and the conscious of this mortal disease. In the studied lot of patients we have not registered cases with relapse, and we cannot predict their future behavior.

CLINICO-PATHOLOGICAL CHARACTERISTICS OF CRC TUMORS	No CASES n (%)
Age	
< 50	12
> 50	81
Gender	
Male	53
Female	40
Tumor localisation	
RC	13
LC	42
RECTUM	38
Stage	
I	23 (24,73%)
II	24 (25,80 %)
III	29 (31,18%)
IV	17 (18,27%)
Lymph nodes status	
N – (N0)	40 (43%)
N +(N1,2,3)	53 (57%)
Histopathological grading	
Well differentiated G1	42
Moderately differentiated G2	33
Poor differentiated G3	18
Total	93

Table 1. Clinico-pathological characteristics of CRC tumors in the study lot

2.3. Immunohistochemical expression by immunofluoresce of the studied proteins

Because the interpretation of immunohistochemistry analyses remains the basic of anatomic pathology, in our study we first evaluated the protein expression of the key point proteins that were taken in our study. Unlike the normal histopathological analyses, our evaluation was based on protein fluorescent signal which, from our point of view, is more specific than classical immunohistochemistry.

The expression of **α-SM** (smooth muscle) was included in our study as a positive control to prove the method accuracy and it is used as a typical marker for myofibroblasts. It is one of the four muscle actin isoforms, a protein involved in supporting basic contractile apparatus in muscle cells. This expression can be found in vascular cells, intestinal muscularis mucosae and muscularis propria, and in the stromal tissue. In normal tissue, the immunofluorescence signal is strong (+3) around tumor crypts, in the vessel walls and stromal smooth muscle fibers. In the crypt epithelial cells the signal is absent (-). In CRC patients the α-SM expression decreases with increasing disease grade, and disappear in most of the advanced CRC, when the tissue is disorganized and a lot of tumor cells are present (Figure 1).

By labeling the **APC** C-terminus, there were observed changes of protein expression in tumor tissue compared with APC expression in normal tissues. In normal tissues, muscle tunic polyps analysis confirmed the expression of target protein in SM from blood vessels and fibers of the smooth muscle shell structure, where it is stored.

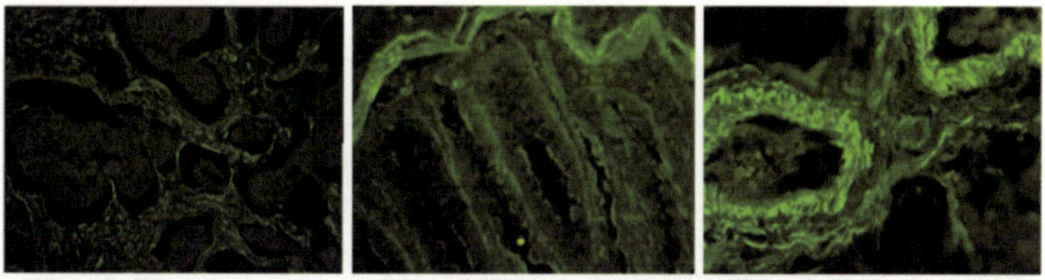

α-SM expression (20×) | α-SM expression (20×) | α-SM expression (40×)

Figure 1. α-SM expression. Smooth muscle, used as a positive marker for immunofluorescence signal, have immunofluorescent signal in blood vessels, intestinal muscularis mucosae and muscularis propria, and in the stromal tissue.

With few exceptions, the intensity of fluorescent signal given by the expression of APC is strong (3+), fluorescent signal obtained overlapping fluorescent signal of α-actin expression given by smooth muscle cells (Figure 2). Adenocarcinomas of the colorectal mucosa analysis revealed APC expression changes. During tumorigenesis process, the mucosa is invaded by stromal tissue, the crypts become large, elongate, their architecture is destroyed and the fluorescent signal intensity of epithelial cells (CE) decreases becoming weak (1+).

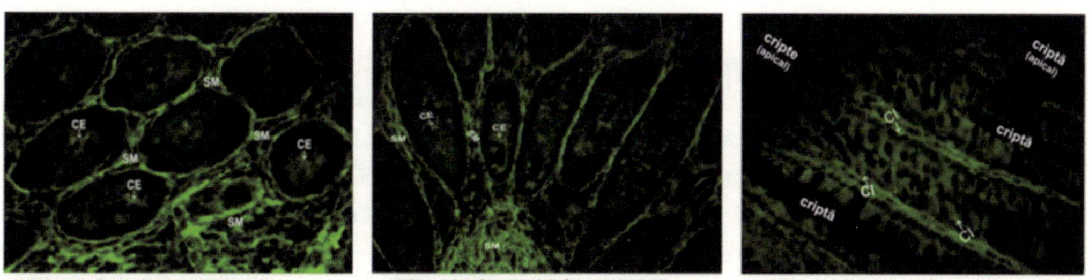

APC expresion (40×) (normal tissue) | APC expression (40×) (adenocarcinoma from patient 8) | APC expression (40×) (adenocarcinoma from patient 3)

Figure 2. APC expression. A normal expression with immunofluorescent signal on the border of the crypts and in SM cells can be observed on 8 patient's section, like in normal tissue. On section obtained from patient 3 we can observe a weak intensity on the apical part of epithelial cells and loss of signal, too.

At the same time we observed an increase of its intensity in neoplastic infiltrated cells (CI). In the apical half of the fluorescent signal crypt, epithelial cells and infiltrated cells disappeared (-). The IHF expression pattern overlaps the APC sequential histopathological changes occurring in the colorectal carcinogenesis, in which β-catenin and APC play the role of so-called "Second Hit".

In normal colorectal tissue, **β-catenin** expression appears on the membrane of epithelial cells. In tumor tissue, can occur either over-expression of β-catenin in the nucleus where it is translocated from the cytoplasm as a result of *APC* mutation, or signal absence when β-catenin changes. In our study, 33.33% (25/ 75) of patients show a similar β-catenin expression to that of normal tissue because the fluorescent signals were obtained on the membrane of epithelial cells. In 33 CRC patients, the β-catenin target protein expression was changed compared with normal tissue (Figure 3).

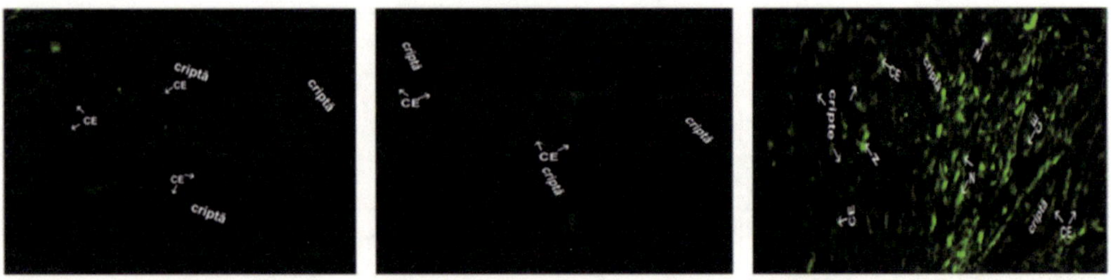

β-Catenin expression (40x) (normal tissue) | β-Catenin expression (40x) (adenocarcinoma from patient 8) | β-Catenin expression (40x) (adenocarcinoma from patient 3)

Figure 3. β-Catenin expression on patient 8. A normal expression with immunofluorescent signal on cytoplasm and on the border of crypts can be observed on the section from patient 8. On section from patient 3 we can observe an over-expression in the cytoplasm/ nucleus of epithelial cells and loss of expression in the membrane.

We can observe how the fluorescent signal on the membrane of epithelial cells gradually decreases in intensity during the tumor progression, along with increased fluorescent signal by over-expression in cytoplasm (in 28 patients) and in the nucleus (in 5 patients).

Regarding **E-cadherin** expression, colorectal tumors showed a heterogeneous type of expression compared to the normal colorectal epithelium in which E-cadherin expression is present on the basolateral membrane to the whole length of the glandular crypts and on the intercellular membranes. An abnormal pattern of expression is observed on CRC tumor sections: i) a reduced expression (2+, 1+) at the membrane level was observed in 20% (15/ 75) of patients; ii) cytoplasmatic expression was observed in 37.33% (28/ 75) of patients and the expression is similar to that observed for β-catenin; iii) loss of expression (-) was observed in 12% (9/ 75) of patients. In 30.66% (23/ 75) of patients, the E-cadherin expression was similar with that observed in normal colon epithelium, in the cell membrane, with strong immunofluorescent signal (3+) and is co-localized with membrane β-catenin (Figure 4).

Comparative analyses of E-cadherin protein expression for CRC tumors with various histological differentiation grades (G1, G2, G3), showed an almost similar expression pattern for all G1, G2 and G3 tumor grades, although the majority of the well differentiated G1 tumors indicated strong membranous signal; the moderately differentiated tumors (G2) showed a heterogeneous membranous signal and some of the poorly differentiated tumors (G3) had no membranous expression for E-cadherin. In the case of lymph nodes analyses,

E-cadherin expression on patient 70 (10x) | E-cadherin expression on patient 74 (10x) | E-cadherin expression on patient 73 (20x)

Figure 4. E-cadherin expression. A normal expression with immunofluorescent signal on the membrane of epithelial cells can be observed on section from patient 70. In the case of patient 74 we can observe a reduced/ loss of expression in the epithelial cell membranes. On patient 73 an over-expression in the cytoplasm of epithelial cells and in some infiltrating cells was noticed.

there is a strong correlation between the presence of the lymph node invasion status and protein expression of E-cadherin. From a total number of 75 cases of CRC, we observed that patients with lymph node invasion N + (N1, N2, N3) have low or no expression of E-cadherin. Thus E-cadherin could be considered a biomarker that can help to determine the risk in patients with CRC, and a strong indicator of the lymph node status. In the group of N0 CRC tumors from 27 cases, only 77.77% (21/ 27) of patients presented E-cadherin membrane expression in different staining grades, scored as 0, 1+, 2+ , while in the group of lymph node invasion N+ tumors (48 cases) only 35.41% (31/ 48) of patients were positive for membranous staining (0,1+, 2+).

In normal colon mucosa the **$sPLA_2$ type IIA** enzyme was detected by a strong staining in muscularis mucosae in a large fraction of SM cells (recognized by α-SM actin antibody) and vascular SM cells (Figure 5). In lamina propria, the PLA_2 type IIA enzyme was detected with a weaker staining (2+), surrounding the crypts (as determined by morphological and histological evaluation), and in vascular smooth muscle. These results show that PLA_2 type IIA enzyme is expressed only in smooth muscle cells from normal colon mucosa. An abnormal pattern for PLA_2 type IIA expression was observed in 27 of the 75 CRC cases (36.00%), which were examined. In muscularis externa and submucosa, the SM cells express PLA_2 type IIA with a strong intensity (3+). The presence of PLA_2 type IIA was not observed (-) in other types of cells.

Beginning with mucosa, the PLA_2 type IIA expression started to be modified. Thus, near the submucosa, the immunofluorescence signal for PLA_2 type IIA was observed in SM cells from lamina propria, but only around crypts, and with a weak signal comparative with the normal pattern (1+). As the crypts get longer with more ramifications, the number of SM cells that express PLA_2 type IIA decrease, although we had a positive signal for α-SM actin from all the SM cells. In this area, PLA_2 type IIA expression was found in epithelial cells, on the border of Lieberkühn crypts. The number of epithelial cells that express PLA_2 type IIA increases during the crypts growing. The immunofluorescence signal is also stronger (3+) than fluorescent signal observed in SM cells. No immunoreaction for PLA_2 (type II) was found in all 11 patients' sections (14.66%) that were analyzed. This may suggest that the malignant cells lose their ability to express PLA_2 type IIA, when invasive carcinoma develops in the adenoma.

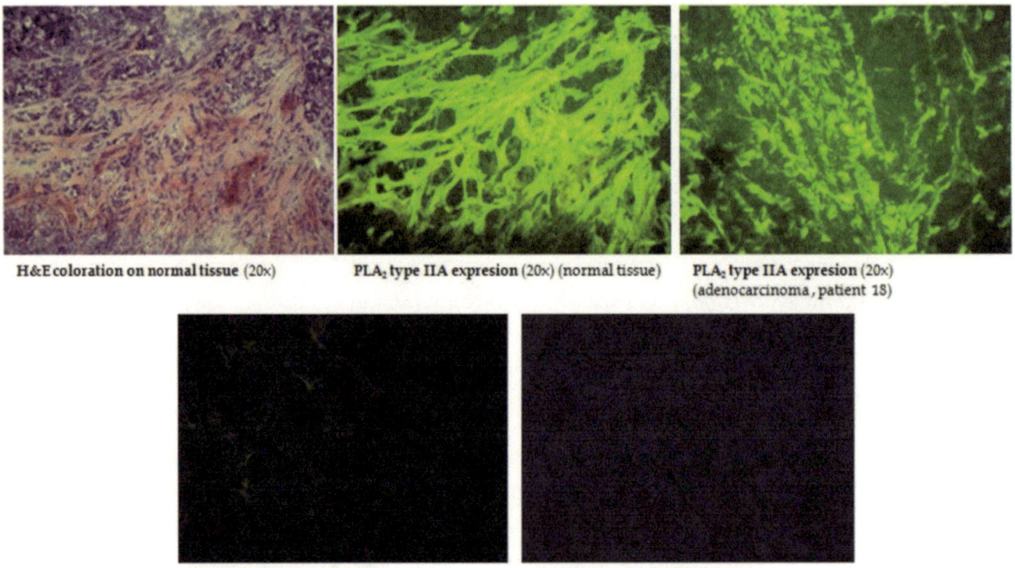

Figure 5. PLA2 type IIA expression. A normal expression with immunofluorescent signal in SM cells can be observed on section from patient 12. On section from patient 18 we observe an over-expression in infiltrated cells. Patient 62 shows a weakly signal on SM cells around the crypts and on vascular smooth muscle. In the case of patient 60 the loss of signal is remarked.

We characterized the expression of **BRCA1** in 75 sporadic colorectal carcinomas. It was found an increased BRCA1 expression in the apical cell pole of epithelial malignant cells and a significant increase in BRCA1 nuclear foci in tumor colorectal specimens in comparison with the corresponding normal tissues, in 10 cases out of 75 (13.33%). These increases in BRCA1 expression may be explained by the fact that colorectal tissue is subject to very active proliferation and differentiation. In 14 cases out 75 (18.66%) we observed the loss of BRCA1 expression (Figure 6).

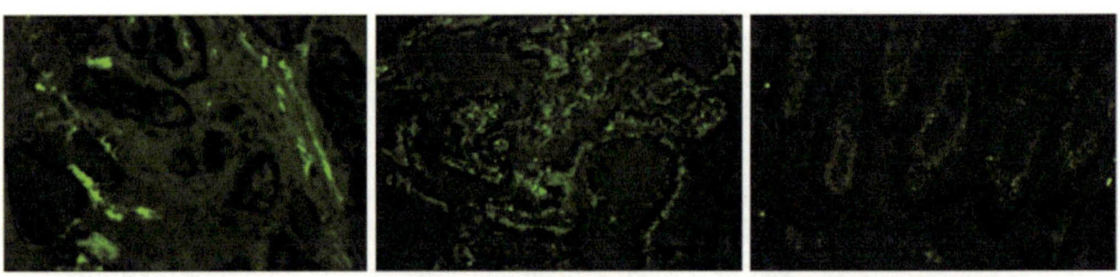

Figure 6. BRCA1 expression. Patient 43 showed loss of expression in nucleus of epithelial cells. On patient 60 we can observe an over-expression on the epithelial cells from the crypt foci. On other sections from patient 60 over-expression was observed only on the apical pole of epithelial cells.

The epidermal growth factor receptor (EGFR) expression had an abnormal pattern in 41.33% (31/ 75) of patients. Out of these, the signal intensity was weak (1+) in 22.58% (7/ 31) of patients and moderate (2+) in 32.25% (10/ 31) of patients. Moreover, in both cases EGFR expression was observed in cytoplasm of tumoral cells (Figure 7). Complete strong circumferential expression (3+) was found in 45.16% (14/ 31) of patients. Normal expression, like signal absence was observed in 58.67% (44/ 75) of patients. In our study (2+) and/ or (3+) were defined for those cases with EGFR expression in 50% or more tumoral cells on the section. By our study we observed that EGFR expression was significantly associated with higher rates of cell proliferation. EGFR activation and intracellular signal can be a result of its roles in transcription, up-regulation, degradation and gene amplification. Our results demonstrate that EGFR over-expression is correlated with higher tumor stage (III and IV) as compared with weaker EGFR expression. Due to the knowledge of EGFR expression in CRC, now it is possible to apply targeted therapy with cetuximab-EGFR monoclonal antibodies in the treatment algorithm of the CRC at the EGFR-positive patients identified by IHC examination. Also, the observed differentiated association between EGFR expression, ganglion EGFR status – N and tumor differentiation degree - G, could significantly assign to the EGFR the role of prognostic marker for disease recurrence. Determination of EGFR status may be used to identify cases of CRC, which could benefit from anti-EGFR therapies and on the other hand would have the potential to be a rigorous mean for monitoring efficacy of anti-EGFR therapy in CRC (Mendelsohn, 2003). Although EGFR remains a controversial prognostic factor, the association between EGFR over-expression and tumor stage may have an important role in the anti-EGFR therapy of patients with CRC.

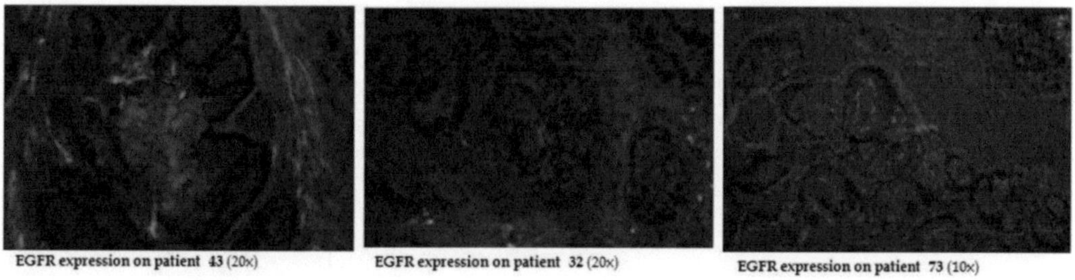

Figure 7. EGFR expression. On patient 43 we can observe an over-expression on the membrane of epithelial cells from the crypt foci. In the case of patient 32 we remarked loss of expression. Patient 73 presented expression in cytoplasm of tumoral cells.

2.4. Deletion/duplication evaluation for the interested genes (MLPA)

MLPA analysis detects large deletions or duplications in the gene. This is a semi quantitative reaction based on PCR identifying copy number variations and contributes for assessing predictive genetic markers giving an intra-individual variation spectrum of the genes included in this study. It is also a useful tool for the diagnosis of genetic diseases characterized by large genomic rearrangements. In order to perform the test on blood and tissue samples in the first step of our analyses we optimized the procedure for the specific genes. For each gene we optimized the range of DNA concentration in order to have a good signal and to obtain the most suitable mix of primers that we have to use. After protocol optimization we went through the technique and in each run we used three DNA samples from blood and tissue for each patient.

According to the microsatellites alteration assay we performed the MLPA analysis of *APC* and *BRCA1* genes and two other genes (*EGFR* and *CDH1*) were included.

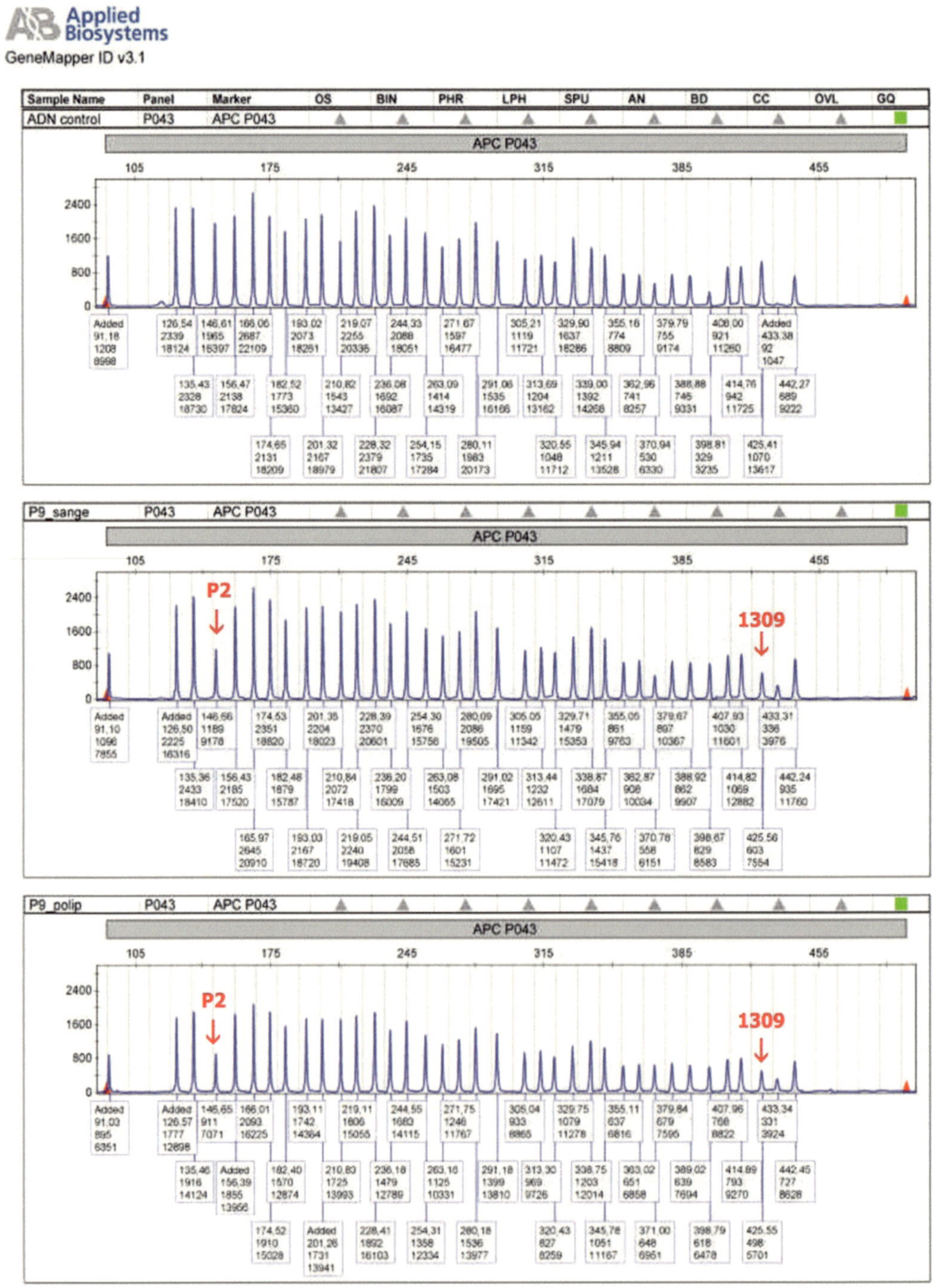

Figure 8. MLPA chromatograms for patient with FAP (patient 15).

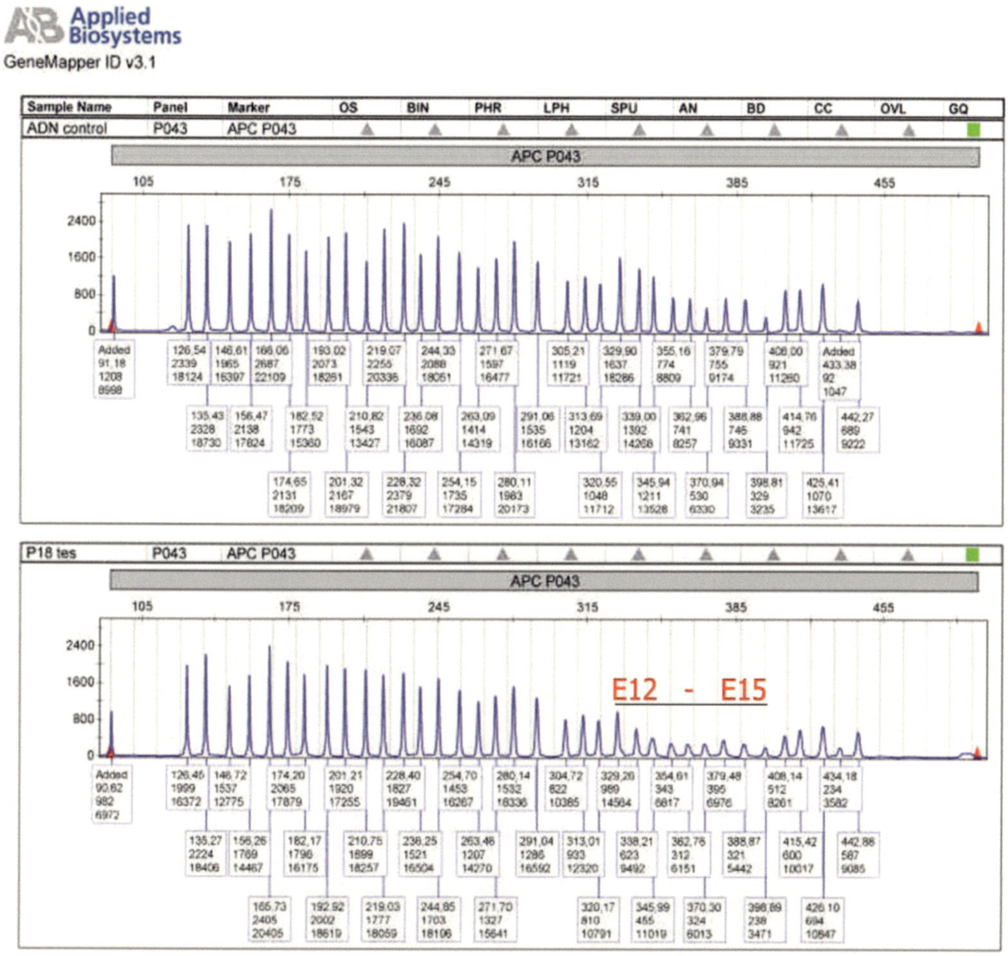

Figure 9. MLPA chromatograms for the patient 31.

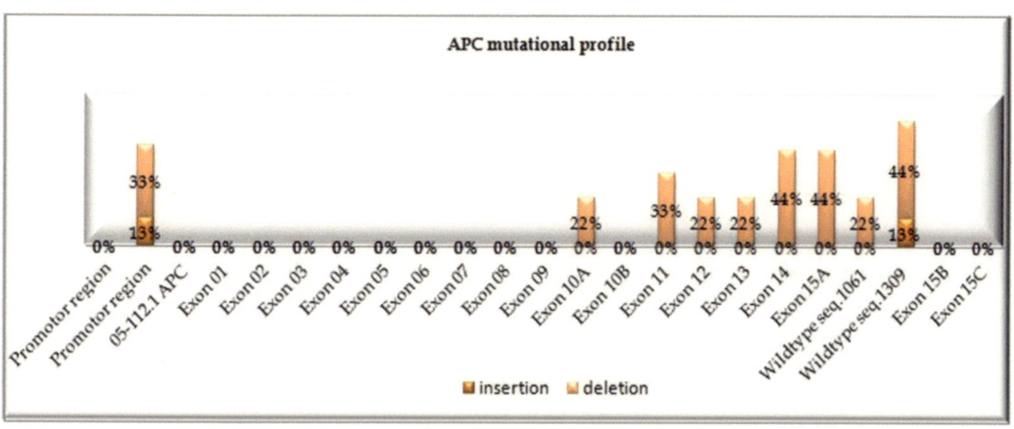

Figure 10. Mutational profile of *APC* by MLPA

The interpretation of the results was made by the help of a specific soft that assesses the reaction products in accordance with their molecular weight and quantitative expression. The GeneMapper results were exported in Coffalyzer software for normalization and the relative probe signals were calculated by dividing each measured peak area by the sum of all peak areas of the sample. A value of 1.0 indicated the presence of two alleles, and values of 0.5 and 1.5 represented a heterozygous deletion or duplication at that locus, respectively.

The mutational analyses at ***APC*** gene indicate that patient 15 diagnosed with FAP (Familial Adenomatous Polyposis) had deletion at the promoter region and also constitutional mutation 1309 (Figure 8) and no positive cases were found in the blood DNA samples.

This patient showed two deletions, in blood and in the tumour, in the promoter 2 and mutation 1309 region, although the individual did not show microsatellite loci alteration. Another example is patient 31 who presents a large deletion in between exon 12 – exon 15 (Figure 9) and by immunohistochemistry we found *APC* loss of expression in epithelial cells. In all studied cases we observed that 12% (9/ 75) of patients had a mutational profile. Deletions appeared frequently at the E12 - E15 level (11.9%) and in 3/ 9 cases in the promotor region 2 (33%); in E15 in 44% (4/ 9) of cases. Insertions were observed in 13% of cases (10/ 75) of cases in the promoter region and 13% (10/ 75) of patients have shown presence of wild type mutation 1309 (Figure 10).

Regarding the ***CDH1*** mutational status we observed that mutational profile appear in 30% (20/ 75) of patients. Insertion was observed at exon 4 in 30% (6/ 20) of patients and in 20% (4/ 20) of patients at exon 10. Loss of heterozygosity was observed at exons 08 and 13 in 20% (4/ 20) of patients for each exon (Figure 11). Without making microsatellite instability analyze, at the *CDH1* gene locus, loss of heterozygosity that was found by MLPA analysis was not necessary overlapped with results of E-cadherin protein expression studied by IHF in the tumors samples.

Mutational analyses at ***BRCA1*** gene indicate that 20% (15/ 75) of patients have mutations like duplication or loss of heterozygosity. Duplication at exon E13B was observed in 40% (6/ 15) of patients and at exon 20 was observed in 20% (3/ 15) of patients. As well as duplication, loss of heterozygosity was observed in principal to exon 13B in 40% (6/ 15) patients (Figure 12).

EGFR mutational status analyzes indicate that mutational profile appears like insertion, in 18.66% (20/ 75) of patients. Out of these, in 50% (10/ 20) of patients we observed insertion at the exon 3, in 20% (4/ 20) of patients at the exon 08, in 40% (8/20) of patients at the exon 17, in 40% (8/ 20) of patients at exon 25 and in 30% (6/ 20) of patients at exon 28 (Figure 13). For each of the following exons 02, 09 – 16, 18 – 24, 26 and 27 we have found insertions in 10% (2/ 20) of patients.

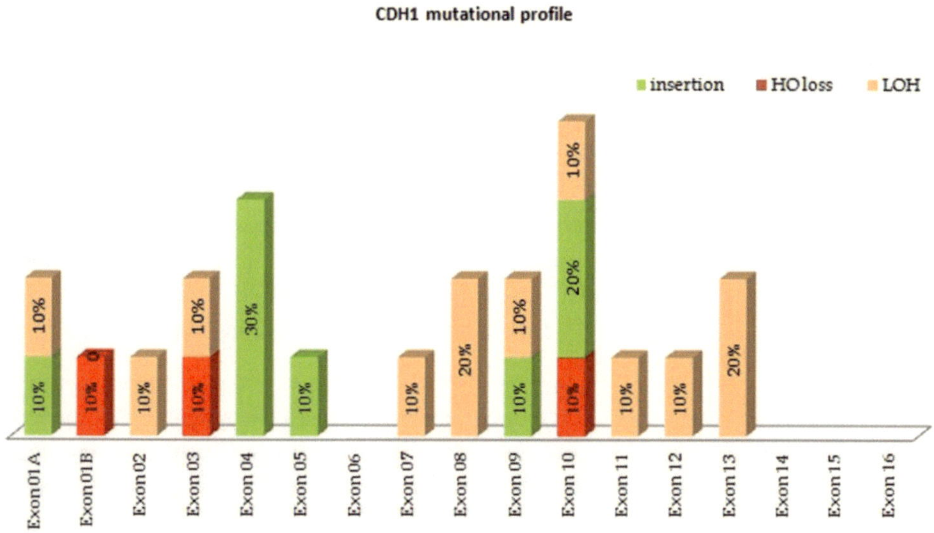

Figure 11. Mutational profile of *CDH1* by MLPA

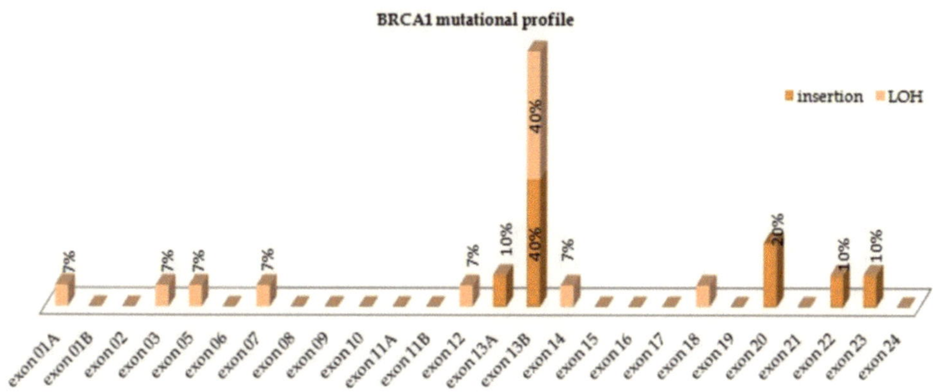

Figure 12. Mutational profile of *BRCA1* by MLPA

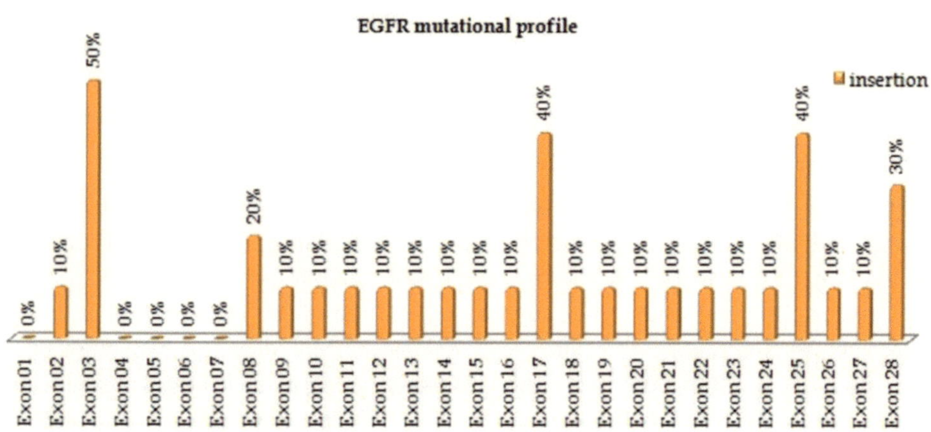

Figure 13. Mutational profile of *EGFR* by MLPA

2.5. Microsatellite instability correlation on *APC, BRCA1* and *PLA2G2A*

During tumorigenesis, loss of wild-type alleles (inherited from the non-mutation-carrying parents) is frequently observed. Loss of heterozygosity (LOH) on tumor suppressor genes play a key role in colorectal cancer transformation, and LOH analysis of sporadic colorectal cancers could help discover unknown tumor suppressor genes (Ahmed B, 2011). For those patients who presented deletion/ duplication at the interested genes, in order to have a more accurate mutational analysis we decided to analyze the microsatellite instability. A panel of microsatellite markers, labeled with FAM, HEX, TET, were used to amplify DNA from normal and tumour tissues for LOH and MSI analyses of chromosomal loci specifics for *APC, PLA2G2A*, and *BRCA1*.

In order to analyze the polymorphic microsatellite markers, a PCR reaction was carried out for 10 ng DNA from normal and tumour tissue. The fluorescent specific-marker amplification PCR products were separated on ABI PRISM™ 310 Genetic Analyzer (Applied Biosystems). Resulted electrophoregrams were analyzed with GeneMapper ID v3.1 software for molecular size and peak heights. Data analysis was done with Sequencing DNA Analysis Software. The allelic imbalance can appear as loss of heterozygosity (LOH) or as microsatellite instability (MSI). LOH was determined using the following ratio: $(T_1:T_2)/\ (N_1:N_2)$, where 1 and 2 are the first and the second peaks of alleles identified in the tumour/ blood DNA samples from patients with colorectal cancer. When the ratio is lower than 0.67 or higher than 1.5, this is revealing the loss of one of the alleles (LOH). The presence of a novel allele in the tumour sample was interpreted as microsatellite instability (MSI).

In case of homozygosity, the two alleles are identical as dimension, and the corresponding picks are overlapped. Thus we cannot make distinction between the two alleles and their height.

Highly polymorphic markers were designed for AI analysis. The designed microsatellite markers for *PLA2G2A* located on chromosome 1, were D1S199, D1S2843, D1S2644 which are located around the gene and D1S234 from the coding region of the gene. For *APC* gene we selected D5S82, D5S489 microsatellite markers which are surrounding the gene, D5S656 which partial overlaps the gene and D5S421 which are localized on the coding region. Another panel of microsatellites loci was used for *BRCA1* gene: D17S855, D17S1322, D17S1323 which are localized on the introns 20, 12 and 19 of the gene and, D17S250, D17S800, D17S856, D17S1327 on chromosome 17q, surrounding the gene.

At the microsatellite loci designed on chromosome 1, LOH/ MSI was observed in 28% (21/ 75) of patients and 68% (17/ 21) of these have had allelic imbalance at the D1S234 locus which covers the *PLA2G2A* locus (Figure 14, Figure 15). MSI was observed in only 6.66% (5/ 75) of patients (Figure 16) and that, make us to suggest that MSI is very rare in sporadic adenocarcinomas and routine screening such lesions for MSI may not be a high priority. Previous studies showed that the 1p36 region frequently present allelic loss in various cancers, such as colon cancer, neuroblastoma, hepatocellular carcinomas, lung cancer, and breast cancer. However, only NB (neuroblastoma) gene was confirmed to be the tumor suppressor gene of neuroblastomas. In 1993, Tanaka *et al.* believed that a normal chromosome 1p36 might contain a tumor suppressor gene of colon carcinogenesis. Due to many genes located in the region of 1p36.33-36.31, additional analyses are necessary in order to confirm our hypothesis.

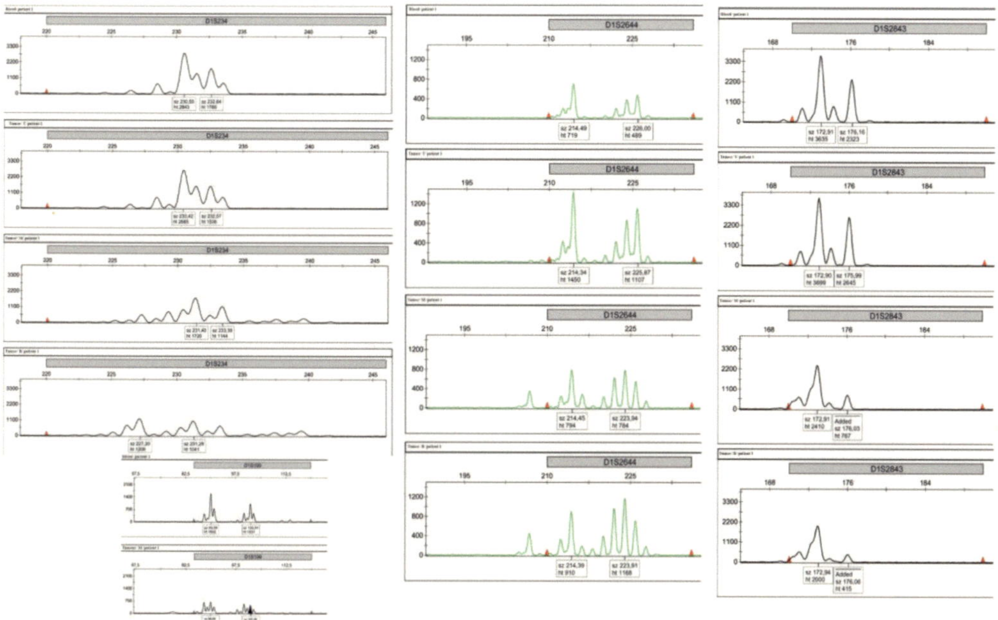

Figure 14. Microsatellite alteration for *PLA2G2A* gene in patient 1. D1S234, D1S 264 and D1S2843

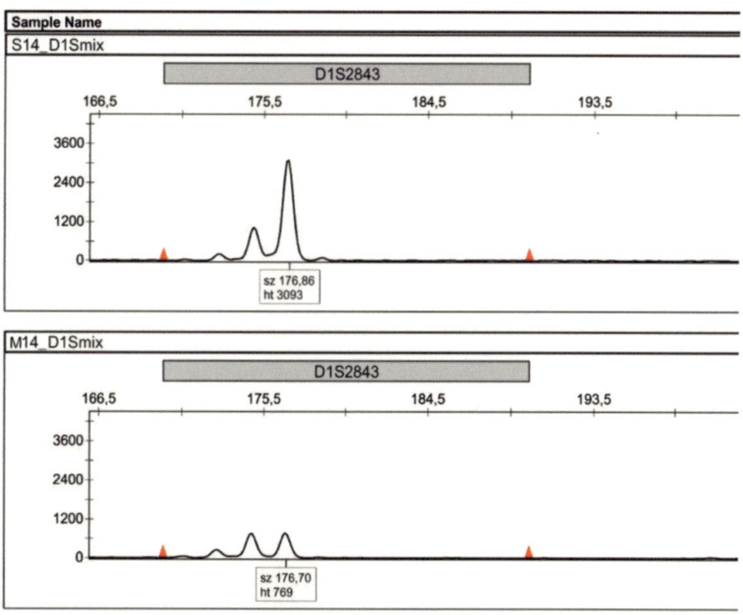

Figure 15. Microsatellite alteration for *PLA2G2A* genes in patient 14. D1S2843 - S14 – Blood (considered as normal); D1S2843 – M14 –MSI with low amplitude signal;

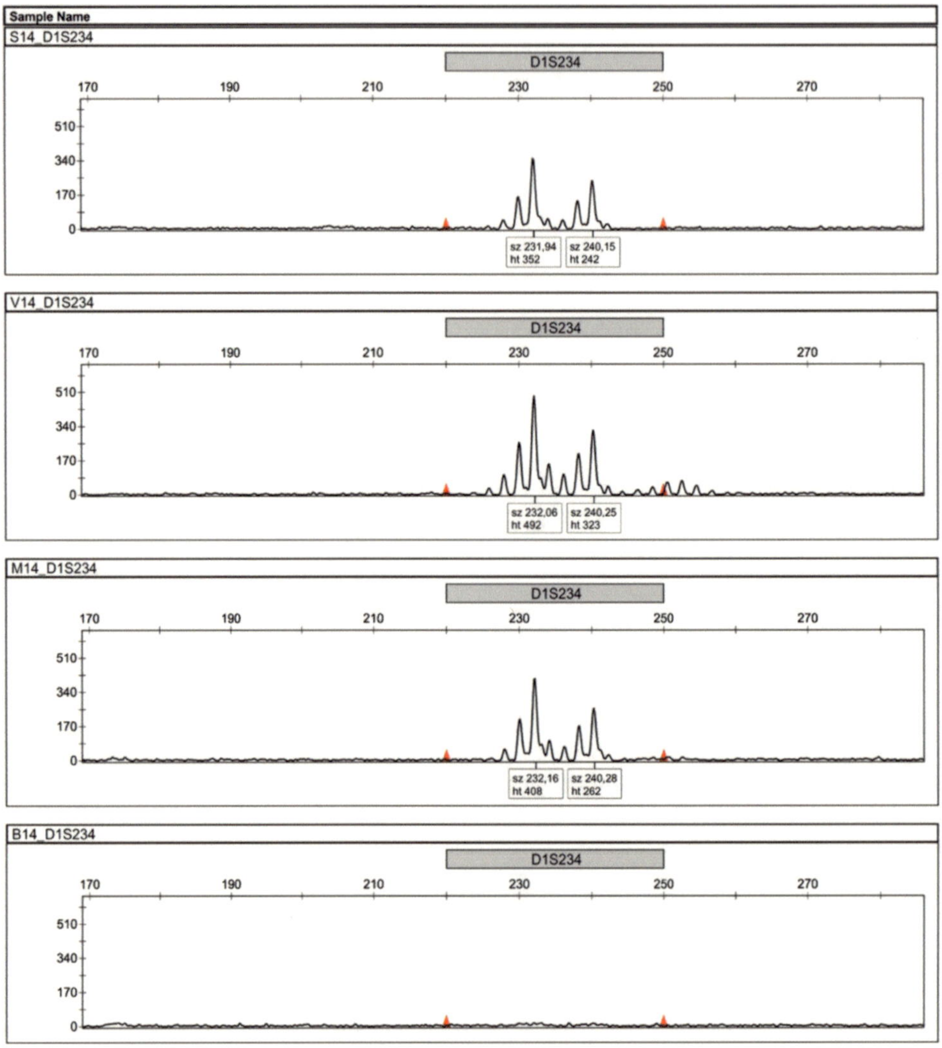

Figure 16. Microsatellite alteration for *PLA2G2A* genes in patient 14. D1S234 - S14 – Blood (considered as normal); D1S234 – Vf14 – with MSI; D1S234 – Mj14 –MSI with low amplitude signal; D1S234 – B14 – the signal could not be detected and was considered not measurable.

On chromosome 5 LOH/ MSI was observed in 38.66% (29/ 75) of patients (Figure 17) and 51.72% (15/ 29) of these have had allelic imbalance at the D5S421 locus which overlap the *APC* locus. MSI was observed only in 6.66% (5/ 75) of patients (Figure 17), similar with the results obtained for *PLA2G2A*. Allelic imbalance/ loss of heterozygosity appear to be a more frequent alteration than microsatellite instability in adenocarcinomas.

Microsatellites loci alterations corresponding to *BRCA1* gene have been found in 29.33% (22/ 75) of patients where D17S855 was the most affected (11 AI). Allelic imbalance analyses at the microsatellite loci D17S1323, D17S1322, and D17S855, which localize to introns 12, 19, and 20, respectively, indicates that 86.36% (19/ 22) of patients have LOH/ MSI in these regions (Figure 18). Another observation is that for microsatellite marker D17S1327, all individuals have a homozygote profile.

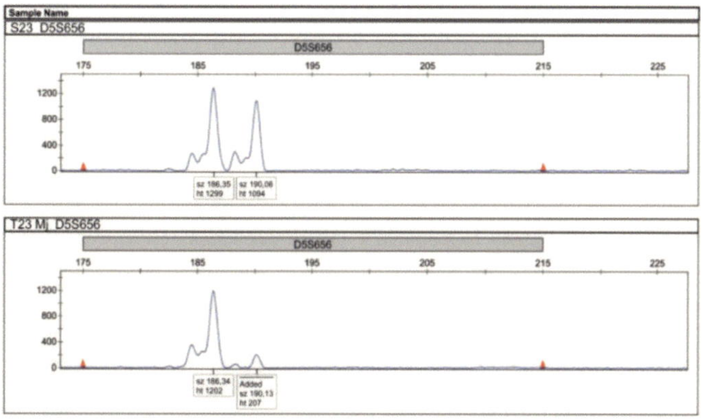

Figure 17. Microsatellite alteration for *APC* genes in patient 23. D5S656 - S23 – Blood (considered as normal); the report between D5S656 – T23_Mj is (1202:207)/ (1299:1094) = 5 which is interpreted as LOH.

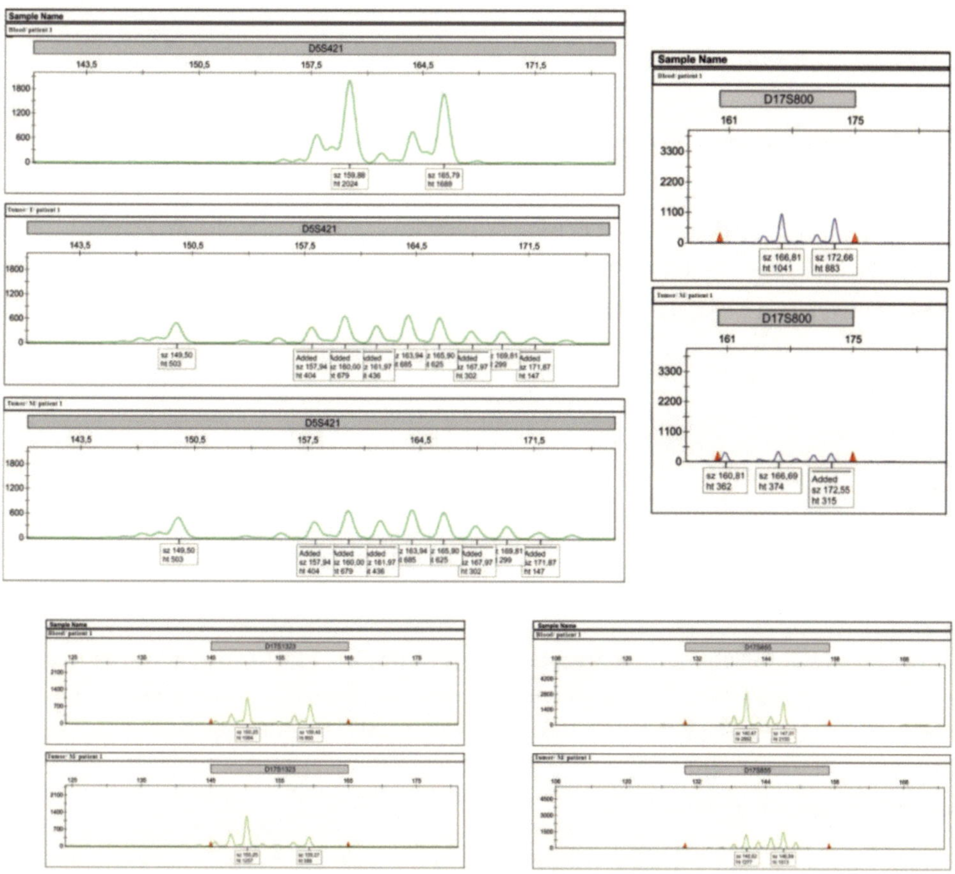

Figure 18. Microsatellite alteration for *APC* and *BRCA1* genes at patient 1.

By examining the allelic imbalance analyses for the three genes included in this study and for all the patients, we can conclude that instability variation was: a) 29.63% on the short arm of chromosome 1; b) 55.56% on the long arm of chromosome 5; c) 37.10% on the long arm of chromosome 17 (Figure 19, Table 2). Because MSI was observed only in 13 patients (14.81%) we suppose that this type of instability is no specific for sporadic colorectal cancer and appears to be a relatively specific pointer for HNPCC. As MSI is very rare in sporadic adenomas, routine screening of such lesions for MSI is not a high priority (Xue-Rong C, 2006). However, MSI analysis in adenomas is likely to be useful in the cases where clinical features or family history suggest hereditary predisposition (Jesus V, 2011). Consequently, these results can be associated with sporadic colon cancer and not with hereditary cancer, like in HNPCC.

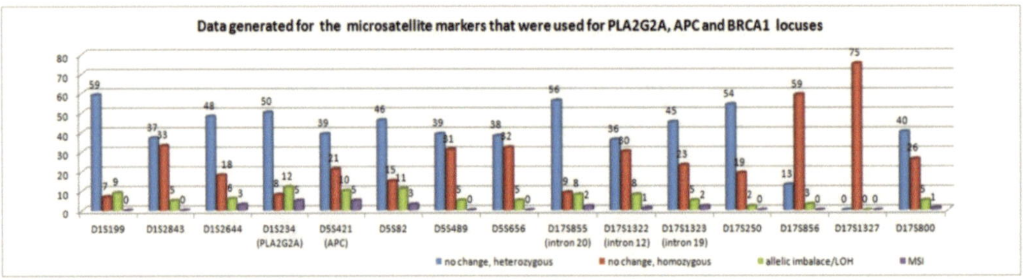

Figure 19. Comparative analyses of the fifteen microsatellites markers

By comparative analysis of all 15 microsatellite markers, we found that: a) 7/ 93 patients have instability on all three genes (7.52%); b) 20/ 93 patients on both *PLA2G2A* and *APC* genes (21.50%); c) 23/ 93 patients on both APC and *BRCA1* genes (24.73%); d) 7/ 93 patients on both *PLA2G2A* and *BRCA1* genes (7.52%) (Table 3).

	PLA2G2A microsatellite markers				APC microsatellite markers				BRCA1 microsatellite markers						
	D1S199	D1S2843	D1S2644	D1S234 (PLA2G2A)	D5S421 (APC)	D5S82	D5S489	D5S656	D17S855 (intron 20)	D17S1322 (intron 12)	D17S1323 (intron 19)	D17S250	D17S856	D17S1327	D17S800
no change, heterozygous	59	37	48	50	39	46	39	38	56	36	45	54	13	0	40
no change, homozygous	7	33	18	8	21	15	31	32	9	30	23	19	59	75	26
allelic imbalace/LOH	9	5	6	12	10	11	5	5	8	8	5	2	3	0	5
MSI	0	0	3	5	5	3	0	0	2	1	2	0	0	0	1
total samples	75	75	75	75	75	75	75	75	75	75	75	75	75	75	72
% Informativity	**90.67**	**56.00**	**76.00**	**89.33**	**72.00**	**80.00**	**58.67**	**57.33**	**88.00**	**60.00**	**69.33**	**74.67**	**21.33**	**0.00**	**63.89**

Table 2. The instability variation at the fifteen microsatellite loci

The frequencies of instability observed at *PLA2G2A* (89.33%) locus makes us not to exclude the possibility that *PLA2G2A* gene plays a key role in colorectal tumorigenesis. Similar to other studies we observed that the region where *PLA2G2A* gene is located is frequently modified in colorectal cancer, and encourages us not to exclude the possibility that it may represent a tumour suppressor gene.

On chromosome 5q, in the region where *APC* gene is located, the informative percent was 72.00%. Despite the construction of D5S421 microsatellite marker, in our analyses we

Pacient code	sPLA2 tip IIA expresion: sPLA2 tip IIA expresion by IHF – SM	sPLA2 tip IIA expresion by IHF – EC	AI on chromosome 1p, around PLA2G2A gene – D1S199	D1S2843	D1S2644	D1S234 PLA2G2A	APC expression: APC expression by IHF – SM	APC expression by IHF – EC	AI on chromosome 5q, around APC gene – APC D5S421	D5S82	D5S409	D5S656	MLPA analize for APC	BRCA1 expression: BRCA1 expression by IHF – nucleus/ citoplasm	AI on chromosome 17q, around BRCA1 gene – D17S855 intron 20 BRCA1	D17S1322 intron 12 BRCA1	D17S1323 intron 15 BRCA1	D17S250	D17S806	D17S1327	D17S800	MLPA analize for BRCA1
1	-	-	++	++	++	++	+	-	MSI	++	+	++	unmodified	++	++	++	++	+	+	+	++	unmodified
2	-	-	++/LOH	++/LOH	MSI	MSI	+	+/Cl	MSI	++	+	++	unmodified	-	++/LOH	++	++/LOH	+	+	+	MSI	deletion E13B
3	-	-	++	++/LOH	MSI	MSI	++	++	++	++	+	++	unmodified	++	++	++	++	+	+	+	++	unmodified
4	++/+	++/+	++	++	++	++	+	+	+	++	++	+	unmodified	+++	+	++	+	+	+	+	+	unmodified
5	++	++	++	++	++	++	+	+	+	++/LOH	++	+	unmodified	+	+	++	+	+	+	+	+	unmodified
6	++	++	++	++	++	++	+	+	+	++/LOH	++	+	unmodified	+	+	++	+	+	+	+	+	unmodified
7	-	+++	++/LOH	+	++	++	+	-	MSI	++	+	++/LOH	unmodified	+	++	+	++	++	+	+	++	unmodified
8	+	+	++	+	++	++/LOH	+	+/Cl	MSI	++	+	++	unmodified	+++	MSI	+	MSI	++	+	+	++	unmodified
9	+	+	++	+	++	++	++	++	nd	++	+	++	unmodified	++	++	+	++	++	+	+	++	unmodified
10	+	+	+	+	++/MSI ?	++	+++	+/Cl	++/MSI ?	++	+	++	unmodified	++	++	++	++	++	+	+	++	unmodified
11	++	++	++	++	++	++	++	++	++	++	+	++	unmodified	++	++	+	++	++	+	+	++	unmodified
12	++	++	++	++	++	++	++	++	++	+	++	++	unmodified	++	++	++	++	++	+	+	++	unmodified
13	++	++	++	++	++	++	++	++	++	+	++	++	unmodified	+++	++	++	++	++	+	+	++	unmodified
14	++	++	++	++	++	++	++	++	++	+	++	++	unmodified	++	++	++	++	++	+	+	++	unmodified
15	++	++	++	++	+	++	-	-	++	++	++	++	partial deletion of P2 and Mut 1309	++	++	+	+	++	+	+	++	unmodified
16	++	++	++	++	+	++	++	++	++	++	++	++	unmodified	++	++	+	+	++	+	+	++	unmodified
17	++	++	++	+	++	++	nd	++	++	++	++	++	unmodified	++	++	+	++	++	+	+	+	unmodified
18	-	+++/C	++	+	++	++	+	+/Cl	++/LOH	++/LOH	++	+	unmodified	-	++	++	++	++	+	+	++	deletion E13B
19	+	nd	++	+	++	++	+	+/Cl	++/LOH	++	++	+	unmodified	-	++	++	++	++	+	+	++	unmodified
20	++	nd	++	+	++	++	++	+	++	++	++	+	unmodified	+	++	++	++	++	+	+	++	unmodified
21	-	+++	+	+	++	++/LOH ?	++/+	++	+	++	++	++	unmodified	++	++	++	++	+	+	+	+	unmodified
22	+	+	+	+	++	++/LOH ?	++	++	+	++	++	++	unmodified	++	++	++	++	+	+	+	+	unmodified
23	nd	nd	+	+	++	++/LOH ?	nd	nd	+	++	++	++	unmodified	++	++	++	++	+	+	+	+	unmodified
24	++	++	++	+	++	++	++	++	+	++	+	+	unmodified	++	++	++	++	++	++	+	++	unmodified
25	-	+++	++	+	+	++/MSI	++/+	++	++	++	+	+	unmodified	++	++	+	+	++	+	+	+	deletion E12
26	+	+	++	+/LOH ?	+	++/MSI	++	++	++	++	+	+	unmodified	++	++	+	+	++	+	+	+	unmodified
27	++	++	++	+	+	++	++	++	++	++/LOH	+	+	unmodified	++	++	+	+	++	+	+	+	unmodified
28	-	+	++	+	++	+	+++	-	++/LOH	++	+	++/LOH	unmodified	-	++/LOH	+	+	+	++/LOH	+	++/LOH	unmodified
29	++	++	++	++	++	++	++	++	++	++	+	++	unmodified	-	++/LOH	++	++	+	+	+	+	unmodified
30	++	++	++	++	++	++	++	++	+	++	+	+	unmodified	++	++	++	++	+	++	+	+	unmodified
31	++/+	++	++	++	++	++	+	-	++	++	++/LOH	++	deletion between E10 - E15	++	++	+	++	++	++	+	++	unmodified
32	++	++	++	++	++	++	+	++	++	++	++	++	unmodified	++	++	+	++	++	++	+	++	unmodified
33	++	++	++	+	++	+	++	++	++	++	++	+	deletion on E10,E11, E14, E15 and Mut at 1061, 1069	++	+	+	+	++	+	+	+	unmodified
34	++/+	nd	++	+	+	++	+	+	+	++/MSI ?	++	+	unmodified	++	++	+	+	++	+	+	++	unmodified
35	nd	nd	++	+	++	++	nd	nd	+	++	++	++	unmodified	++	++	++	++	+	++	+	++	unmodified
36	+	+	++	+	++	++	++	++	+	++	++	++	unmodified	-	++/LOH	++	++	+	++	+	++	unmodified
37	+	+	++	+	++	++	++	++	+	++	++	++	unmodified	++	++	++/LOH	++	+/LOH ?	++	+	++	unmodified
38	++/+	++	+	++	+	++	+	-	++	+	+	++	unmodified	+++	++	+	+	++	+	+	++	unmodified
39	++/+	++	+	++	+	++	+	+/Cl	++/LOH	MSI	+	++/LOH	deletion between E12 - E19 and mutation at 1061 and 1309	-	++/LOH	+	+	++	+	+	++/LOH	deletion E18, E19
40	++	++	+	++	+	++	+	+	++	+	+	++	unmodified	++	++	+	+	nd	+	+	++	unmodified
41	-	-	++/LOH	+	++/LOH	++/LOH	++/+	++/+	+	+	++	+	unmodified	+++	+	+	+	++	+	+	++	unmodified
42	-	-	++/LOH	+	++/LOH	++/LOH	++/+	++	+	+	++	+	unmodified	++	+	+	+	++	+	+	++	unmodified
43	-	-	++/LOH	+	++/LOH	++/LOH	++	++	+	+	++/LOH	+	unmodified	++	+	+	+	++	+	+	++	unmodified
44	++/+	++	++	+	++	++	+	+	+	++/MSI	++/LOH	+	unmodified	++	++	+	+	++	+	+	++	unmodified
45	nd	nd	++	+	++	++	++	++	++	++	++	+	unmodified	++	++	++/LOH	++	++	++	+	+	unmodified
46	++	++	++	+	++	++	++	++	++	++	++	+	unmodified	-	++	++/LOH	++	+	++	+	+	unmodified
47	++	++	++	+	++	++	nd	nd	++	++	++	+	unmodified	++	++	++/LOH	++	++	++	+	+	unmodified
48	++	++	++	+	++	++	++	++	++/LOH	++/LOH	+	+	unmodified	-	++/LOH	++/LOH	++	++	+	+	++/LOH	deletion between E10-E14
49	++	++	++	+	++	++	++/+	++/+	++	++/LOH	+	+	unmodified	+++	++	++/LOH	++	++	+	+	++/LOH	unmodified
50	++	++	++	+	++	++	++	++	++	++/LOH	+	+	unmodified	-	++	++/LOH	++	++	+	+	++	unmodified
51	-	+	++	++	++	++	++	++	++	++	++	++	unmodified	++	++/LOH	++	++	++	+	+	++	unmodified
52	+	+	++/LOH	++	++	++	++	+	++	++	++/LOH	++	partial deletion of P2 and Mut 1309	++	++	++	++	++	+	+	++	unmodified
53	++	++	++	++	++	++	++	+	++	++	++	++	unmodified	+	++	++	++	++	+	+	++	unmodified
54	+	+++	++	++	+	+	+	-	++	++/LOH	+	++/LOH	unmodified	++	++	++	++	++	++	+	++	unmodified
55	+	+++	++	++	+	+	+	+/Cl	++/LOH	++/LOH	+	++/LOH	partial deletion of P2 and Mut 1309	+++	++	++	++	++	++	+	++	unmodified
56	++	++	++	++	+	+	++	++	++	++	+	++	unmodified	++	++	++	++	++/LOH	++	+	++	unmodified
57	++/+	++	++	++	++	++	++/+	++	++	+	++	+	unmodified	++	++	+	+	++	++	+	+	unmodified
58	nd	nd	++	++	++/LOH	++	nd	nd	++	+	++	+	unmodified	++	++	+	+	++	++	+	+	unmodified
59	++	++	++	++	++	++	++	++	++	+	++	+	unmodified	++	++	+	+	++	++	+	+	unmodified
60	-	-	++/LOH	++	++	++/LOH	-	-	++/LOH	nd	+	++	unmodified	-	++	+	+	nd	++	+	+	unmodified
61	-	-	++	++	++	++/LOH	-	-	+	nd	+	+	unmodified	++	MSI	MSI	++/LOH	nd	++	+	++	unmodified
62	+	-	++	++	++	+	+	+	++/LOH	+	+	+	deletion E15	+	++	+	++	+	+	+	+	unmodified
63	++	++	++	++	++	++	++	++	++	++	+	+	unmodified	++	++	++	++	++	++	+	+	deletion E1A, E3-E7
64	+	+	++	+	+	+	++	++	+	++	+	+	unmodified	+++	++	++	++	+	++	+	++	unmodified
65	-	-	++/LOH	++/LOH	++	+	++	++	++	++	++	++	unmodified	++	++	+	++	++	+	+	+	deletion E13B
66	++	++	++	++	++	++	++	++	++	++	+	+	unmodified	nd	+	++/LOH	++/LOH	nd	++	+	nd	unmodified
67	++	++	++	+	+	++/LOH	-	-	++/LOH	+	++	++	unmodified	-	++	+	+	+	++	+	+	unmodified
68	+	+	++	++	+	+	++	++	+	++	++	++	unmodified	++	++	+	+	++	++/LOH	+	++	unmodified
69	++	++	++	++	++	++	nd	nd	++	+	++	++	unmodified	+++	++	+	++/LOH	++	+	+	++	deletion E13B, E19
70	++	++	++	++	++	++	++	++	++	++	++	++	unmodified	+/+++	+	++	++/LOH	++	+	+	+	deletion E13B
71	+	-	++	++	+	++/MSI	++	-	+	++/LOH	++	++	partial deletion E11, E14, E16	-	++	++	++	++	++	+	++	unmodified
72	-	-	++/LOH	++/LOH	++/LOH	++/LOH	-	-	+	++/LOH	++/LOH	++	deletion E15	++	++	+	+	++	+	+	++	unmodified
73	-	-	++	++	++/LOH	++/LOH	+	+/-	++/LOH	+	++	++	unmodified	+++	++	+	+	++	+	+	++/LOH	unmodified
74	++	++	++	++	++	++	++	++	++	++	++	++	unmodified	-	++	++	+	++	++/LOH	+	+	unmodified
75	++	++	++	++	++	++	+	-	++	++	+	+	unmodified	++	++/LOH	++	MSI	+	+	+	nd	unmodified

Table 3. Comparative analyses of protein and genetic expression of PLA2 type IIA, APC and BRCA1

observed that the informative percent of the larger D5S82 (5q15 – 5q21) marker is at higher level (80.00%), and makes us to suppose that, probably, other genes around *APC* can be also mutated in colorectal cancer. According to our expectation, the other two markers located under D5S82 marker, have also a good informative percent: 58.67% for D5S489 (5q21) and 57.33% for D5S656 (5q21.3). On the other hand, the higher percentage of modifications encountered at the level of the microsatellites in the *PLA2G2A* gene region, demonstrates that the alterations at its level are much more frequent than those of the *APC* gene.

By comparing *APC* and *PLA2G2A* genes with the allelic imbalance observed at the *BRCA1* locus, the informative percent was 69.33%. Among all 7 microsatellites designed for the *BRCA1* gene, only one marker – D17S1327 is non-informative because it constantly appears as homozygote meaning that it has no variable number repeat. The most altered microsatellite marker was D17S855 (17q21), designed for intron 20 of *BRCA1* gene, for which the informative percent was 88.00%. For the other two markers designed into the *BRCA1* gene, namely D17S1322 for intron 12 and D17S1323 for intron 19, the informative percent was 56.00% and 64.00% respectively.

3. Conclusions

In order to improve the "personalized" therapeutic strategy in CRC, by our study we have comparatively evaluated the protein and gene expression for several key point biomarkers (APC, PLA2G2A, CDH1, BRCA1, and EGFR). Our *in vivo* experiment involved diagnosis testing of CRC patients and molecular biology testing on biological samples in order to clarify the cross-talk of interested genes and to better understand the CRC typology among Romanian patients.

We observed a close relationship in between different proteins and genes, which depends on the tumor type, cell grade and staging. For LOH/ MSI evaluation, our investigations were undertaken at the chromosomal regions where *APC*, *PLA2G2A* and *BRCA1* genes are located. We used microsatellite markers, in a series of sporadic CRCs with unknown status with respect to mutations in germline *PLA2G2A*, *APC* and *BRCA1*. Mutational status of 1p35-36.1, 5q and 17q21 chromosomal regions was evaluated and correlated with immunohistochemical and MLPA expression.

Regarding the *APC* MLPA analyses, our results are in accordance with those obtained by Sieber and Lamlum (2000), according to which, occasionally, in certain tumors in patients with germline mutations at the level of codon 1309, either the MCR (mutational cluster region) locus or the 3′ and 5′ region of *APC* gene, do not associate with the allelic loss at the level of adenomas. This same fact is observed in the case of patient 19 whose deletion, detected through MLPA at the E12 - E15 level, a region also including the MCR situ, is not supported by an allelic loss in any of the other microsatellite markers assayed. Although in this case no germline mutations were identified, we could extrapolate the same argument as Lamlum, starting from the premise that *APC* is often cited as the first tumor suppressor gene affected both by familial and sporadic tumours. Regarding the PLA_2 type IIA expression our results suggest that the malignant cells lose their ability to express PLA_2 type IIA when invasive carcinoma develops in the adenoma. Our results are in line with the findings of Avoranta et al., who reported elevated gene and protein expression of PLA_2 type IIA in colorectal adenomas from FAP patients. The lack of PLA_2 type IIA expression is very common among colorectal cancer patients and, accordingly to the other studies, it seems that during tumor progression, malignant cells lose their ability to express PLA_2 type IIA. These patients have a better prognosis than the patients with positive tumours (Buhmeida A., 2009) in contrast to normal mucosa. Most of the cell types that over-express PLA_2 type IIA are apoptotic and necrotic, and this expression can be associated with the role of PLA_2 type IIA in promoting death of cancer cells. Regarding BRCA1 expression, previous studies indicate a higher rates of CRC in families linked to the *BRCA1* gene than in other families (Porter D.E., 1994) and mutations on this gene in stomach and colon cancers are associated with the microsatellite mutator phenotype. After several studies in which controversial importance of BRCA1 expression and mutator phenotype is still in debate, in 13.33% (10/ 75) of patients we observed a correlation between IHF and AI analyses. Considering that 3/7 microsatellites are intragenic to *BRCA1*, hypermethylation of *BRCA1* can be an event that has been described in breast and ovarian tumours. Because LOH was not observed in the microsatellites surrounding the *BRCA1* locus, the loss of the large part of chromosome 17q is not necessary to be considered. Somatic mutation can be taken in account because by MLPA analyses in 13.33% (10/ 75) of patients we observed deletion at different exons, especially on exon 13B. Our results suggest that BRCA1 can be an independent prognostic factor in patients with CRC, and it may be used to identify patient subgroups at high risk that might benefit from adjuvant chemotherapy. In conclusion, the comparative analyses between immunohistochemical expression and mutational status of *APC*, *PLA2G2A* and *BRCA1* genes suggest that at the *APC* level, 10% (7/ 75) samples have loss of heterozygosity without any presence of a deletion on MLPA. A complete loss is correlated with reduction of APC protein expression. The mutational status of the studied genes correlated with the protein and MLPA expression provides us useful data about the most common type of modification that can appear in individuals with colorectal cancer and how they can be group in order to receive a proper therapy.

Without making microsatellite instability analyze, at the *CDH1* gene locus, loss of heterozygosity that was found by MLPA analysis was not necessary overlapped with results of E-cadherin protein expression studied by IHF in the tumors samples. We can suppose that abnormal E-cadherin protein expression could be a result of some type of mutation at *CDH1* level or to others genes that are involved by association in its regulatory functions (some members of ECCU complex such α-cadherin or β-catenin), probably, as a consequence of tumor progression status. At the locus of *EGFR* gene, the mutational profile indicates only the presence of insertions, which can be interpreted as frame-shift mutations. The insertions founded at the exons E18, E19 and E21 are in relation with the catalytic domain of the *EGFR* gene. Future analyzes have to be done in order to reveal some specific somatic mutations that are generally associated with the target therapy in CRCs.

Author details

Mihaela Tica
University of Medicine and Pharmacie "Carol Davila", Bucharest, Romania

Valeria Tica, Mihaela Uta, Ovidiu Vlaicu and Elena Ionica
University of Bucharest, Department of Biochemistry and Molecular Biology, Bucharest, Romania

Alexandru Naumescu
Emergency University Hospital, Bucharest, Romania

Acknowledgement

This work has been supported by the Government of Romania, through National Plan of Research II, grant no. 137/ and 42-158/ 2008. We are grateful to all our partners from Bucharest Emergency Clinical Hospital Bucharest, Romania and Department of Biochemistry and Molecular Biology from the University of Bucharest, for their excellent technical support.

4. References

Aleksandra S, Rafal S., Lubomir B., Wojciech O., Marzena C., Wojciech K., Cezary S., Tadeusz P., Maciej W. & Monika LP. (2011). Prognostic Significance of Wnt-1, β-catenin and E-cadherin Expression in Advanced Colorectal Carcinoma, *Pathol. Oncol. Res.*, Vol. 17, Issue 4, pp. 955–963, ISSN 1219-4956

Arteaga CL. (2001). The epidermal growth factor receptor: from mutant oncogene in nonhuman cancers to therapeutic target in human neoplasia. *J Clin Oncol.*, Vol. 19 (18 suppl), Issue 18, pp. 32S– 40S, ISSN 0732-183X

Avoranta T., Sundström J., Korkeila E., Syrjänen K., Pyrhönen S. and Laine J. (2010). The expression and distribution of group IIA phospholipase A2 in human colorectal tumours, *Virchows Arch.*, Vol. 457, Issue 6, pp. 659–667, ISSN 0945-6317

Bos JL. (1989). Ras oncogene in human cancer: a review. *Cancer Res.,* Vol. 49, Issue 17, pp. 4682– 4689, ISSN 0008-5472

Bryant D.M., Stow J.L. (2004). The ins and outs of E-cadherin trafficking. *Trends Cell Biol.* Vol. 14, Issue 8, pp. 427–434, ISSN 0962-8924

Buhmeida A, Bendardaf R, Hilska M, Laine J, Collan Y, Laato M, Syrjänen K. and Pyrhönen S. (2009). PLA2 (group IIA phospholipase A2) as a prognostic determinant in stage II colorectal carcinoma. *Ann Oncol.*, Vol. 20, Issue 7, pp. 1230–1235, ISSN 0923-7534

Friedenson Bernard, (2004). BRCA1 and BRCA2 Founder Mutations and the Risk of Colorectal Cancer. *Journal of the National Cancer Institute,* Vol. 96, Issue 15, pp. 1185 – 1186, ISSN 0027-8874

Goodwin M, Yap A.S. (2004) Classical cadherin adhesion molecules: coordinating cell adhesion, signaling and the cytoskeleton. *J Mol Histol.* Vol. 35, Issue 8, pp. 839–844, ISSN 1567-2379

Haapamaki M.M., Gronroos, J M; Nurmi, H; Alanen, K; Kallajoki, M; Nevalainen, T J. (1997). Gene expression of group II phospholipase A2 in intestine in ulcerative colitis. *Gut,* Vol. 40, Issue 1, pp. 95 – 101, ISSN 0017-5749

Hardy R.G., Meltzer S.J. and Jankowski J.A. (2000). ABC of colorectal cancer: Molecular basis for risk factors. *BMJ*, Vol. 321, Issue 7265, pp. 886-889, ISSN 0959-8146

Ishiguro Y., Ochiai M. and Sugimura T (1999). Strain differences of rats in the susceptibility to aberrant crypt foci formation by 2-amino-1-methyl-6phenylimidazo-[4,5-b]pyridine: no implication of Apc and Pla2g2a genetic polymorphisms in differential susceptibility. *Carcinogenesis,* Vol. 20, pp. 1063–1068.

Jhawer M, Goel S, Wilson AJ, Montagna C, Ling YH, Byun DS, Nasser S, Arango D, Shin J, Klampfer L, Augenlicht L.H, Soler R.P, Mariadason J.M. (2008). PIK3CA mutation/PTEN expression status predicts response of colon cancer cells to the epidermal growth factor receptor inhibitor cetuximab. *Cancer Res.*, Vol. 68, Issue 6, pp. 1953-1961, ISSN 0008-5472

Knudson A.G., (2001).Two genetic hits (more or less) to cancer, *Nat Rev Cancer.*, Vol. 1, Issue 2, pp. 157 – 162

Sieber O.M., Tomlinson I.P. and Lamlum H. (2000). The adenomatous polyposis coli (APC) tumour suppressor – genetics, function and disease. *Molecular Medicine Today,* Vol. 6, Issue 12, pp. 462-469, ISSN: 1357-4310

Lee J.J. and Chu E. (2007). First-line use of anti-EGFR monoclonal antibodies in the treatment of metastatic colorectal cancer. *Clin Colorectal Cancer,* Vol. 6 (suppl 2), pp. S42–S46, ISSN: 1533-0028

Mendelsohn J.and Baselga J. (2003) Status of epidermal growth factor receptor antagonist in the biology and treatment of cancer. *J Clinical Oncology,* Vol. 21, pp. 2787-2799, ISSN 0732-183X

Mihalcea A., Tica V., Georgescu S.E., Tesio C., Dinischiotu A, Condac E., Costache M. and Ionica E. (2005). Allelic imbalance on chromosomes 1 and 5 in colorectal carcinoma. *Plovdiv University Press,* pp. 568-575.

Mihalcea (Chitu) A., Stefan (Berlin) I., Tica V., Costache M and Ionica E. (2009). The detection of mutations in the APC gene of Romanian patients with colorectal cancer through two independent techniques. *Rom. Biotechnol. Lett.*, Vol. 14, Issue. 5, pp. 4747-4755, ISSN 1224-5984

Mounier C.M., Wendum D., Greenspan E. Flejou J., Rosenberg D.W. and Lambeau, G. (2008). Distinct expression pattern of the full set of secreted phospholipases A2 in human colorectal adenocarcinomas: sPLA2-III as a biomarker candidate. *Br J Cancer.*, Vol. 98, Issue 3, pp. 587–595, ISSN 0007-0920

Muhammad W.S., and Edward C. (2010). Biology of Colorectal Cancer, *Cancer J.*, Vol. 16, Issue 3, pp. 196 –201, ISSN 1528-9117

Narayan S. and Roy D. (2003). Role of APC and DNA mismatch repair genes in the development of colorectal cancers. *Molecular cancer,* Vol. 2, Issue 1, pp. 1 – 15, ISSN 1476-4598

Nevalainen T.J., Gronroos J.M. and Kallajoki M. (1995). Expression of group II phospholipase A2 in the human gastrointestinal tract. *Lab Invest.*, Vol. 72, Issue 2, pp. 201–208, ISSN 0023-6837

Nevalainen T.J. and Haapanen T.J. (1993). Distribution of pancreatic (group I) and synovial type (group II) phospholipases A2 in human tissues. *Inflammation,* Vol. 17, Issue 4, pp. 453–464, ISSN 0360-3997

Ogawa M., Yamashita S., Sakamoto K. and Ikei S. (1991). Elevation of serum group II phospholipase A2 in patients with cancers of digestive organs. *Res Commun Chem. Pathol Pharmacol.*, Vol. 74, Issue 2, pp. 241–244, ISSN 0034-5164

Porter D.E., Cohen B.B., Wallace M.R., Smyth E., Chetty U., M. Dixon J., Steel C.M., Carter D.C. (1994). Breast cancer incidence, penetrance and survival in probable carriers of BRCA1 gene mutations in families linked to BRCA1 on chromosome 17q12–21. *Br J Surg*, Vol. 81, Issue 10, pp 1512–1515, Online ISSN: 1365-2168

Rizzo P., Osipo C., Foreman K., Golde T., Osborne B. and Miele, L., (2008). Rational targeting of Notch signaling in cancer. *Oncogene*, Vol. 27, Issue 38, pp. 5124-5131, ISSN 0950-9232

Roukos D., (2010). Novel clinico–genome network modeling for 27 revolutionizing genotype–phenotype-based personalized cancer care. *Expert Rev. Mol. Diagn.*, Vol. 10, Issue 1, pp. 33–48, ISSN 1473-7159

Samowitz W.S., Powers M.D., Spirio L.N., Nollet F., Frans van Roy, Slattery M.L. (1999). β-Catenin mutations are more frequent in small colorectal adenomas than in larger adenomas and invasive carcinomas. *Cancer Res.*, Vol. 59, pp. 1442 - 1444, ISSN 0008-5472

Senda T., Shimomura A., and Iizuka-Kogo A. (2005). Adenomatous polyposis coli (APC) tumor suppressor gene as a multifunctional gene. *Anat Sci Int.*, Vol. 80, Issue 3, pp. 121-131, ISSN 0022-7722

Spano J.P., Lagorce C., Atlan D., Milano G., Domont J., Benamouzig R., Attar A., Benichou J., Martin A., Morere J.F., Raphael M., Penault-Llorca F., Breau, J.L., Fagard R., Khayat D., and Wind P. (2005). Impact of EGFR expression on colorectal cancer patient prognosis and survival. *Annals of Oncology*, Vol. 16, Issue 1, pp. 102-108, ISSN 0923-7534

Spirio L.N., Kutchera W., Winstead M.V., Pearson B., Kaplan C., Robertson M., Lawrence E., Burt R.W., Tischfield J.A., Leppert M.F., Prescott S.M. and White R. (1996). Three secretory phospholipase A(2) genes that map to human chromosome 1P35-36 are not mutated in individuals with attenuated adenomatous polyposis coli. *Cancer Res.*, Vol. 56, Issue 5, pp. 955–958, ISSN 0008-5472

Stanczak A., Stec R., Bodnar L., Olszewski W., Cichowicz M., Kozlowski W., Szczylik C., Pietrucha T., Wieczorek M. and Lamparska-Przybysz M. (2011). Prognostic Significance of Wnt-1, β-catenin and E-cadherin Expression in advanced colorectal carcinoma. *Pathol Oncol Res.*, Vol.17, Issue 4, pp. 955-63, ISSN 1219-4956

Thorstensen L., Ovist H., Heim S., Jan-Liefers G., Nesland J.M., Giercksky K.E. and Löthe, R. (2000). Evaluation of 1p losses in primary carcinomas, local recurrences and peripheral metastases from colorectal cancer patients. *Neoplasia*, Vol. 2, Issue 6, pp. 514-522, ISSN 1522-8002

Valle J., Menendez M., Izquierdo A., Campos O., Velasco A., Feliubadalo L., Brunet J., Tornero E., Capella G., Darder E., Blanco I.and Lazaro C., (2011). Identification of a new complex rearrangement affecting exon 20 of BRCA1, *Breast Cancer Res Treat.*, Vol. 130, pp. 341–344, ISSN 0167-6806

Ng K. and Zhu A.X. (2006). Anti Targeting the epidermal growth factor receptor in metastatic colorectal cancer. *Critical Reviews in Oncology/Hematology*, Vol. 65, Issue 1, pp. 8-20, ISSN: 1040-8428

Xue-Rong C., Wei-Zhong Z., Xing-Qiu L. and Jin-Wei W., (2006). Genetic instability of BRCA1 gene at locus D17S855 is related to clinicopathological behaviors of gastric cancer from Chinese population, *World J Gastroenterol.*, Vol. 12, Issue 26, ISSN 1007-9327

Chapter 6

Genetic Causes of Syndromic and Non-Syndromic Congenital Heart Disease

Akl C. Fahed and Georges M. Nemer

Additional information is available at the end of the chapter

http://dx.doi.org/10.5772/48477

1. Introduction

Congenital heart disease (CHD) is the most common human congenital defect, and a leading cause of death in infants. With an incidence that varies between 0.8 to 2% in neonates, congenital heart disease contributes to a much larger fraction of stillbirths.(Goldmuntz 2001; Loffredo 2000) Additionally, undiagnosed mild malformations of the heart often appear later in adulthood or remain undiagnosed for life. If these are included, some expect a prevalence of CHD that is up to 4% among all newborns.(Loffredo 2000) An additional contributor to the rising prevalence of CHD among adults is the advance in diagnostics and medical and surgical treatments of children with CHD, which is allowing them, in the majority of cases, to get their heart defect, fixed and sustain a normal life into adulthood.(van der Bom and others 2011) Management of the increasing number of adult patients living with CHD is becoming more and more complicated due to the fact that many patients with mild cardiac lesions are missed during childhood and later appear with complications due to these defects such as heart failure, but even more due to the improvements in diagnosis and surgical care of pediatric patients which are allowing them to survive to adulthood and have their own children.

The majority of CHD is thought to result from gene mutations. This was suggested by early observations of Mendelian inheritance of CHD in families. Another evidence came from congenital syndromes due to micro and macro deletions of chromosomal regions that would result in CHD together with several other manifestations. Over the past few decades, and with the advent of gene sequencing and other techniques it became possible to identify the genetic causes of CHD.(Goldmuntz 2001) In syndromic cases, although it was possible to identify the chromosomal deletions causing the disease, in many cases the gene responsible for the heart phenotype remains undefined. Other syndromes were found to be due to single gene defects; however, for the majority, the downstream pathophysiology linking the gene defect to the development of disease remains obscure. In parallel, extensive *in-vitro* and *in-vivo* studies widened our understanding of the molecular basis of heart development. It is thought that perturbations during embryonic heart development are at the origin of CHD. These studies resulted in large sets of candidate genes and molecular pathways involved in heart development. It is hypothesized that mutations in these genes cause CHD. This was confirmed by sequencing of genes encoding cardiac-enriched transcription factors such as *GATA4, NKX2-5,* and *TBX5* in non-syndromic cases of CHD, and finding mutations that segregate with the disease. This prompted excitement in the field; however, screening of large cohorts of isolated CHD cases brought some disappointment as these genes explained only a minority of the cases.

The understanding of how defects in these genes cause CHD turned out to be more complicated that initially expected. It became evident that not all CHD manifests true Mendelian inheritance. It is possible that combinations of mutations in different genes result in a particular phenotype, or combination of a gene mutation with a particular environmental exposure results in a CHD phenotype. Mutations might have low penetrance and only serve to increase the risk of CHD. Other mutations might yield totally defective proteins, yet be compensated for by other proteins in interlinked pathways. Copy Number Variations (CNVs), altered transcription, somatic mutations, and microRNA (miRNA) are also additional mechanisms through which the molecular basis of CHD can be explained. Current research explores all of these mechanisms with a wide array of technologies that are better than ever, and hence the future decade promises a near complete understanding of heart development and the genetic basis of Congenital Heart Disease.

This chapter covers the genetics of syndromic and non-syndromic congenital heart disease. It discusses all genes that have been associated with congenital heart disease in humans with depiction of the spectrum of mutations and the genotype-phenotype correlations for each. The chapter also covers the roles of CNVs, epigenetics, somatic mutations, and miRNA in CHD. Current technologies and strategies used to understand the genetics of congenital heart disease are also discussed. The chapter ends with an explanation of how these technologies can unravel the genetics of CHD and allow the application of research findings for the benefit of patients.

2. Classifications, anatomy, and clinical significance

Congenital heart disease encompasses a broad category of anatomic malformations, which can range from a small septal defect or leaky valve to a severe malformation requiring extensive surgical repair or leading to death such as a single ventricle. Several classification systems exist for describing congenital heart disease. The most common classification used to describe CHD is purely clinical whereby CHD is cyanotic if the malformation results in deoxygenated blood bypassing the lung and causes cyanosis (blue patient), or non-cyanotic if the malformation does not result in cyanosis. The most common cyanotic heart defects are Tetralogy of Fallot (TOF), Hypoplastic Left Heart Syndrome (HLHS), Transposition of the Great Arteries (TGA), Truncus Arteriosus (TA), and Total Anomalous Pulmonary Venous

Connection (TAPVC). Congenital heart defects can also be simple or complex. A complex malformation includes several simple malformations occurring together. The most typical example is Tetralogy of Fallot, which -as its name implies- includes four malformations: Pulmonary Stenosis (PS), an overriding aorta, Ventricular Septal Defect (VSD), and right ventricular hypertrophy. Because of the wide diversity in the anatomy of the cardiac malformations, several detailed morphological classifications were also developed. The most widely recognized one is the International Pediatric and Congenital Cardiac Code (IPCCC), which was developed by the International Society for Nomenclature of Paediatric and Congenital Heart Disease (ISNPCHD). Table 1 shows the categories of CHD classifications of the IPCCC with the most common diagnoses within each category. The detailed version could be downloaded from the IPCCC website (www.ipccc.net). Other classification systems are radiologic based on echocardiography or magnetic resonance imaging, hemodynamic based on shunts and circulations in the heart, or embryological based on the presumed origin during heart development. CHD can occur as part of a syndrome and as such is labeled as syndromic or nonsyndromic, both of which are discussed in this chapter. In syndromic and non-syndromic cases, CHD can be isolated, that is occurring in a single patient, or familial afflicting many members within the same family. The recurrence rate of CHD after an isolated case is 2.7%. (Gill and others 2003)

This anatomical heterogeneity of CHD has been one major reason why we know little about its genetics. Beyond the anatomical classification described in the IPCCC, different combinations of malformations and variations to described malformations can occur. Pediatric cardiologists often end up using different terminologies to describe similar defects because of their complexity. Extremely rare complex malformations are also sometimes described and run in families while their cause remains unknown.(Herrera and others 2008; Jaeggi and others 2008) Genotype-phenotype correlations are hard to establish due to this heterogeneity. In the majority of familial cases of CHD, there are different types of structural malformations within the same family. The same single gene mutation has been shown to cause a variety of cardiac defects, even within the same family.(Goldmuntz 2001) Whenever mouse knockout models were developed to recapitulate a human CHD phenotype, the mouse phenotype was not always similar to that seen in humans.(Bruneau 2008) All these issues raised the hypothesis of a multifactorial and perhaps polygenetic origin of CHD. The genetic background of the individual, in-utero environment, epigenetic changes, and embryological hemodynamics and physiology are all possible causes of this phenotypic heterogeneity.

Being a leading cause of deaths in the first year of life, CHD has prompted a large wave of development in surgical and interventional procedures to treat CHD. As such, CHD is mostly corrected with surgical and interventional procedures when the malformation causes symptoms or can cause heart failure such as a large septal defect or a cyanotic heart disease. Small malformations such as tiny septal defects that are expected to correct on their own or to not cause any complication are simply observed. With the recent advances in treatment, the mortality from CHD has decreased tremendously and most CHD patients survive a normal life throughout adulthood.(van der Bom and others 2011) This prompted a whole new subspecialty in adult cardiology to take care of adult patients with CHD.(Moodie 1994) As these adults with CHD are planning to have children of their own, the recurrence risk became a problem, and this was yet another force to identify the genetic causes behind the disease, given that genetic counseling and pre-implantation genetic diagnosis (PGD) can be useful tools for these parents.

Classification Category	Most Common Diagnoses
Abnormalities of position and connection of the heart	Dextrocardia Atrial Situs Inversus Double Inlet Left Ventricle (DILV); Double Inlet Right Ventricle (DIRV) Transposition of the Great Arteries (TGA) Double Outlet Left Ventricle (DORV); Double Outlet Right Ventricle (DORV) Common Arterial Trunk (CAT), aka Truncus Arteriosus (TA)
Tetralogy of Fallot and variants	Tetralogy of Fallot (TOF) Pulmonary Atresia (PA) and Venticular Septal Defect (VSD)
Abnormalities of great veins	Supervior Vena Cava (SVC) Abnormality Inferior Vena Cava (SVC) Abnormality Coronary Sinus Abnormality Total Anomalous Pulmonary Venous Connection (TAPVC) Partially Anomalous Pulmonary Venous Connection (PAPVC)
Abnormalities of atriums and atrial septum	Atrial Septal Defect (ASD) Patent Foramen Ovale (PFO)
Abnormalities of AV valves and AV septal defect	Tricuspid Regurgitation (TR) Tricuspid Stenosis (TS) Ebstein's Anomaly Mitral Regurgitation (MR) Mitral Stenosis (MS) Mitral Valve Proplapse (MVP) Atrioventricular Septal Defect (AVSD)
Abnormalities of ventricles and ventricular septum	Single Ventricle Ventricular imbalance: dominant LV +hypoplastic RV, or dominant RV+hypoplastic RV Aneurysm (RV, LV, or septal) Hypoplastic Left Heart Syndrome (HLHS) Double Chambered Right Ventricle (DCRV) Ventricular Septal Defect (VSD)
Abnormalities of VA valves and great arteries	Aortopulmonary Window (AP Window) Pulmonary Stenosis (PS), valvar or subalvar Pulmonary Artery Stenosis (PAS) Aortic Stenosis (AS), valvar or suvalvar Aortic Insufficiency (AI) Bicuspid Aortic Valve (BAV) Supravalvar Aortic Stenosis (SVS) Coarctation of the Aorta (COA) Interrupted Aortic Arach (IAA)
Abnormalities of coronary arteries, arterial duct and pericardium; AV fistulae	Anomalous Origin of Coronary Artery from Pulmonary Artery (ALCAPA) Patent Ductus Arteriosus (PDA)

Table 1. IPCCC Classification of Congenital Heart Disease and Most Common Diagnoses

3. Developmental genetics of congenital heart disease

Heart development is crucial to understand because its molecular basis is evolutionary conserved as depicted by studies in several model organisms. Heart development is a complex process regulated by combinatorial interactions of transcription factors and their regulators, ligands and receptors, signaling pathways, and contractile protein genes among others. The differential expression of each of these genes at unique stages of development and in different areas of the heart is responsible for the normal development of the heart. Any disruption in these genes will result in congenital malformations of the heart. This molecular program for heart development has been a heavy field of research, yet our knowledge is far from being complete.

The heart is the first organ to develop in the embryo at the second week of gestation when pre-cardiac lateral plate mesoderm cells migrate towards the midline of the embryo and form two crescent-shaped primordia, which fuse to form a beating heart tube at week 3. Within only few days the heart tube folds on itself in a process known as looping. This is the first event in the organogenesis of the embryo that manifests left-right asymmetry and is believed to be at the origin of the laterality program of the embryo. Subsequently, the four chambers of the heart are formed. This requires the differentiation of myocytes into two different subtypes, atrial and ventricular. Finally, valves and septa form through divisions within the heart to form the mature four-chambered heart. Valvulogenesis and septogenesis both require interaction between endocardial and myocardial cells, and valvoseptal malformations are the most common CHDs. In addition, development of the conduction system occurs into pacemakers and purkinjie cells, as well as vascularization from neural crest cells, and coronary arteries from epicardial precursor cells. As such, heart development requires a complex interplay of cell-commitment, migration, proliferation, differentiation, and apoptosis. Any perturbation in this program can result in congenital heart disease.

Transcription factors regulate this tight program of gene expression, which is chamber-, and stage-specific. Protein interactions and formation of complexes that regulate downstream targets cardiac targets with convergent and divergent pathways have made the understanding of the molecular basis of CHD complicated. In-vitro and in-vivo studies have been crucial in widening our understanding of the molecular program for heart development. Major transcription factor families involved in heart development include the GATA, T-box, homeobox, and basic Helix-Loop-Helix (bHLH) among others. Screening of human CHD patients for gene mutations within these transcription factor families as well as other cardiac-enriched genes implicated in heart development has not been as rewarding. Mutations in *TBX5, GATA4, NKX2-5* have been implicated in many CHD families and genetic tests became clinically available. Several other genes have been clearly established to cause syndromic cases of CHD such as *JAG1* and *ELN*. Deletions of chromosomal regions have also been established to cause several CHD syndromes, the most famous of which is DiGeorge Syndrome, which is caused by the 22q11.2 deletion. Despite all this progress, the majority of gene mutations discovered in a family with CHD have not been confirmed in other families, or in only a few. Also screening of large cohorts of isolated CHD cases for mutations in a large set of cardiac-enriched candidate genes consistently results in a low yield of genetic causality.

This gap has prompted novel directions in understanding the genetics of CHD. One of the hypotheses is the multifactorial and polygenetic nature of CHD, with gene mutations acting on a certain genetic background or acting within a particular susceptible environment within a developmental window. There have been efforts towards a new systems biology approach to understanding CHD. In addition to germline DNA sequencing which comprises the majority of the literature, somatic DNA sequencing, RNA sequencing, study of microRNAs (miRNAs), and Copy Number Variations (CNVs) analysis are becoming more popular tools to study CHD. Also with the advent of next-generation sequencing and the decreased cost of both sequencing and array comparative genomic hybridization (array-CGH), more data are becoming available, and the molecular biology approach of the past few decades is shifting into a bioinformatics approach to help decipher the genetics of this complex disease. The subsequent sections of the chapter will dwell into the genetics of CHD from the oldest and most known to the most recent and least known. The below section discusses syndromic CHD, which comprises entities where the genetic causes is the most well established. Then the genes implicated in non-syndromic CHD in humans will be discussed with the degree of evidence for each. The most recent but least developed technologies to understand CHD mentioned above will be discussed at the end of the chapter.

4. Syndromic congenital heart disease

Cardiac malformations are among the most prevalent malformations in congenital syndromes. A large list of syndromes with congenital heart disease as a common manifestation has known genetic defects. CHD syndromes can be either due chromosome dosage disorders, large chromosomal deletions, small micro-deletions, or single gene defects. Table 2 shows a list of CHD syndromes within each of these categories with the corresponding genetic defect. This section will discuss the most common syndromes that include congenital heart disease as a primary manifestation. Within each syndrome, the phenotypic diversity as well as the spectrum of mutations and chromosomal defects that have been reported will be discussed.

4.1. Down Syndrome (trisomy 21)

Down Syndrome is the most common disorder of chromosome dosage with an incidence of 1 in 700 to 1 in 800 live births. The incidence is known to increase tremendously with increased maternal age, particularly above the age of 35. The main clinical manifestations of Down Syndrome are characteristic dysmorphic facies, mental retardation, premature ageing, congenital heart disease, hearing loss, and increased risk of hematologic malignancies.(Pueschel 1990)

Syndrome with CHD	Genetic Cause for CHD
Disorders of Chromosome Dosage	
Trisomy 21 (Down Syndrome)	Unknown
Turner	Unknown
Chromosomal Microdeletions	
Di Georges Syndrome	22q11.2 deletion resulting in absent *TBX1* gene
Williams-Beuren Syndrome	Microdeletion of *ELN* gene; Mutations in *ELN* gene
Single Gene Defects	
Holt-Oram Syndrome	*TBX5* mutations
Alagille Syndome	*JAG1* or *Notch1* mutations; Microdeletion or rearrangement at 20p12 resulting in absent *JAG1* gene
Noonan Syndrome	Mutations in *PTPN11, SOS1, RAF1, KRAS, BRAF, MEK1, MEK2*, and *HRAS*
CHARGE Association	Mutations in *CHD7* and *SEMA3E*; Microdeletion at 22q11.2
Char Syndrome	Mutations in *TFAP2B*
Ellis-can Creveld Syndrome	Mutations in *EVC* or *EVC2*
Cardiofaciocutaneous Syndrome	Mutations in *KRAS, BRAK, MEK1*, or *MEK2*; Microdeletion at 12q21.2-q22
Costello Syndrome	Mutations in *HRAS* (overlap with Noonan and Cardiofaciocutaneous Syndrome)
Marfan Syndrome	Mutations in *Fibrillin-1*

Table 2. Syndromes Manifesting Congenital Heart Disease and their Genetic Cause

Congenital Heart Disease occurs in 40 to 50% of Down Syndrome patients. The most common abnormality is Atrioventricular Septal Defect (AVSD).(Marino 1993) Other malformations include VSD and TOF among others. Some CHD phenotypes are not seen in Down Syndrome patients such as Transposition of the Great Arteries (TGA) and Situs Inversus.(Marino 1993) Adult patients with Down Syndrome are also predisposed to Mitral Valve Prolapse (MVP) and fenestrations in the cusps of the aortic and pulmonary valves. (Hamada and others 1998)

Given the complexity of the phenotype in Down Syndrome, there has been tremendous effort to build a phenotype map and identify the genetic cause behind each phenotype.(Delabar and others 1993; Korenberg and others 1994) Although successful for other features of Down Syndrome, the cause of the cardiac malformations in Down Syndrome are still unclear. Knowing that *CRELD1* gene mutations have been associated with AVSD, one screening of 39 Down Syndrome patients identified two missense *CRELD1* mutations and suggested that CRELD1 mutations might cause AVSD in Down Syndrome.(Maslen and others 2006) However other complex hypotheses have been suggested such as epigenetic mechanisms. Despite considerable process for molecular genetic analysis of Down Syndrome has been achieved using mouse models, to date no clear cause for CHD is known.

4.2. Turner Syndrome

Turner syndrome is a condition in females where all or part of one sex chromosome is absent. It is estimated to occur in 1 of 2500 females.(Bondy 2009) It manifests most commonly with characteristic physical features such as short stature, webbed necks, broad chest, low hairline, and low set ears, gonadal dysfunction, and cognitive deficits.(Bondy 2009) Clinical features are highly variable and can sometimes be very mild. Congenital heart disease is found in 20% to 50% of Turner Syndrome patients. The most common malformation is a Coarctation of the Aorta (COA) of the postductal type, which comprises 50% to 70% of CHD in Turner Syndrome.(Doswell and others 2006) Other cardiac malformations seen in Turner Syndrome include Bicuspid Aortic Valve (BAV), Partial Anomalous Pulmonary Venous Connection (PAPVC), and Hypoplastic Left Heart (HLH). In addition, a higher frequency of cardiac conduction abnormalities, hypertension, and aortic dilation has been reported in Turner Syndrome patients.(Doswell and others 2006; Lopez and others 2008) The molecular mechanisms leading to the cardiac malformations in Turner Syndrome are not clear.

4.3. Di George Syndrome

Di George Syndrome (DGS) is also known as Velocardiofacial Syndrome (VCFS) or Chromosome 22q11.2 Deletion Syndrome. It is caused by a 1.5 to 3.0-Mb hemizygous deletion on chromosome 22 q11, which can be inherited in an autosomal dominant fashion, but most commonly arises *de novo*.(Emanuel 2008) The clinical manifestations are highly variable owing to incomplete penetrance. When the disease is fully penetrant, clinical manifestations include cardiac outflow tract defects, parathyroid gland hypoplasia resulting in hypocalcaemia, thymus gland aplasia resulting in immunodeficiency, and neurologic and facial abnormalities.(Emanuel 2008) Cardiac outflow tact defects in DGS include TOF, type B Interrupted Aortic Arch (IAA), Truncus Arteriosus, Right Aortic Arch, and aberrant right subclavian artery.(Momma 2010) (Yagi and others 2003) The molecular mechanisms leading to the phenotype in DGS are more known than for Down and Turner Syndromes. The microdeletion results in haploinsufficiency of the *TBX1* gene, which is responsible for neural crest migration into the derivatives of the pharyngeal arches and pouches in the developing embryo.(Emanuel 2008) Target genes downstream of *TBX1* are not yet elucidated, however they are most likely to explain the different phenotypes in DGS.

4.4. Williams-Beuren Syndrome

Williams-Beuren Syndrome (WBS) results from a hemizygous deletion of 1.5 to 1.8 Mb on chromosome 7q11.23, an area that encompasses 28 genes. Its prevalence is estimated to be 1 in 7500.(Stromme and others 2002) Clinically, patients have Supravalvular Aortic Stenosis (SVAS), mental retardation, characteristic facial features, distinctive dental anomalies, infantile hypercalcemia, and peripheral pulmonary artery stenosis.(Beuren and others 1962; Grimm and Wesselhoeft 1980; Williams and others 1961) The cardiac phenotype of vascular stenosis is caused by haploinsufficiency of the Elastin (*ELN*) gene and is found in at least 70% of the patients.(Pober 2010) Mutations of the *ELN* gene also result in familial cases of SVAS without the syndromic features of Williams-Beuren.(Curran and others 1993; Metcalfe and others 2000) Although SVAS is the most common lesion in WBS patients, vascular stenoses can occur in any medium or large artery due to the thick media layer. Lesions have been described in aortic arch, descending aorta, pulmonary, coronary, renal artery, mesenteric arteries, and intracranial arteries.(Pober 2010) Half of Williams-Beuren patients also suffer form hypertension, and cardiovascular disease is the most common cause of death in these patients.(Pober 2010; Pober and others 2008)

4.5. Holt-Oram Syndrome

Holt-Oram Syndrome (HOS) is also known as Heart-Hand Syndrome, and it manifests as congenital heart disease and upper limb dysplasia. The heart manifestations are mostly septal malformations and include secundum ASD, VSD, patent ductus arteriosus, and conduction system abnormalities. The upper limb malformations are widely variable but are typically bilateral and asymmetric in severity. They can range from a small abnormality such as a distally-placed thumb to phocomelia or hypoplasia of the shoulders and clavicles. Sometimes the upper limb dysplasia can go unnoticed and will be seen only after radiological imaging. Congenital heart malformations occur in 85% of HOS patients.(Basson and others 1994; Boehme and Shotar 1989)

Genetically, HOS is an autosomal dominant disease caused by mutations in the *TBX5* gene, a member of the T-box family of transcription factors. (Basson and others 1997; Li and others 1997b) Haploinsufficiency of *TBX5* was shown to be at the origin of the HOS. *TBX5* interacts with other cardiac-specific transcription factors *GATA4* and *NKX2-5* to regulate the expression of downstream genes such as *ID2,* which are essential in septation of the cardiac chambers as well as development of the conduction system. The functional mechanisms through which the three transcription factors *TBX5, GATA-4,* and *Nkx2-5* interact to mediate processes in heart development have been heavily studied, and there is a very complex network of interactions among these and other transcription factors and downstream genes that exists but that is still partially understood (Figure 1).

Genotype-phenotype correlations were also performed in HOS, and it has been shown that *TBX5* mutations that create null alleles result in more severe abnormalities in both upper limbs and the heart as compared to missense mutations.(Basson and others 1999) Some mutations caused very severe cardiac malformations but only subtle upper limb deformities. From a clinical perspective, it is important to look for subtle upper limb malformations in patients with septal deformities, because a diagnosis of HOS can increase the recurrence risk in a sibling from 3% to 50% given that this is an autosomal dominant disease. Clinical genetic testing for *TBX5* has also become available in some laboratories across the world.

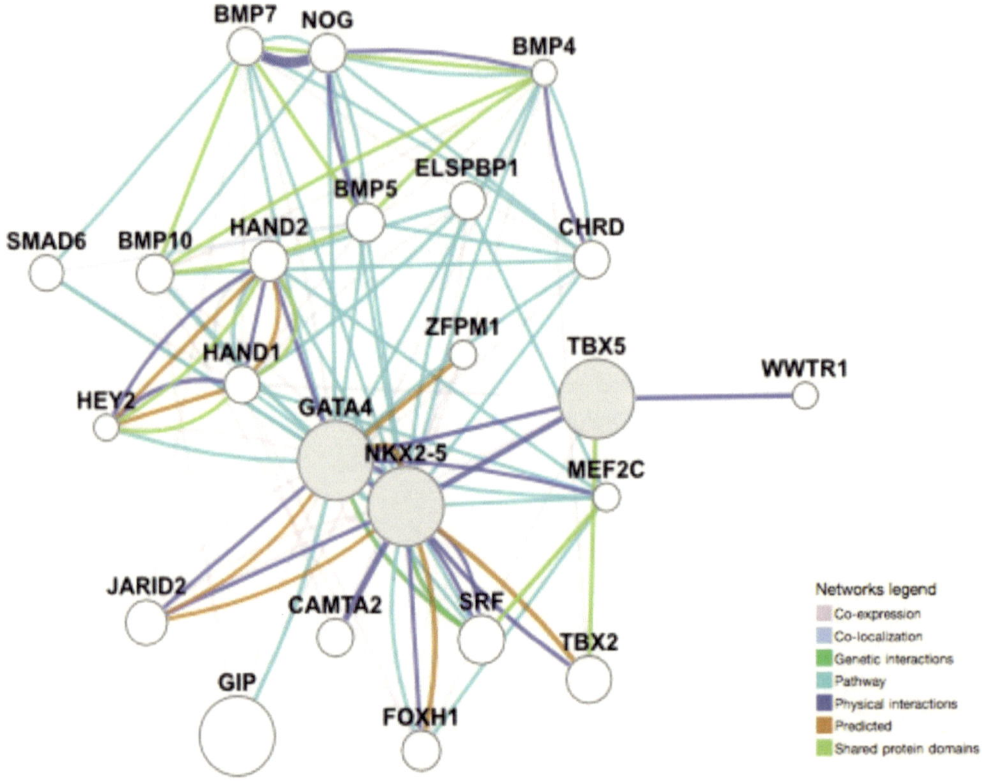

Figure 1. Complex Genetic Interactions of *TBX5, GATA4,* and *Nkx2-5* (Network created using www.genemani.org)

4.6. Alagille Syndrome

Alagille Syndrome is inherited in an autosomal dominant fashion and is defined in the presence of intrahepatic bile duct paucity that usually manifests as cholestasis, congenital heart disease, distinctive facies, skeletal, ocular, renal, and neurological abnormalities. (Kamath and others 2011; Li and others 1997a) CHD is found in more than 90% of patients with Alagille Syndrome and the most common lesion is Pulmonary Atery Stenosis (PAS) or hypoplasia. Other common lesions include TOF, pulmonary valve stenosis (PS), and ASD.(McElhinney and others 2002) The prevalence of the disease is estimated at around one in 700,000 neonates when presence of jaundice is used to ascertain cases (Danks and others 1977), but in fact the disease has a tremendous variability in the phenotype and variable penetrance in families so that the actual prevalence is expected to be much higher.

Alagille Syndrome is caused by mutations in the *JAG1* gene.(Li and others 1997a; Oda and others 1997) The gene encodes a ligand to the Notch1 receptor. Jagged-Notch cell-cell interactions are crucial in determining cell fates during early developmental processes. The mutations spectrum of *JAG1* in Alagille Syndrome encompasses frameshift mutations, nonsense mutations, splice site mutations, or deletion of the whole gene.(Yuan and others

1998) Mutations have also been identified in patients with a predominantly cardiac phenotype.(Li and others 1997a) Some families do have variable penetrance of the mutation as well as variant expressivity of the disease within the same family, such as facial dysmorphism only, or subtle liver disease only within members of the family carrying the same mutation.(El-Rassy and others 2008) JAG-1 mutations are present in 94% of patients that are clinically diagnosed with Alagille Syndrome. A small number of cases are also explained by mutations in the *Notch1* gene, the JAG-1 receptor.(McDaniell and others 2006).

Clinical testing for *JAG-1* mutations is available. If patients are clinically diagnosed, a *JAG-1* mutation could confirm the diagnosis, and indicate the need for multisystem assessment to look for other subclinical abnormalities and possibly prevent them. It would also allow for similar assessment of family members. Due to the high variability of the disease, patients with suspicious right-sided heart lesions such as PAS, TOF, and PS who do not necessarily fulfill the criteria for Alagille Syndrome could also be tested for *JAG-1* mutations.

4.7. Noonan Syndrome

Noonan Syndrome (NS) is a dysmorphic cardiofacial syndrome inherited mostly in an autosomal dominant fashion, with some cases occurring sporadically. Its incidence ranges between 1 in 1000 to 1 in 2500 live births.(Tartaglia and others 2010) The characteristic physical features are downward eyeslanting of the eyes, hypertelorism, low-set ears, short stature, short and webbed neck, and epicanthic folds.(Tartaglia and others 2010) Congenital Heart Disease is found in 80 to 90% of patients with Noonan Syndrome and valvar pulmonary stenosis (PS) and Hypertrophic Cardiomyopathy (HCM) are the two most common cardiac manifestations. A large set of cardiac malformations can also occur including secundum ASD, AVSD, TOF, COA, VSD, PDA, and mitral valve disease.(Marino and others 1999; Noonan 1994) Patients might also have deafness, cryptorchidism, motor delay, and bleeding diathesis.(Tartaglia and others 2010)

NS is a genetically heterogeneous syndrome with at least 8 genes that have been associated with the disease so far: *PTPN11, SOS1, RAF1, KRAS, BRAF, MEK1, MEK2,* and *HRAS*.(Tidyman and Rauen 2009) Mutations in *PTPN11* are most common and explain 50% of the Noonan Syndrome cases, the other 7 genes explain roughly 25% of the cases, and in about 25% of the cases no mutation is found.(Tartaglia and others 2010) All the genes implicated in NS encode proteins that are part of the Ras/Raf/MEK/ERK signaling pathway, an important regulator of cell proliferation, differentiation, and survival. *PTPN11* encodes SHP-2, a protein tyrosine phosphatase that plays an important role in the signal transduction to medial the biological processes described above.

Disease penetrance is almost complete with *PTPN11* mutations, but there is a wide variability in the phenotype. Clinical testing for some of the genes involved in NS such as *PTPN11, SOS1,* and *KRAS* is available. Clinical diagnosis might be helpful might be helpful in borderline cases given the variability in the phenotype.

5. Nonsyndromic congenital heart disease

Isolated congenital heart disease is the most prevalent form of CHD. Evidence for the genetic basis of isolated CHD comes from familial clustering of cases as well as higher recurrence rate of CHD. Mutations in many genes have been associated with several CHD phenotypes, yet the evidence is variable for each gene. Gene mutations can best be classified as highly penetrant mutations in disease-causing genes, low-penetrance mutations in susceptibility genes, and common variants in CHD risk-genes. Transcription factor genes are the most common group of genes implicated in CHD. Other genes are part of signaling transduction pathways and structural components of the heart. Evidence for each gene comes from family studies and segregation analyses using direct sequencing. As mentioned earlier, one of the biggest challenges in the genetics of nonsyndromic CHD is that sequencing for all genes implicated in CHD explains the genetic cause of only a small percentage of patients. Most gene mutations have been described in one or few cases, while only a small number of genes have been duplicated in many cohorts and families.

Table 3 lists all genes in which mutations have been found in different nonsyndromic CHD phenotypes. Most of these are based on only few cases and hence remain to be ascertained; however some have been duplicated in several families such as the phenotypes associated with *NKX2-5* or *GATA4* mutations. The table lists all the genes in which mutations have ever been described for each phenotype. The corresponding PubMed IDs are provided for the published studies where these gene mutations are reported so that readers can make their own assessment regarding the strength of the association.

Phenotype	Implicated Genes	PubMed ID
Dextrocardia	*ACVR2B, NODAL, ZIC3*	9916846, 19064609, 14682828
Tricuspid Atresia	*MYH6*	15643620, 15389319
Mitral Atresia	*FLNA*	20730588
Transposition of the Great Arteries (TGA)	*NODAL, FOXH1, CFC1, THRAP2, GDF1, ACVR2B, ZIC3, NKX2-5, MYH6*	9916847, 14638541, 17924340, 11799476, 18538293, 19553149, 19933292, 19064609, 17295247, 19933292, 14681828, 18538293, 1460745420656787
Double Outlet Right Ventricle (DORV)	*NODAL, FOG2, GDF1, CFC1, ACVR2B, NKX2-5*	9916847, 17924340, 11799476, 19553149, 14681828, 20807224, 14607454
Common Arterial Trunk (CAT)	*GATA6, NKX2-5, Nkx2-6*	19666519, 14607454, 15649947

Tetralogy of Fallot (TOF)	*Nkx2-5, NODAL, CFC1, FOXH1, GATA4, FOG2, GDF1, HAND2, ALDH1A2, GATA6, TDGF1, JAG1*	20437614, 19886994, 17924340, 16470721, 18538293, 20581743, 19553149, 18538293, 18538293, 20819618, 14517948, 14607454
Total Anomalous Pulmonary Venous Connection (TAPVC)	*NODAL, PDGFRA, ANKRD1, ZIC3*	20071345, 18273862, 19064609, 14681828
Partial Anomalous Pulmonary Venous Connection (PAPVC)	*GATA4*	18076106
ASD	*NKX2-5, GATA4, GATA6, TBX20, CFC1, CITED2*	18159245, 1480002, 15689439, 12845333, 17072672, 19853937, 19666519, 16287139, 17668378, 9651244, 15810002, 15689439,14607454
Ebstein 's Anomaly	*MYH7*	21127202
Atrioventricular Septal Defect (AVSD)	*NODAL, GATA4, ACVR1, CRELD1, CFC1, LEFTY2*	12845333, 20670841, 19064609, 19506109, 12632326, 15857420, 18538293, 10053005
Hypoplastic Left Heart Syndrome (HLH)	*NOTCH1, NKX2-5, GJA1, ZIC3*	18593716, 14607454, 20456451, 11470490, 14681828
VSD	*NKX2-5, GATA4, CFC1, IRX4, ZIC3, TDGF1, CITED2, TBX20*	21544582, 12845333, 17253934, 18055909, 19853937, 14681828, 19853938, 16287139, 17668378, 12074273, 9651244, 10587520
Pulmonary Valve Stenosis (PS)	*ELN, GATA4, ACVR2B, ZIC3, GATA6*	21080980, 9916847, 12845333, 19666519, 14681828
Pulmonary Artery Stenosis (PAS)	*ELN, JAG1*	16944981, 11175284, 10942104, 20437614
Aortic Valve Stenosis (AS)	*NOTCH1, ELN, MYH6*	21080980, 16025100, 20656787
Bicuspid Aortic Valve (BAV)	*NOTCH1*	16729972, 160251100
Supravalvar Aortic Stenosis (SVAS)	*ELN*	9215670, 16944981, 11175284
Coarcation of the Aorta	*VEGF, NOTCH1, NKX2-5,*	20420808, 10053005,

(COA)	*LEFTY2*	18593716, 14607454
Interrupted Aortic Arch (IAA)	*CFC1, LEFTY2, NKX2-5*	18538293, 10053005, 14607454
Patent Ductus Arteriosus (PDA)	*MYH11, TFAP2B*	16444274, 17956658, 18752453

Table 3. Implicated Genes in Different Nonsyndromic CHD Phenotypes

In the remaining part this section, the most common genes implicated in nonsyndromic CHD are discussed in details. For each gene, the mutational spectrum, function, associated CHD phenotypes, and mechanism of disease (if known) are provided. The three large groups of cardiac specific transcription factors, the GATA (*GATA4, GATA5,* and *GATA6*), Homebox (*Nkx2-5* and *Nkx2-6*), and T-box (*TBX1, TBX5,* and *TBX20*) are first discussed in detail each in a separate subsection. These three categories of genes comprise the majority of the known genetic causes of CHD. Genes from all three categories interact to regulate downstream gene expression in the developing heart. Other transcription factor genes are discussed in a separate section. Different signaling pathway genes such as the NODAL signaling genes and the Notch signaling pathway are discussed separately. Contractile protein genes, in addition to their well-established role in cadiomyopathy, have been associated with CHD and are mentioned under one section. All remaining genes with minimal evidence for causing CHD comprise are clustered under the final subtitle of this section of the chapter.

5.1. GATA transcription factors (*GATA4, GATA5, GATA6*)

GATA-binding proteins are a family of transcription factors that regulate gene expression and are involved in cell differentiation, survival, and proliferation in many tissues. GATA proteins are evolutionary conserved proteins containing two zinc-finger motifs. They recognize and bind to a "GATA" consensus sequence, which is an important *cis*-element of the promoters of many genes.

GATA4, GATA5, and *GATA6* are involved in the developing heart, and knockout studies in mice have shown that all three are essential for normal cardiac development. Silencing of GATA genes can result in cardiac malformations ranging from valvoseptal defects to acardia. However, mutations in humans with CHD have been described only in *GATA4* and *GATA6* but not *GATA5*.

GATA genes are also among the earliest transcription factors to be expressed in the developing heart. They are expressed in different but overlapping time and tissue patterns in the embryonic heart and manifest complex combinatorial interactions. These characteristics seem to be essential for proper embryonic and postnatal cardiac development.

GATA4 mutations are a well-established cause of CHD in humans. They are inherited in an autosomal dominant fashion in familial cases and are also seen in isolated cases. Haploinsufficiency of the *GATA4* gene causes CHD, which is highly penetrant as observed in familial studies. The most common phenotypes were causative *GATA4* mutations are found are ASD, VSD, TOF, and AVSD.(Garg and others 2003; Nemer and others 2006) Findings of *GATA4* mutations have been duplicated in many familial studies.(Chen and others 2010; Garg and others 2003) Multiple phenotypes are often seen within the same family segregating the same mutation. In isolated studies of CHD cohorts with phenotypes within the spectrum of phenotypes obtained from *GATA4* knockout mice, the frequency of *GATA4* mutations ranges between 0.8% and 3.7%.(Peng and others 2010; Rajagopal and others 2007; Tomita-Mitchell and others 2007; Zhang and others 2006) The spectrum of mutations in *GATA4* includes missense mutations as well as mutations that truncate the protein such as nonsense, frameshift, or splice site variants. Disease-causing missense mutations often disturb the cooperative binding of *GATA4* to other transcription factors such as *Nkx2-5* and *TBX5* (Figure 1), a process which is essential for modulating downstream gene expression during cardiac development.

Animal studies have shown that while *Gata4*$^{+/-}$ and *Gata6*$^{+/-}$ mice survive normally, compound heterozygous *Gata4*$^{+/-}$ *Gata6*$^{+/-}$ mice die at embryonic day 13.5 due to severe cardiac malformations.(Xin and others 2006) Also when both genes are knocked out completely, mice fail to develop any heart.(Zhao and others 2008) These studies have shown that both *Gata4* and *Gata6* are essential for cardiac development and that they interact to regulate downstream targets during heart development. Inactivating *Gata6* in specific vascular cells using transgenic mice has also shown that *Gata6* is involved in the migration of neural crest cells and differentiation of terminal smooth muscle cells, late processes in cardiac development.(Lepore and others 2006) Sequencing of patients with CHD corroborated animal findings by identifying heterozygous *GATA6* mutations in outflow tract defects, mainly Common Arterial Trunk (CAT).(Kodo and others 2009) Subsequent studies showed that *GATA6* mutations also cause ASD and TOF.(Lin and others 2010) Like for *GATA4*, the mutational spectrum of *GATA6* includes missense as well as truncating variants, and genotype-phenotype correlations are not established as the same mutation can cause different phenotypes. In many laboratories around the world, clinical genetic testing is commonly available for *GATA4*, but not for *GATA6*.

5.2. Homeobox transcription factors (*NKX2-5, NKX2-6*)

Homeobox-containing genes are transcription factors that play crucial roles in cardiac development through regulating essential processes such as the spatio-temporal specificity of gene expression required for normal cardiac tissue differentiation. This transcription factor is evolutionary conserved and essential for cardiac development. The "*Tinman*" gene in drosophila is a homeobox-containing gene that is essential for development of the dorsal vessel, a structure analogous to the human heart. *NKX2-5* is the "*Tinman*" homologue in mouse and is highly expressed in the mouse embryologic heart and essential for its development.(Reamon-Buettner and Borlak 2010) The *NKX2-5* gene was cloned in 1996 (Turbay and others 1996), and since then it was shown to be one of the most common known genetic causes of human CHD.

NKX2-5 plays critical roles in later stages of cardiac development, namely septation and development of the conduction system. It physically interacts with *TBX5* to form a complex that cooperatively regulates downstream gene expression that is essential for proper septation and formation of the conduction system.(Habets and others 2002; Moskowitz and others 2007) Mutations in *NKX2-5* gene cause congenital heart disease in an autosomal dominant fashion and with high penetrance.(Kasahara and others 2000) Many families have been described. The most common phenotype is ASD with Atrioventricular (AV) Block. However *NKX2-5* mutations have also been associated with many other CHD phenotypes such as VSD, TOF, subvalvar AS, Ebstein's Anomaly, cardiomyopathy, ventricular hypertrophy or non-compaction, and arrythmias other than the common AV block.(Reamon-Buettner and Borlak 2010) Also in families, different CHD phenotypes can be observed with the same *NKX2-5* mutations making genotype-phenotype correlations difficult. In cohorts of isolated CHD, *NKX2-5* mutations are found in around 2%.(Reamon-Buettner and Borlak 2010) The mutational spectrum is wide with missense and truncating mutations being heavily described. Sequencing for *NKX2-5* is clinically available for genetic testing. Identifying family members through cascade screening might allow the diagnosis of fatal arrythmias or silent ASD's that can otherwise lead to heart failure.

NKX2-6 is another homeobox transcription factor that shares great homology with *NKX2-6* but whose downstream targets are unknown. Mouse in which *NKX2-6* was knocked out did not have any cardiac phenotype, but one mutation has been associated with CAT in one family.(Heathcote and others 2005) More mutations in *NKX2-6* remain to be detected in CHD patients with high throughput screening before its causality to CHD could be established.

5.3. T-Box transcription factors (*TBX1, TBX5, TBX20*)

The T-box family of binding proteins also consists of important transcription factors in cardiac development. T-box genes are evolutionary conserved and share a T-binding domain. All family members are involved in regulating developmental processes such as the initiation and potentiation of cardiac development.(Hariri and others 2011)

The crucial role of *TBX5* in heart development and its interactions with *GATA4* and *NKX2-5* has been discussed earlier in this chapter. Apart from Holt-Oram Syndrome, *TBX5* has not been implicated in nonsyndromic CHD, although some *TBX5* mutations can cause a heart-predominant phenotype with very subtle upper limbs disease. *TBX1* was also discussed earlier as the cause of cardiac malformations in Di George Syndrome. A large deletion of 57bp in the *TBX1* gene was found in one non-syndromic patient with TOF.(Griffin and others 2010) Apart from this single report, findings of *TBX1* mutations have not been duplicated in non-syndromic CHD patients.

Another member of the family that has been implicated in non-syndromic CHD is *TBX20*. $Tbx20^{+/-}$ mice have dilated cardiomyopathy and $TBX20^{-/-}$ mice die at midgestation due to grossly abnormal heart.(Stennard and others 2005) Mutations in *TBX20* are found in less than 1% of patients with CHD phenotypes such as septal defects, left ventricular outflow tract abnormalities, and HLH syndrome.(Kirk and others 2007; Posch and others 2010) Both missense and nonsense heterozygous mutations are described. Functional studies suggest that both loss of function and gain of function mutations in the *TBX20* gene can cause CHD.(Posch and others 2010)

5.4. Other transcription factors (*CITED2, ANKRD1, FOG2, ZIC3*)

The above three families of transcription factors are the most heavily studied in heart development, however a large set of other transcription factors have also been implicated in CHD, yet with lower degrees of evidence, or for some lower penetrance. This section will briefly discuss each of these transcription factors.

CITED2 codes for CBP/p300-Interacting Transactivator with E/D-rich c-terminal Domain Type 2, a transcriptional co-activator several transcriptional responses such as *TFAP2*, the known cause of Char Syndrome. *CITED2* null mouse embryos die embryologically and manifest septal, outflow tract, and aortic arch defects.(Bamforth and others 2004) CITED2 mutations were detected in about 1% of sporadic cases of CHD. Phenotypes include ASD, VSD, and TAPVC.(Sperling and others 2005)

Ankyrin Repeat Domain 1 (*ANKRD1*) is a transcription factor that interacts with cardiac sarcomere proteins. One balanced translocation and one missense mutation in *ANKRD1* gene were detected in two separate cases of TAPVC.(Cinquetti and others 2008)

Friend of GATA 2 (*FOG2*) is, as its name implies, a cofactor of *GATA4*. *FOG2* knockout mice have TOF-like phenotype,(Tevosian and others 2000) and *FOG2* mutations have been described in TOF patients however with reduced penetrance.(Pizzuti and others 2003)

ZIC3 encodes for a zinc finger transcription factor that is implicated in left-right axis development. It is a known gene in human *situs* abnormalities and is inherited in an X-linked fashion. Mutations in *ZIC3* have been identified in families and cohorts of heterotaxy.(Gebbia and others 1997) Additionally, there has been one reported family with TGA carrying a transversion in the *ZIC3* gene, yet with incomplete penetrance.(Megarbane and others 2000)

5.5. NODAL signaling genes (NODAL, GDF1, FOXH1, CFC1, ACVR2B, LEFTY2)

The NODAL family of proteins is member of the TGF-beta superfamily of secreted signaling molecules. NODAL signaling is responsible for dorso-ventral patterning in vertebrate development as well as mesoderm and endoderm generation. Mutations in different genes in the NODAL signaling cascade are believed to occur and cumulatively decrease NODAL signaling leading to CHD phenotypes.(Roessler and others 2009) NODAL mutations have been reported in patients with heterotaxy, TGA, and conotruncal defects,(Gebbia and others 1997; Mohapatra and others 2009) but as mentioned earlier simple heterozygosity is not enough to cause the phenotype in the majority of cases. Mutations in other pathway genes such as *GDF1, FOXH1, CFC1,* and *LEFTY2* are often necessary to cause disease.

CFC1 (Cryptic) is a cofactor of NODAL signaling and its acts through activin receptors. *CFC1* mutations have been initially reported in laterality defects.(Bamford and others 2000) However, outflow tract defects such as TGA and DORV have also been associated with CFC1 mutations.(Goldmuntz and others 2002) Similar associations with CHD phenotypes apart from *situs* abnormalities have been observed for *GDF1,* another member of the TGF-beta superfamily involved in NODAL signaling.(Karkera and others 2007) *FOXH1* mutations have been associated with CHD however only within the context of reduced NODAL signaling due to mutations in more than one gene in the cascade.(Roessler and others 2008) Therefore, sequencing of all NODAL signaling genes together would give a better picture of the genetic cause of a particular CHD phenotype rather than identifying a variant in one of the genes.

5.6. Notch signaling genes (*NOTCH1, JAG1, NOTCH2*)

The Notch-Jagged signaling pathway is an important regulatory mechanism of cell differentiation processes during embryonic and adult life. In the heart, it is particularly important in cardiac valve development. *JAG1* and *NOTCH2* mutations are known causes of Alagille Syndrome. However mutations in both can cause non-syndromic CHD.(Bauer and others 2010; McDaniell and others 2006) *NOTCH1* has been also implicated in non-syndromic CHD. Mutations can cause BAV, AS, COA, and HLH.(Garg and others 2005; McBride and others 2008; Mohamed and others 2006)

5.7. Contractile protein genes (*MYH6, MYH7, MYH11, MYBPC3, ACTC1*)

Mutations in contractile protein genes are common causes of Hypertrophic Cardiomyopathy (HCM) and other cardiomyopathies. However, some of these genes have also been implicated in a minority of CHD cases. One *MYH6* (Alpha Myosin Heavy Chain) mutation has been described in a family with ASD. (Ching and others 2005) Mutations in *MYH7* (Beta Myosin Heavy Chain) can cause Ebstein's Anomaly and septal defects.(Budde and others 2007) Heterozygous *MYBPC3* mutations are a very frequent cause of HCM, however there have been reports of ASD and PDA in addition to severe HCM in patients with homozygous truncating mutations in the Myosin Binding Protein C gene *MYBPC3*.(Xin and others 2007; Zahka and others 2008) Similarly, mutations in Alpha-Cardiac Actin *ACTC1,* another sarcomere protein gene, cause ASD together with HCM.(Monserrat and others 2007) Finally, Myosin Heavy Chain 11 (MYH11) has a role in smooth muscles, and mutations in *MYH11* have been implicated in familial thoracic aortic aneurysm with PDA due to decreased elasticity of the aortic wall and the ductus arteriosus.(Zhu and others 2006)

5.8. Miscellaneous genes (*ELN, GJA1, FLNA, THRAP2*)

Elastin (*ELN*) deletion or mutations are implicated in Williams-Beuren syndrome, however have also been reported in many cases of isolated SVAS and PS. (Arrington and others 2006;

Metcalfe and others 2000) *GJA1* encodes Connexin-43, a gap junction protein that maintains cell-cell adhesion and communication. Mutations in *GJA1* were reported in a case of HLH and another report of heterotaxia patients. (Britz-Cunningham and others 1995; Dasgupta and others 2001) Filamin A (FLNA) cross-links actin filaments in the cytoplasm and anchors them to the rest of the cytoskeleton. *FLNA* is an X-linked gene in which mutations are associated with valvular dystrophy. (Kyndt and others 2007) Finally, mutations in the *THRAP2* gene, which encodes a TRAP-complex protein, have been associated with TGA in one study.(Muncke and others 2003)

6. Other genetic mechanisms of CHD

Despite the large number of genes implicated in non-syndromic CHD, the genetic cause of the majority of isolated cases of CHD is still poorly understood. This has led researchers to investigate genetic mechanisms other than gene mutations that can contribute to inherited or isolated CHD. Copy Number Variations (CNVs), micro RNA (miRNA), somatic mutations, and epigenetics are all active areas of research into the genetics of CHD.

6.1. Copy Number Variations

Copy Number Variations (CNVs) are structural alterations to the genomic DNA that result in the cell having abnormal copies of large sections of its DNA. They can be inherited or occur *de novo*. Over the past decade, the role of CNVs in disease has been heavily studied, mostly in different types of cancers. In the heart, CNV analysis has explained an additional small fraction of the genetics of syndromic CHD (3.6%), but more of the non-syndromic CHD (19%).(Breckpot and others 2011) Submicroscopic deletions have been discovered using array-CGH in large CHD cohorts. CNVs occured in regions harboring known CHD candidate genes but were also capable of identifying new CHD loci in TOF, HLH, heterotaxy, and other CHD phenotypes.(Fakhro and others 2011; Greenway and others 2009; Payne and others 2012) One of the most commonly used strategies in CNV analysis is trio analysis, which allows the determination of de novo CNVs in CHD patients. Comparison with control groups is also helpful in assessing the likelihood of causality of CNVs using statistical methods. Despite several successful examples, the use of CNVs in understanding CHD remains challenging, particularly in proving the causality of the CNVs and assessing the magnitude that these CNVs have on the phenotype.

6.2. Micro RNA

Micro RNAs (miRNAs) are small (around 22 nucleotides long) single stranded noncoding RNAs and are encoded by miRNA genes. miRNAs serve as regulators of gene expression. Since cardiac development involves tremendous spatio-temportal specificity of gene expression, it is believed that miRNAs are involved in cardiac development and they can potentially cause CHD. miRNAs are important players in cellular proliferation, differentiation, and migration all of which are essential processes for proper cardiac development. In fact, cardiac specific miRNAs were discovered such as miR-133 and miR-1-2, both of which when knocked out in mice cause cardiac defects, specifically VSD and dilated cardiomyopathy.(Ikeda and others 2007) miR-208a and miR-208b are also cardiac-enriched, and they are encoded within the introns of *MYH6* and *MYH7*.(Callis and others 2009; van Rooij and others 2007) Current research focuses on sequencing miRNA to identify potential mutations that can cause CHD. Definite evidence in humans is still unavailable but might be underway.

6.3. Somatic mutations

Another direction of research to assess CHD is the study of somatic mutations using surgically discarded tissues from CHD patients who undergo surgical repair. Both DNA and RNA can be extracted and sequenced. Previous studies have focused on sequencing *GATA4* and *Nkx2-5* in somatic DNA of patients with septal defects, and yielded controversial findings as to whether somatic mutations contribute significantly to these genes.(Draus and others 2009; Esposito and others 2011; Reamon-Buettner and Borlak 2004) In the current era of high throughput DNA sequencing, and development of new analytical frameworks for RNA sequencing, the contribution of somatic mutations to CHD will become clearer soon, however no significant data in this field is published yet.

6.4. Epigenetics

The multifactorial causality of CHD has long been hypothesized to explain the complexity of the genetics of cardiac malformations. Epigenetics is one model where gene-environment interaction can affect gene expression and disturb developmental processes in the embryonic heart. Histone modifications and chromatin remodeling both play important roles in cardiac development and physiology(Han and others 2011; Lange and others 2008; Ohtani and Dimmeler 2011), and recent studies shoed that they can directly interact with some classes of transcription factors like the T-box family.(Miller and Weinmann 2009) It is possible that epigenetic mechanisms contribute to the etiology of CHD, however more evidence remains to be established.

7. Current tools for the genetic evaluation of CHD

Different techniques are currently available to interrogate the genetic causes of CHD. Karyotyping and Fluorescent In-Situ Hybridization (FISH) analysis remain the best tools to assess chromosomal deletions or rearrangements. They are often the starting point for the genetic assessment of a CHD patient. Whenever candidate genes are suspected, for instance in the setting of a clinically diagnosed syndrome, Sanger sequencing is performed on the candidate gene to look for disease-causing mutations. For many years, together with positional mapping through linkage analysis, these were the only tools that drove genetic discovery in CHD in humans. Current technology makes use of array-comparative genomic hybridization (array-CGH) for linkage analysis, Genome Wide Association Studies (GWAS), CNV analysis, homozygosity mapping, and transcriptome analysis. More importantly was the introduction of next-generation sequencing in 2005 and the tremendous decrease in the cost of sequencing over the past several years, which is allowing the massive sequencing of the exome and even genome of huge numbers of patients. Next-generation RNA sequencing is also beginning to be used to sequence cardiac transcripts from CHD patients who have underwent surgery. The rapid pooling of high throughput data is expected to massively increase our understanding of CHD within the coming two years. To deal with these large amounts of data, bioinformatics and modeling of genetic variants determine function is becoming the standard and many molecular biology labs are forced to become genetics and bioinformatics labs to make use of current technology. A systems biology approach is needed nowadays to integrate high throughput data from the many possible sources.

8. From the bench to the bedside

With the advances in sequencing and bioinformatics, gene discovery in CHD is escalating. This advance in research is directly translated to clinical testing to provide genetic counseling for adult patients with CHD who plan to have children. From a technical aspect, our capability to identify genetic variants in CHD genes has magnified. Nonetheless, making functional significance and even clinical sense of the large number of gene mutations remains a big challenge. Given the complexity of CHD, definite gene mutations remain uncommon. At this time when the genetic inflow of information is very fast, physician-scientists must be very careful in communicating genetic information that is not validated to patients, in order to avoid psychological and emotional harm. On a different angle, with sequencing of the exome or genome, the chances of detecting incidental findings that indicate disease risk or prognosis becomes very high. All such unintentionally detected serious genetic findings are termed the incidentalome.(Kohane and others 2006) Since CHD is mostly surgically treated and people who undergo genetic testing are often already cured, caregivers need to be cautious before rushing next-generation sequencing into the CHD clinic.

9. Future prospects

Current trends in CHD genetics research are making use of the rapidly developing technology, particularly high throughput sequencing. This trend will continue over the coming few years. The challenge is in integrating the increasing amounts of data to answer the questions that need to be answered. Systems biology and innovative bioinformatics tools are crucial to integrate data from different sources and build a pipeline that can unravel the mysteries that molecular biologists have been trying to answer for many years.

Eventually, more validated genetic information will be available in the clinic to allow accurate genetic counseling and prenatal screening. Understanding heart development will also allow for possible therapeutic applications given the many-shared molecular pathways between embryologic heart development and adult heart disease, particularly tissue death and regeneration in the setting of ischemic heart disease.

Author details

Akl C. Fahed
Department of Genetics, Harvard Medical School, Boston, Massachusetts, USA

Georges M. Nemer
Departent of Biochemistry and Molecular Genetics, American University of Beirut, Beirut, Lebanon

10. References

Arrington CB, Nightengale D, Lowichik A, Rosenthal ET, Christian-Ritter K, Viskochil DH. (2006). Pathologic and molecular analysis in a family with rare mixed supravalvar aortic and pulmonic stenosis. Pediatr Dev Pathol 9,297-306.

Bamford RN, Roessler E, Burdine RD, Saplakoglu U, dela Cruz J, Splitt M, Goodship JA, Towbin J, Bowers P, Ferrero GB and others. (2000). Loss-of-function mutations in the EGF-CFC gene CFC1 are associated with human left-right laterality defects. Nat Genet 26,365-9.

Bamforth SD, Braganca J, Farthing CR, Schneider JE, Broadbent C, Michell AC, Clarke K, Neubauer S, Norris D, Brown NA and others. (2004). Cited2 controls left-right patterning and heart development through a Nodal-Pitx2c pathway. Nat Genet 36,1189-96.

Basson CT, Bachinsky DR, Lin RC, Levi T, Elkins JA, Soults J, Grayzel D, Kroumpouzou E, Traill TA, Leblanc-Straceski J and others. (1997). Mutations in human TBX5 [corrected] cause limb and cardiac malformation in Holt-Oram syndrome. Nat Genet 15,30-5.

Basson CT, Cowley GS, Solomon SD, Weissman B, Poznanski AK, Traill TA, Seidman JG, Seidman CE. (1994). The clinical and genetic spectrum of the Holt-Oram syndrome (heart-hand syndrome). N Engl J Med 330,885-91.

Basson CT, Huang T, Lin RC, Bachinsky DR, Weremowicz S, Vaglio A, Bruzzone R, Quadrelli R, Lerone M, Romeo G and others. (1999). Different TBX5 interactions in heart and limb defined by Holt-Oram syndrome mutations. Proc Natl Acad Sci U S A 96,2919-24.

Bauer RC, Laney AO, Smith R, Gerfen J, Morrissette JJ, Woyciechowski S, Garbarini J, Loomes KM, Krantz ID, Urban Z and others. (2010). Jagged1 (JAG1) mutations in patients with tetralogy of Fallot or pulmonic stenosis. Hum Mutat 31,594-601.

Beuren AJ, Apitz J, Harmjanz D. (1962). Supravalvular aortic stenosis in association with mental retardation and a certain facial appearance. Circulation 26,1235-40.

Boehme DH, Shotar AO. (1989). A complex deformity of appendicular skeleton and shoulder with congenital heart disease in three generations of a Jordanian family. Clin Genet 36,442-50.

Bondy CA. (2009). Turner syndrome 2008. Horm Res 71 Suppl 1,52-6.

Breckpot J, Thienpont B, Arens Y, Tranchevent LC, Vermeesch JR, Moreau Y, Gewillig M, Devriendt K. (2011). Challenges of interpreting copy number variation in syndromic and non-syndromic congenital heart defects. Cytogenet Genome Res 135, 251-9.

Britz-Cunningham SH, Shah MM, Zuppan CW, Fletcher WH. (1995). Mutations of the Connexin43 gap-junction gene in patients with heart malformations and defects of laterality. N Engl J Med 332,1323-9.

Bruneau BG. (2008). The developmental genetics of congenital heart disease. Nature 451,943-8.

Budde BS, Binner P, Waldmuller S, Hohne W, Blankenfeldt W, Hassfeld S, Bromsen J, Dermintzoglou A, Wieczorek M, May E and others. (2007). Noncompaction of the ventricular myocardium is associated with a de novo mutation in the beta-myosin heavy chain gene. PLoS One 2,e1362.

Callis TE, Pandya K, Seok HY, Tang RH, Tatsuguchi M, Huang ZP, Chen JF, Deng Z, Gunn B, Shumate J and others. (2009). MicroRNA-208a is a regulator of cardiac hypertrophy and conduction in mice. J Clin Invest 119,2772-86.

Chen Y, Han ZQ, Yan WD, Tang CZ, Xie JY, Chen H, Hu DY. (2010). A novel mutation in GATA4 gene associated with dominant inherited familial atrial septal defect. J Thorac Cardiovasc Surg 140,684-7.

Ching YH, Ghosh TK, Cross SJ, Packham EA, Honeyman L, Loughna S, Robinson TE, Dearlove AM, Ribas G, Bonser AJ and others. (2005). Mutation in myosin heavy chain 6 causes atrial septal defect. Nat Genet 37,423-8.

Cinquetti R, Badi I, Campione M, Bortoletto E, Chiesa G, Parolini C, Camesasca C, Russo A, Taramelli R, Acquati F. (2008). Transcriptional deregulation and a missense mutation define ANKRD1 as a candidate gene for total anomalous pulmonary venous return. Hum Mutat 29,468-74.

Curran ME, Atkinson DL, Ewart AK, Morris CA, Leppert MF, Keating MT. (1993). The elastin gene is disrupted by a translocation associated with supravalvular aortic stenosis. Cell 73,159-68.

Danks DM, Campbell PE, Jack I, Rogers J, Smith AL. (1977). Studies of the aetiology of neonatal hepatitis and biliary atresia. Arch Dis Child 52,360-7.

Dasgupta C, Martinez AM, Zuppan CW, Shah MM, Bailey LL, Fletcher WH. (2001). Identification of connexin43 (alpha1) gap junction gene mutations in patients with hypoplastic left heart syndrome by denaturing gradient gel electrophoresis (DGGE). Mutat Res 479,173-86.

Delabar JM, Theophile D, Rahmani Z, Chettouh Z, Blouin JL, Prieur M, Noel B, Sinet PM. (1993). Molecular mapping of twenty-four features of Down syndrome on chromosome 21. Eur J Hum Genet 1,114-24.

Doswell BH, Visootsak J, Brady AN, Graham JM, Jr. (2006). Turner syndrome: an update and review for the primary pediatrician. Clin Pediatr (Phila) 45,301-13.

Draus JM, Jr., Hauck MA, Goetsch M, Austin EH, 3rd, Tomita-Mitchell A, Mitchell ME. (2009). Investigation of somatic NKX2-5 mutations in congenital heart disease. J Med Genet 46,115-22.

El-Rassy I, Bou-Abdallah J, Al-Ghadban S, Bitar F, Nemer G. (2008). Absence of NOTCH2 and Hey2 mutations in a familial Alagille syndrome case with a novel frameshift mutation in JAG1. Am J Med Genet A 146,937-9.

Emanuel BS. (2008). Molecular mechanisms and diagnosis of chromosome 22q11.2 rearrangements. Dev Disabil Res Rev 14,11-8.

Esposito G, Butler TL, Blue GM, Cole AD, Sholler GF, Kirk EP, Grossfeld P, Perryman BM, Harvey RP, Winlaw DS. (2011). Somatic mutations in NKX2-5, GATA4, and HAND1 are not a common cause of tetralogy of Fallot or hypoplastic left heart. Am J Med Genet A 155A,2416-21.

Fakhro KA, Choi M, Ware SM, Belmont JW, Towbin JA, Lifton RP, Khokha MK, Brueckner M. (2011). Rare copy number variations in congenital heart disease patients identify unique genes in left-right patterning. Proc Natl Acad Sci U S A 108,2915-20.

Garg V, Kathiriya IS, Barnes R, Schluterman MK, King IN, Butler CA, Rothrock CR, Eapen RS, Hirayama-Yamada K, Joo K and others. (2003). GATA4 mutations cause human congenital heart defects and reveal an interaction with TBX5. Nature 424, 443-7.

Garg V, Muth AN, Ransom JF, Schluterman MK, Barnes R, King IN, Grossfeld PD, Srivastava D. (2005). Mutations in NOTCH1 cause aortic valve disease. Nature 437,270-4.

Gebbia M, Ferrero GB, Pilia G, Bassi MT, Aylsworth A, Penman-Splitt M, Bird LM, Bamforth JS, Burn J, Schlessinger D and others. (1997). X-linked situs abnormalities result from mutations in ZIC3. Nat Genet 17,305-8.

Gill HK, Splitt M, Sharland GK, Simpson JM. (2003). Patterns of recurrence of congenital heart disease: an analysis of 6,640 consecutive pregnancies evaluated by detailed fetal echocardiography. J Am Coll Cardiol 42,923-9.

Goldmuntz E. (2001). The epidemiology and genetics of congenital heart disease. Clin Perinatol 28,1-10.

Goldmuntz E, Bamford R, Karkera JD, dela Cruz J, Roessler E, Muenke M. (2002). CFC1 mutations in patients with transposition of the great arteries and double-outlet right ventricle. Am J Hum Genet 70,776-80.

Greenway SC, Pereira AC, Lin JC, DePalma SR, Israel SJ, Mesquita SM, Ergul E, Conta JH, Korn JM, McCarroll SA and others. (2009). De novo copy number variants identify new genes and loci in isolated sporadic tetralogy of Fallot. Nat Genet 41,931-5.

Griffin HR, Topf A, Glen E, Zweier C, Stuart AG, Parsons J, Peart I, Deanfield J, O'Sullivan J, Rauch A and others. (2010). Systematic survey of variants in TBX1 in non-syndromic tetralogy of Fallot identifies a novel 57 base pair deletion that reduces transcriptional activity but finds no evidence for association with common variants. Heart 96, 1651-5.

Grimm T, Wesselhoeft H. (1980). [The genetic aspects of Williams-Beuren syndrome and the isolated form of the supravalvular aortic stenosis. Investigation of 128 families (author's transl)]. Z Kardiol 69,168-72.

Habets PE, Moorman AF, Clout DE, van Roon MA, Lingbeek M, van Lohuizen M, Campione M, Christoffels VM. (2002). Cooperative action of Tbx2 and Nkx2.5 inhibits

ANF expression in the atrioventricular canal: implications for cardiac chamber formation. Genes Dev 16,1234-46.

Hamada T, Gejyo F, Koshino Y, Murata T, Omori M, Nishio M, Misawa T, Isaki K. (1998). Echocardiographic evaluation of cardiac valvular abnormalities in adults with Down's syndrome. Tohoku J Exp Med 185,31-5.

Han P, Hang CT, Yang J, Chang CP. (2011). Chromatin remodeling in cardiovascular development and physiology. Circ Res 108,378-96.

Hariri F, Nemer M, Nemer G. (2011). T-box factors: Insights into the evolutionary emergence of the complex heart. Ann Med.

Heathcote K, Braybrook C, Abushaban L, Guy M, Khetyar ME, Patton MA, Carter ND, Scambler PJ, Syrris P. (2005). Common arterial trunk associated with a homeodomain mutation of NKX2.6. Hum Mol Genet 14,585-93.

Herrera P, Caldarone CA, Forte V, Holtby H, Cox P, Chiu P, Kim PC. (2008). Topsy-turvy heart with associated congenital tracheobronchial stenosis and airway compression requiring surgical reconstruction. Ann Thorac Surg 86,282-3.

Ikeda S, Kong SW, Lu J, Bisping E, Zhang H, Allen PD, Golub TR, Pieske B, Pu WT. (2007). Altered microRNA expression in human heart disease. Physiol Genomics 31,367-73.

Jaeggi E, Chitayat D, Golding F, Kim P, Yoo SJ. (2008). Prenatal diagnosis of topsy-turvy heart. Cardiol Young 18,337-42.

Kamath BM, Podkameni G, Hutchinson AL, Leonard LD, Gerfen J, Krantz ID, Piccoli DA, Spinner NB, Loomes KM, Meyers K. (2011). Renal anomalies in Alagille syndrome: A disease-defining feature. Am J Med Genet A.

Karkera JD, Lee JS, Roessler E, Banerjee-Basu S, Ouspenskaia MV, Mez J, Goldmuntz E, Bowers P, Towbin J, Belmont JW and others. (2007). Loss-of-function mutations in growth differentiation factor-1 (GDF1) are associated with congenital heart defects in humans. Am J Hum Genet 81,987-94.

Kasahara H, Lee B, Schott JJ, Benson DW, Seidman JG, Seidman CE, Izumo S. (2000). Loss of function and inhibitory effects of human CSX/NKX2.5 homeoprotein mutations associated with congenital heart disease. J Clin Invest 106,299-308.

Kirk EP, Sunde M, Costa MW, Rankin SA, Wolstein O, Castro ML, Butler TL, Hyun C, Guo G, Otway R and others. (2007). Mutations in cardiac T-box factor gene TBX20 are associated with diverse cardiac pathologies, including defects of septation and valvulogenesis and cardiomyopathy. Am J Hum Genet 81,280-91.

Kodo K, Nishizawa T, Furutani M, Arai S, Yamamura E, Joo K, Takahashi T, Matsuoka R, Yamagishi H. (2009). GATA6 mutations cause human cardiac outflow tract defects by disrupting semaphorin-plexin signaling. Proc Natl Acad Sci U S A 106,13933-8.

Kohane IS, Masys DR, Altman RB. (2006). The incidentalome: a threat to genomic medicine. JAMA 296,212-5.

Korenberg JR, Chen XN, Schipper R, Sun Z, Gonsky R, Gerwehr S, Carpenter N, Daumer C, Dignan P, Disteche C and others. (1994). Down syndrome phenotypes:

the consequences of chromosomal imbalance. Proc Natl Acad Sci U S A 91,4997-5001.

Kyndt F, Gueffet JP, Probst V, Jaafar P, Legendre A, Le Bouffant F, Toquet C, Roy E, McGregor L, Lynch SA and others. (2007). Mutations in the gene encoding filamin A as a cause for familial cardiac valvular dystrophy. Circulation 115,40-9.

Lange M, Kaynak B, Forster UB, Tonjes M, Fischer JJ, Grimm C, Schlesinger J, Just S, Dunkel I, Krueger T and others. (2008). Regulation of muscle development by DPF3, a novel histone acetylation and methylation reader of the BAF chromatin remodeling complex. Genes Dev 22,2370-84.

Lepore JJ, Mericko PA, Cheng L, Lu MM, Morrisey EE, Parmacek MS. (2006). GATA-6 regulates semaphorin 3C and is required in cardiac neural crest for cardiovascular morphogenesis. J Clin Invest 116,929-39.

Li L, Krantz ID, Deng Y, Genin A, Banta AB, Collins CC, Qi M, Trask BJ, Kuo WL, Cochran J and others. (1997a). Alagille syndrome is caused by mutations in human Jagged1, which encodes a ligand for Notch1. Nat Genet 16,243-51.

Li QY, Newbury-Ecob RA, Terrett JA, Wilson DI, Curtis AR, Yi CH, Gebuhr T, Bullen PJ, Robson SC, Strachan T and others. (1997b). Holt-Oram syndrome is caused by mutations in TBX5, a member of the Brachyury (T) gene family. Nat Genet 15, 21-9.

Lin X, Huo Z, Liu X, Zhang Y, Li L, Zhao H, Yan B, Liu Y, Yang Y, Chen YH. (2010). A novel GATA6 mutation in patients with tetralogy of Fallot or atrial septal defect. J Hum Genet 55,662-7.

Loffredo CA. (2000). Epidemiology of cardiovascular malformations: prevalence and risk factors. Am J Med Genet 97,319-25.

Lopez L, Arheart KL, Colan SD, Stein NS, Lopez-Mitnik G, Lin AE, Reller MD, Ventura R, Silberbach M. (2008). Turner syndrome is an independent risk factor for aortic dilation in the young. Pediatrics 121,e1622-7.

Marino B. (1993). Congenital heart disease in patients with Down's syndrome: anatomic and genetic aspects. Biomed Pharmacother 47,197-200.

Marino B, Digilio MC, Toscano A, Giannotti A, Dallapiccola B. (1999). Congenital heart diseases in children with Noonan syndrome: An expanded cardiac spectrum with high prevalence of atrioventricular canal. J Pediatr 135,703-6.

Maslen CL, Babcock D, Robinson SW, Bean LJ, Dooley KJ, Willour VL, Sherman SL. (2006). CRELD1 mutations contribute to the occurrence of cardiac atrioventricular septal defects in Down syndrome. Am J Med Genet A 140,2501-5.

McBride KL, Riley MF, Zender GA, Fitzgerald-Butt SM, Towbin JA, Belmont JW, Cole SE. (2008). NOTCH1 mutations in individuals with left ventricular outflow tract malformations reduce ligand-induced signaling. Hum Mol Genet 17,2886-93.

McDaniell R, Warthen DM, Sanchez-Lara PA, Pai A, Krantz ID, Piccoli DA, Spinner NB. (2006). NOTCH2 mutations cause Alagille syndrome, a heterogeneous disorder of the notch signaling pathway. Am J Hum Genet 79,169-73.

McElhinney DB, Krantz ID, Bason L, Piccoli DA, Emerick KM, Spinner NB, Goldmuntz E. (2002). Analysis of cardiovascular phenotype and genotype-phenotype correlation in individuals with a JAG1 mutation and/or Alagille syndrome. Circulation 106,2567-74.

Megarbane A, Salem N, Stephan E, Ashoush R, Lenoir D, Delague V, Kassab R, Loiselet J, Bouvagnet P. (2000). X-linked transposition of the great arteries and incomplete penetrance among males with a nonsense mutation in ZIC3. Eur J Hum Genet 8, 704-8.

Metcalfe K, Rucka AK, Smoot L, Hofstadler G, Tuzler G, McKeown P, Siu V, Rauch A, Dean J, Dennis N and others. (2000). Elastin: mutational spectrum in supravalvular aortic stenosis. Eur J Hum Genet 8,955-63.

Miller SA, Weinmann AS. (2009). An essential interaction between T-box proteins and histone-modifying enzymes. Epigenetics 4,85-8.

Mohamed SA, Aherrahrou Z, Liptau H, Erasmi AW, Hagemann C, Wrobel S, Borzym K, Schunkert H, Sievers HH, Erdmann J. (2006). Novel missense mutations (p.T596M and p.P1797H) in NOTCH1 in patients with bicuspid aortic valve. Biochem Biophys Res Commun 345,1460-5.

Mohapatra B, Casey B, Li H, Ho-Dawson T, Smith L, Fernbach SD, Molinari L, Niesh SR, Jefferies JL, Craigen WJ and others. (2009). Identification and functional characterization of NODAL rare variants in heterotaxy and isolated cardiovascular malformations. Hum Mol Genet 18,861-71.

Momma K. (2010). Cardiovascular anomalies associated with chromosome 22q11.2 deletion syndrome. Am J Cardiol 105,1617-24.

Monserrat L, Hermida-Prieto M, Fernandez X, Rodriguez I, Dumont C, Cazon L, Cuesta MG, Gonzalez-Juanatey C, Peteiro J, Alvarez N and others. (2007). Mutation in the alpha-cardiac actin gene associated with apical hypertrophic cardiomyopathy, left ventricular non-compaction, and septal defects. Eur Heart J 28,1953-61.

Moodie DS. (1994). Adult congenital heart disease. Curr Opin Cardiol 9,137-42.

Moskowitz IP, Kim JB, Moore ML, Wolf CM, Peterson MA, Shendure J, Nobrega MA, Yokota Y, Berul C, Izumo S and others. (2007). A molecular pathway including Id2, Tbx5, and Nkx2-5 required for cardiac conduction system development. Cell 129,1365-76.

Muncke N, Jung C, Rudiger H, Ulmer H, Roeth R, Hubert A, Goldmuntz E, Driscoll D, Goodship J, Schon K and others. (2003). Missense mutations and gene interruption in PROSIT240, a novel TRAP240-like gene, in patients with congenital heart defect (transposition of the great arteries). Circulation 108,2843-50.

Nemer G, Fadlalah F, Usta J, Nemer M, Dbaibo G, Obeid M, Bitar F. (2006). A novel mutation in the GATA4 gene in patients with Tetralogy of Fallot. Hum Mutat 27,293-4.

Noonan JA. (1994). Noonan syndrome. An update and review for the primary pediatrician. Clin Pediatr (Phila) 33,548-55.

Oda T, Elkahloun AG, Pike BL, Okajima K, Krantz ID, Genin A, Piccoli DA, Meltzer PS, Spinner NB, Collins FS and others. (1997). Mutations in the human Jagged1 gene are responsible for Alagille syndrome. Nat Genet 16,235-42.

Ohtani K, Dimmeler S. (2011). Epigenetic regulation of cardiovascular differentiation. Cardiovasc Res 90,404-12.

Payne AR, Chang SW, Koenig SN, Zinn AR, Garg V. (2012). Submicroscopic Chromosomal Copy Number Variations Identified in Children With Hypoplastic Left Heart Syndrome. Pediatr Cardiol.

Peng T, Wang L, Zhou SF, Li X. (2010). Mutations of the GATA4 and NKX2.5 genes in Chinese pediatric patients with non-familial congenital heart disease. Genetica 138,1231-40.

Pizzuti A, Sarkozy A, Newton AL, Conti E, Flex E, Digilio MC, Amati F, Gianni D, Tandoi C, Marino B and others. (2003). Mutations of ZFPM2/FOG2 gene in sporadic cases of tetralogy of Fallot. Hum Mutat 22,372-7.

Pober BR. (2010). Williams-Beuren syndrome. N Engl J Med 362,239-52.

Pober BR, Johnson M, Urban Z. (2008). Mechanisms and treatment of cardiovascular disease in Williams-Beuren syndrome. J Clin Invest 118,1606-15.

Posch MG, Gramlich M, Sunde M, Schmitt KR, Lee SH, Richter S, Kersten A, Perrot A, Panek AN, Al Khatib IH and others. (2010). A gain-of-function TBX20 mutation causes congenital atrial septal defects, patent foramen ovale and cardiac valve defects. J Med Genet 47,230-5.

Pueschel SM. (1990). Clinical aspects of Down syndrome from infancy to adulthood. Am J Med Genet Suppl 7,52-6.

Rajagopal SK, Ma Q, Obler D, Shen J, Manichaikul A, Tomita-Mitchell A, Boardman K, Briggs C, Garg V, Srivastava D and others. (2007). Spectrum of heart disease associated with murine and human GATA4 mutation. J Mol Cell Cardiol 43,677-85.

Reamon-Buettner SM, Borlak J. (2004). Somatic NKX2-5 mutations as a novel mechanism of disease in complex congenital heart disease. J Med Genet 41,684-90.

Reamon-Buettner SM, Borlak J. (2010). NKX2-5: an update on this hypermutable homeodomain protein and its role in human congenital heart disease (CHD). Hum Mutat 31,1185-94.

Roessler E, Ouspenskaia MV, Karkera JD, Velez JI, Kantipong A, Lacbawan F, Bowers P, Belmont JW, Towbin JA, Goldmuntz E and others. (2008). Reduced NODAL signaling strength via mutation of several pathway members including FOXH1 is linked to human heart defects and holoprosencephaly. Am J Hum Genet 83,18-29.

Roessler E, Pei W, Ouspenskaia MV, Karkera JD, Velez JI, Banerjee-Basu S, Gibney G, Lupo PJ, Mitchell LE, Towbin JA and others. (2009). Cumulative ligand activity of NODAL mutations and modifiers are linked to human heart defects and holoprosencephaly. Mol Genet Metab 98,225-34.

Sperling S, Grimm CH, Dunkel I, Mebus S, Sperling HP, Ebner A, Galli R, Lehrach H, Fusch C, Berger F and others. (2005). Identification and functional analysis of CITED2 mutations in patients with congenital heart defects. Hum Mutat 26,575-82.

Stennard FA, Costa MW, Lai D, Biben C, Furtado MB, Solloway MJ, McCulley DJ, Leimena C, Preis JI, Dunwoodie SL and others. (2005). Murine T-box transcription factor Tbx20 acts as a repressor during heart development, and is essential for adult heart integrity, function and adaptation. Development 132,2451-62.

Stromme P, Bjornstad PG, Ramstad K. (2002). Prevalence estimation of Williams syndrome. J Child Neurol 17,269-71.

Tartaglia M, Zampino G, Gelb BD. (2010). Noonan syndrome: clinical aspects and molecular pathogenesis. Mol Syndromol 1,2-26.

Tevosian SG, Deconinck AE, Tanaka M, Schinke M, Litovsky SH, Izumo S, Fujiwara Y, Orkin SH. (2000). FOG-2, a cofactor for GATA transcription factors, is essential for heart morphogenesis and development of coronary vessels from epicardium. Cell 101, 729-39.

Tidyman WE, Rauen KA. (2009). The RASopathies: developmental syndromes of Ras/MAPK pathway dysregulation. Curr Opin Genet Dev 19,230-6.

Tomita-Mitchell A, Maslen CL, Morris CD, Garg V, Goldmuntz E. (2007). GATA4 sequence variants in patients with congenital heart disease. J Med Genet 44,779-83.

Turbay D, Wechsler SB, Blanchard KM, Izumo S. (1996). Molecular cloning, chromosomal mapping, and characterization of the human cardiac-specific homeobox gene hCsx. Mol Med 2,86-96.

van der Bom T, Zomer AC, Zwinderman AH, Meijboom FJ, Bouma BJ, Mulder BJ. (2011). The changing epidemiology of congenital heart disease. Nat Rev Cardiol 8, 50-60.

van Rooij E, Sutherland LB, Qi X, Richardson JA, Hill J, Olson EN. (2007). Control of stress-dependent cardiac growth and gene expression by a microRNA. Science 316,575-9.

Williams JC, Barratt-Boyes BG, Lowe JB. (1961). Supravalvular aortic stenosis. Circulation 24,1311-8.

Xin B, Puffenberger E, Tumbush J, Bockoven JR, Wang H. (2007). Homozygosity for a novel splice site mutation in the cardiac myosin-binding protein C gene causes severe neonatal hypertrophic cardiomyopathy. Am J Med Genet A 143A,2662-7.

Xin M, Davis CA, Molkentin JD, Lien CL, Duncan SA, Richardson JA, Olson EN. (2006). A threshold of GATA4 and GATA6 expression is required for cardiovascular development. Proc Natl Acad Sci U S A 103,11189-94.

Yagi H, Furutani Y, Hamada H, Sasaki T, Asakawa S, Minoshima S, Ichida F, Joo K, Kimura M, Imamura S and others. (2003). Role of TBX1 in human del22q11.2 syndrome. Lancet 362,1366-73.

Yuan ZR, Kohsaka T, Ikegaya T, Suzuki T, Okano S, Abe J, Kobayashi N, Yamada M. (1998). Mutational analysis of the Jagged 1 gene in Alagille syndrome families. Hum Mol Genet 7,1363-9.

Zahka K, Kalidas K, Simpson MA, Cross H, Keller BB, Galambos C, Gurtz K, Patton MA, Crosby AH. (2008). Homozygous mutation of MYBPC3 associated with severe infantile hypertrophic cardiomyopathy at high frequency among the Amish. Heart 94,1326-30.

Zhang L, Tumer Z, Jacobsen JR, Andersen PS, Tommerup N, Larsen LA. (2006). Screening of 99 Danish patients with congenital heart disease for GATA4 mutations. Genet Test 10,277-80.

Zhao R, Watt AJ, Battle MA, Li J, Bondow BJ, Duncan SA. (2008). Loss of both GATA4 and GATA6 blocks cardiac myocyte differentiation and results in acardia in mice. Dev Biol 317,614-9.

Zhu L, Vranckx R, Khau Van Kien P, Lalande A, Boisset N, Mathieu F, Wegman M, Glancy L, Gasc JM, Brunotte F and others. (2006). Mutations in myosin heavy chain 11 cause a syndrome associating thoracic aortic aneurysm/aortic dissection and patent ductus arteriosus. Nat Genet 38,343-9.

Chapter 7

The Prototype of Hereditary Periodic Fevers: Familial Mediterranean Fever

Afig Berdeli and Sinem Nalbantoglu

Additional information is available at the end of the chapter

http://dx.doi.org/10.5772/51378

1. Introduction

Autoinflammatory disorders are multisystem periodic fever syndromes, and characterized with recurrent unprovoked inflammation of the serosal membranes. Unlike autoimmune disorders, autoinflammatory disorders lack the production of high-titer autoantibodies or antigen-specific T cells. These diseases primarily include hereditary syndromes (**Table 1**); Familial Mediterrenean fever (FMF), TNF receptor-associated periodic fever syndrome (TRAPS), hyperimmunoglobulinaemia D and periodic fever syndrome (HIDS), and the cryopyrin-associated periodic syndrome (CAPS) which involves familial cold autoinflammatory syndrome (FCAS), Muckle–Wells syndrome (MWS) and neonatal onset multi-system inflammatory disease (NOMID)/chronic infantile neurological cutaneous and articular syndrome (CINCA). Familial mediterrenean fever has been considered as the most prevalent of innate immune system disorders involving systemic autoinflammatory reaction effecting joints, skin, bones and the kidney. Systemic amyloidosis is the most severe manifestation of the disease, commonly effecting the kidneys (11% of cases), and sometimes the adrenals, intestine, spleen, lung, and testis (1). As an innate immune system disorder, FMF is characterized by recurrent episodes of unseemingly unprovoked inflammation and fever with lasting 1- to 3-day attacks accompanied by sterile peritonitis, pleurisy, rash, arthritis, and in some cases amyloidosis leading to renal failure. this (Sohar et al., 1967). Apart from the typical implications of the disease, there is increasing evidence about the expanding clinical spectrum of FMF that embraces unusual clinical characters (2-4). These are the rare presentations of the disease and therefore undescores the role of molecular analysis in particular for the suspicious and probable cases.

FMF is classically transmitted with autosomal recessive inheritance, and has been common among Mediterranean populations; however, previous reports have confirmed its presence worldwide. It has been described in Mediterranean populations, including

Italian, Spanish (5), Portuguese, French, and Greek, as well as in patients from Northern Europe and Japan. Nevertheless, only rare occurrences have been reported throughout the general population because of the low frequency of the causative alleles (6). Among susceptible ethnic groups, FMF prevalence is between 1/500-1/2000, and the carrier rate is between 16-22%. Contrary to the traditionally known monogenic inheritance of the disease, it has been previously evidenced that there have been a number of patients who have the typical FMF phenotype or FMF related symptoms with only one MEFV heterozygous mutation and/or even without any MEFV mutations (5-7), indicating the presence of clinical phenotype not only in homozygous patients, but also similarly in the heterozygous patients with mild disease.

Syndrome (MIM)	State of Inheritance	Gene (GenBank no)	Protein	Age at disease onset
FMF (249100)	Autosomal Recessive (dominant forms are rarely presented)	MEFV (NM_000243) Ch-16	Pyrin (marenostrin)	Childhood
HIDS (260920; 251170)	Autosomal Recessive	MVK (M88468) Ch-12	Mevalonate kinase	Infancy
TRAPS (142680; 191190)	Autosomal Dominant	TNFRSF1A (NM_001065) Ch-12	TNF-receptor type I (p55)	Childhood
CAPS (606416) - MWS - FCAS - CINCA/ NOMID	Autosomal Dominant	NLRP3 Ch-1	Cryopyrin	-Childhood -Infancy -Neonatal
PAPA Syndrome	Autosomal Dominant	PSTPIP1 Ch-15	PSTPIP1	Childhood
Blau Syndrome	Autosomal Dominant	NOD2/CARD15 Ch-16	NOD2/CARD15	Childhood

*CINCA, chronic infantile neurological, cutaneous, and articular syndrome; FCAS, familial cold autoinflammatory syndrome; FMF, familial Mediterranean fever; MWS, Muckle-Wells syndrome; NOMID, neonatal onset multisystem inflammatory disease; PAPA, pyogenic sterile arthritis, pyoderma gangrenosum, and acne; CAPS, cryopyrin-associated periodic syndrome; TRAPS, tumour necrosis factor receptor-associated periodic syndrome.

Table 1. Hereditary autoinflammatory syndromes with identified gene loci (adapted from Lachmann and Hawkins, 2009: 36).

16p13.3 chromosomally located MEFV (Mediterranean Fever) gene has been found responsible for FMF disease, and the protein product, Pyrin, is a 781-amino-acid protein (8-11). Evolutionary conserved domains of pyrin protein involves N-terminal pyrin domain, a B-box zinc-finger, a coiled coil and a C-terminal B30.2 PrySpry domains. Pyrin protein has been reported as a component of the inflammasome complex with both pro-inflammatory and anti-inflammatory role in the cytokine regulation (10-13). Thus, a proapoptotic or antiapoptotic role have been still not precise for the pyrin protein in NF-kB activation and apoptosis (11-16). By means of its PYD and B30.2 interacting domains, pyrin has been shown to bind different proteins of autoinflammatory disease genes. Each interacting protein that binds through the pyrin domains (PYD) consists of PSTPIP1 (17), 14-3-3 (18), Caspase-1 (19), ASC (20), and Siva (21).

In 1997, The International FMF Consortium and The French FMF Consortium reported four missense disease associated mutations in the MEFV gene involving M694V, M680I, V726A, and M694I. Major and minor mutations of MEFV gene are well documented in INFEVERS, the database of hereditary autoinflammatory disorder mutations, and exons 2 and 10 comprises the hot-spots (22). To date, mutations have been mostly identified in exons 2, 3, 5, and 10 of the MEFV gene. According to previous reports by Touitou I. (2001), and by the Turkish FMF study group (2005), the most common MEFV mutation in Turkey is M694V (57.0 and 51.4%, respectively), followed by M680I (16.5 and 14.4%, respectively), and V726A (13.9 and 8.6%, respectively). Moreover, no correlation has been reported between various MEFV gene mutations and the severity of the phenotype in various populations supporting the genotypic and phenotypic heterogeneity present for FMF (5, 23-25).

According to INFEVERS (22), the database of hereditary autoinflammatory disorder mutations, To date, approximately 222 sequence variants including both missense mutations (only one nonsense mutation; Y688X) and polymorphisms have been defined in the FMF gene (MEFV), INFEVERS, 100 of them was clinically associated with the phenotype, 33 of them was not associated with the disease and the remaining was of uncertain pathogenicity. The remarkably wide clinical variability of the disease, as indicated by previous reports, has been linked to the MEFV allelic heterogeneity that underlies genotypic and phenotypic heterogeneity (23, 26, 27), and this has made detailed mutation screening critically important. In particular, Turkish FMF patients are characterized by an increased genetic heterogeneity due to various mutation frequencies from different regions, explained by the intrapopulation differentiation.

With respect to our mutation screenings, a previous comprehensive study was performed with 3430 Turkish individuals from all regions of Turkey (ages range from 2 months to 67 years; 2101 females and 1329 males) including first and second-degree relatives of individuals with FMF clinical diagnoses (including suspicious, possible, and definitive cases) who referred to the Molecular Medicine Laboratory for genetic diagnosis between years May, 2005 and December, 2010. The Tel-Hashomer and Livneh criteria were used for the clinical diagnosis of FMF based on the model of major, minor, and supportive criteria, which stipulates the presence of either 1 major or 2 minor criteria or 1 minor and 5 supportive criteria for a diagnosis. A simple set of criteria for the diagnosis of FMF required

1 or more major and/or 2 or more minor criteria (28). None of the patients with FMF had an immunological disorder or another rheumatic disease. Active clinical presentations (fever, abdominal pain, arthritis, and myalgia) and laboratory parameters (high levels of serum amyloid A [SAA], C-reactive protein [CRP], fibrinogen, white blood cell [WBC] counts and erythrocyte sedimentation rates [ESR]) were determined for each patient. For the detection of all coding and non-coding sequence variations along the MEFV gene, we performed bidirectional DNA sequencing analysis in all 10 coding exons and exon-intron boundaries of the respective gene, and reported frequencies of common and rare nucleotide substitutions and synonymous and non-synonimous single nucleotide polymorphisms obtained in the Turkish population (7).

2. Methods

2 ml peripheral blood was collected into ethylenediaminetetraacetic acid (EDTA)-anticoagulated tubes by the standard venipuncture method and DNA was extracted using the QIAamp DNA Blood Isolation kit (Qiagen GmbH, Hilden, Germany) following the manufacturer's instructions. The extracted DNA concentration was determined using a Thermo Scientific NanoDrop spectrophotometer (Wilmington, USA). The quality assessment of the extracted DNA was determined by 2% agarose gel electrophoresis.

2.1. FMF strip asay - Reverse hybridization multiplex PCR

Reverse hybridization assay (FMF StripAssay, Viennalab Labordiagnostika GmbH) was used to investigate the mutations. According to the manufacturer's instructions, in a first step multiplex PCR was performed using biotinylated primers for exons 2, 3, 5, 10 amplification. PCR products were selectively hybridized to a test strip presenting a paralel array of allele-specific oligonucleotide probes which includes 12 MEFV mutations [E148Q, P369S, F479L, M680I (G/C), M680I (G/A), I692del, M694V, M694I, K695R, V726A, A744S, R761H]. Hybridizations were illuminated by the reaction of streptavidin-alkaline phosphatase and color substrate.

2.2. DNA sequencing strategy

Hot-spots, exons 10, and 2; with 3 and 5, and when necessary exons 1, 4, 6, 7, 8 and 9 of the MEFV gene were analyzed for MEFV mutations by PCR amplification followed by automated DNA sequence analysis. One microliter (100 ng) of genomic DNA was added to Polymerase Chain Reaction (PCR) amplification buffer containing 20 mM Tris (pH 8.3); 50 mM KCl; 1.5 mM $MgCl_2$; 0.2 mM each of dATP, 2′-deoxycytidine 5′-triphosphate, dGTP, and 2′-deoxythymidine 5′-triphosphate; 10 pmol each of reverse and forward primers provided by Invitrogen; and 1.0 U of PlatiniumTaq DNA Polymerase (Invitrogen, Carlsbad, CA) in a total volume of 25 µl. The cycling conditions included a hot-start denaturation step at 95°C for 10 min, followed by 35 amplification cycles of denaturation at 95°C for 30 s, annealing at 61°C for exon 10, 58°C for exons 2 and 3, or 57°C for exon 5 for 40 s, and elongation at 72°C for 45 s; a final extension was performed at 72°C for 7 min (the oligonucleotide sequences are available upon request). Prior to sequencing, PCR products were purified using an ExoSAP-IT PCR Product Clean-Up kit. BigDye Terminatorv3.1 Cycle Sequencing Kit (Applied Biosystems, San Diego, CA, USA) was used in cycle sequencing reactions. Cycle sequencing PCR products followed purification with the BigDyeXT kit(Applied Biosystems,) and the data were analyzed using an ABI3130xl Genetic Analyzer (Applied Biosystems). DNA sequencing was performed in both directions, initiated from the forward and reverse primers that were used in the initial PCR reaction. SeqScape 2.0 sequence analysis software (Applied Biosystems, San Diego, CA, USA) was employed for sequence evaluation.

2.3. Restriction fragment length polymorphism analysis (RFLP)

A RFLP was identified in the mutation site and was utilized for mutation detection. Amplicons encompassing exon 5 were digested with the restriction enzyme Tsp509I, and electrophoresed on a 1% agarose gel.

3. Results

We found that M694V accounted for the majority of FMF chromosomes (44%), followed by E148Q (19%), V726A (10%), M680I (10%), P369S (4%), R408Q (3%), K695R (2%), M694I and R761H (1.6%), A744S (1.4%), and F479L (0.09%) (**Tables 2, 3**). Missense disease-causing mutations and synonymous polymorphisms accounted for 38% and 54% of MEFV chromosomes, respectively. Among the Turkish general population, the most frequent healthy heterozygous carrier mutation was found E148Q (6.9%), and the carrier rate was found 16%, with a mutation frequency of 8% (Berdeli et al., 2011). Except for the known major FMF mutations, by DNA sequencing, we frequently detect additional rare and novel mutations and critical SNPs about which we have only limited information in Turkish FMF patients. Remarkable consequences of sequencing analysis have been found relative to mutation-SNP combination underlying the combined existence of nucleotide variations in the same haplotype.

For patients whose MEFV gene does not contain mutations of exons 2, 3, 5, and 10, we performed bidirectional DNA sequencing also in exons 1, 4, 6, 7, 8, and 9. However, we could not find any disease related mutation except for an exon 9 homozygous SNP, P588P, which is thought to be symptomatic with disease relation. This SNP was always in homozygous state and was not seen in combination with any of the major and minor mutations or any of the SNPs in the entire coding and non-coding regions of the gene. Relative to our experiences, this SNP has a disease relation to a minor degree, however possible validation of other autoinflammatory disease gene mutations should need to be considered. Single P588P SNP was associated with continuously high SAA levels and musculoskeletal complications which has a good response to colchicine in a three-member family who did not have any sequence variations along other coding and non-coding regions of the MEFV gene.

Genotype					
MEFV Mutation				Number of Patients	Genotype Frequency
Exon 2	Exon 3	Exon 5	Exon 10	No	(%)
			M680IG-C/Wt	69	5.24
			M680IG-A/Wt	5	0.37
			M680IG-C/M680I	12	0.91
			M680IG-C/V726A	23	1.74
			M680IG-C/ M694V	42	3.19
E230K			M680IG-C/ M694V	2	0.15
			M680IG-C/A744S	1	0.12
			M680IG-C/ R761H	2	0.15
E148Q			M680IG-C	4	0.3
E167D		F479L	M680IG-C	1	0.07
E167D		F479L		2	0.15
		F479L/Wt		1	0.12
			M694V/Wt	322	24.4
			M694V/M694V	91	6.91
			M694V/V722M*	1	0.12
			M694V/V726A	42	3.19
			M694V/R761H	5	0.37
			M694V/K695R	2	0.15
			M694V/A744S	1	0.12
R241K			M694V/	1	0.12
E230K			M694V/	3	0.22
E148Q	P369S		M694V	1	0.12
E148Q/S179N*			M694V	1	0.12
E148Q/Wt				237	18
E148Q/E148Q				19	1.44
E148Q			M694V	42	3.19
E148Q			L709R	1	0.12
E148Q	P369S			4	0.3
E148Q			V726A	7	0.53
E148Q			A744S	1	0.12
E148Q			M694I	7	0.53
E148Q			K695N	1	0.12
E148Q			R761H	4	0.3
E148Q			I72OM	2	0.15
E148Q/L110P				6	0.45
E148Q/R151S				1	0.12

Genotype					
MEFV Mutation				Number of Patients	Genotype Frequency
Exon 2	Exon 3	Exon 5	Exon 10	No	(%)
E148Q			K695R	2	0.15
E148Q/T267M				1	0.12
E148Q/E230K				4	0.3
E148Q/T267I				1	0.12
E148Q/L110P			M694I	1	0.12
E148Q	P369S/R408Q			18	1.36
E148Q	P369S/R408Q		M680I	1	0.12
			M694I/A744S	1	0.12
			V726A/Wt	111	8.43
			V726A/V726A	4	0.3
E167D			V726A	3	0.22
			V726A/M694I	2	0.15
			V726A/R761H	3	0.22
			V726A/R761H/ M680IG-C	1	0.12
			V726A/K695R	1	0.12
		F479L	V726A	3	0.22
			K695R/Wt	38	2.88
			A744S/Wt	19	1.44
	P369S/Wt			7	0.53
	P369S/R408Q			40	3.03
	P369S/R408Q		M694V	4	0.3
			M694I/Wt	10	0.75
			R761H/Wt	31	2.35
			R761H/ A744S	1	0.12
			R653H/Wt	1	0.12
			E685K/E685K	1	0.12
L110P/L1010P				1	0.12
E230K/E230K				1	0.12
E230K/ Wt				1	0.12
T267M/Wt				3	0.22
R241K/R241K				1	0.12
E148V/Wt				5	0.37
E148L/Wt				2	0.15
E167D/Wt				2	0.15
	P350R/Wt			1	0.12
	P350R		A744S	2	0.15

Genotype					
MEFV Mutation				**Number of Patients**	**Genotype Frequency**
Exon 2	**Exon 3**	**Exon 5**	**Exon 10**	**No**	**(%)**
		G456A/Wt		1	0.12
		S503C/Wt		2	0.15
		I506V/Wt		1	0.12
		Y471X/Wt		1	0.12
	G340R/Wt			1	0.12
S141I/Wt				3	0.22
S166L/Wt				2	0.15
		A511V/Wt		1	0.12
	R354W/Wt			1	0.12
	S339F/Wt			4	0.3
	R329H/Wt			3	0.22
	R329H/		M694V	1	0.12
E148Q	R329H/			1	0.12
Heterozygotes				885	67.2
Compound heterozygotes				271	20.5
Homozygotes				130	9.87
Complex genotypes				30	2.27
Total number of patients with mutations				1316	38.36
No mutation or SNPs identified				231	6.7
Total number of patients with only SNPs (+**R202Q**)				1883	54.8
Total number of patients				3430	100

*, novel mutations

Table 2. DNA sequencing results of MEFV genotyping among 3430 Turkish patients.

Mutation	Number of Alleles (No)	Allelic Frequency (%)
M694V	908	44.7
E148Q	386	19
V726A	204	10
M680IG-C	170	8.3
P369S	75	3.69
R408Q	63	3.1
K695R	43	2.11
M694I	21	1
R761H	47	2.31
A744S	26	1.28
E148V	5	0.24
E167D	8	0,39
T267M	4	0.19
L110P	8	0.39
R241K	3	0.14
I720M	2	0.09
E230K	12	0.59
M680IG-A	5	0.24
E148L	2	0.09
F479L	7	0.34
E685K	2	0.09
R653H	1	0.04
T267I	1	0.04
V722M	1	0.04
S141I	3	0.14
S339F	4	0.19
R151S	1	0.04
I506V	1	0.04
S503C	2	0.09
L709R	1	0.04
K695N	1	0.04
P350R	3	0.14
G340R	1	0.04
G456A	1	0.04
Y471X	1	0.04
R329H	5	0.24
S166L	2	0.09
S179N	1	0.04
A511V	1	0.04
R354W	1	0.04
Total	**2033**	**100**

Table 3. Allelic frequencies of totally 40 MEFV mutations involving major, rare and, novel sequence changes among the detected mutations in 1316 mutation positive patients group (mutation frequency for the studied mutations; complex alleles excluded).

Additionally, sequence analysis revealed that there was a single FMF-associated mutation in the MEFV coding region of 76% of the Turkish individuals studied, and 80% of these individuals initiated colchicine treatment following molecular diagnosis. The prevalence of a single mutation in patients experiencing a pathogenic effect in Turkey (76%) is contrary to the expected pattern of autosomal recessive inheritance and does not support the "heterozygous advantage" selection theory. However, the expression of the FMF phenotype may be influenced by other candidate modifier gene loci, autoinflammatory pathway genes or FMF-like diseases (29-31). For this reason, genome-wide association studies involving more patients should be performed and the data included in future investigations covering critical coding and noncoding gene SNPs for Turkish FMF patients.

As an ancestral population of FMF, Turkey was one of the regions which involves most of the rare and novel mutations. As referenced in INVEFERS, most of the rare mutations in view of the ethnic origins were found to be symptomatic. Novel Y471X mutation found in the present study was the second nonsense mutation in FMF era. Among the newly identified mutations, involving R151S, S166N, S179N, and G340R; P350R, G456A, Y471X, S503C, I506V, L709R and K695N; Y471X, R151S, L709R, and K695N were observed as pathogenic reflecting the typical FMF character. The main clinical characteristics of the patients were as follows: abdominal pain (92.1%), fever (93.9%), thoracic pain (59%), myalgia (67.8%), arthritis (55.1%), erysipelas like erythema (ELE) (21.8%). None of the patients developed amyloidosis. This finding verifies the importance of molecular diagnosis and detailed sequencing which is recommended to perform in particular for the ancestral populations of FMF.

In this report, from a large scaled heterogeneous group of patients, we describe a 44-year-old Turkish patient from Western Turkey with clinical diagnosis of periodic fever. The case presented here is a 44-year-old Turkish woman, from western Turkey. The course of the patient includes short and rare episodes of fever, ongoing abdominal pain, temporary myalgia and arthralgia since her childhood. Physical examination revealed no pathology except for arthritis on the right knee. Her weight, height, and blood pressure were normal. Primarily, she had diagnosed as having conditions secondary to FMF. Although family and relatives screening are of great importance, her family (parents are dead in an accident) and past history were noncontributory and unhappy. She had undergone antibiotherapy, steroid treatment and appendectomy. Laboratory tests revealed the acute phase reactants as follows; ESR 81 mm/h, SAA 76 mg/dl, CRP 3.46 mg/dl, and fibrinogen 526 mg/dl. Renal function tests and other biochemical parameters were normal. No molecular genetic diagnosis was done except for Strip Assay in other centers. The clinical figure associated with her was not much contributed to the start of colchicine not fulfilling most of the clinical criteria, so in our laboratory, FMF strip assay was used as the first stage of mutation detection method involving 12 common mutations. However, no particular mutation was identified. Thereafter, DNA sequence analysis revealed the responsible nonsense mutation, p.Y471X, in MEFV gene (**Figure 1**). By means of the molecular diagnosis, colchicine therapy (1.5 mg/day) was started properly. She had no symptoms after the colchicine therapy and had a good response to 1,5 mg/d, and the acute phase reactants were completely normal in the last 3 years. So, other autoinflammatory genes, MVK, TNFRSF1A, CIAS1, were not considered to evaluate as the suspicious genes in this case and were not evaluated as molecular diagnostics.

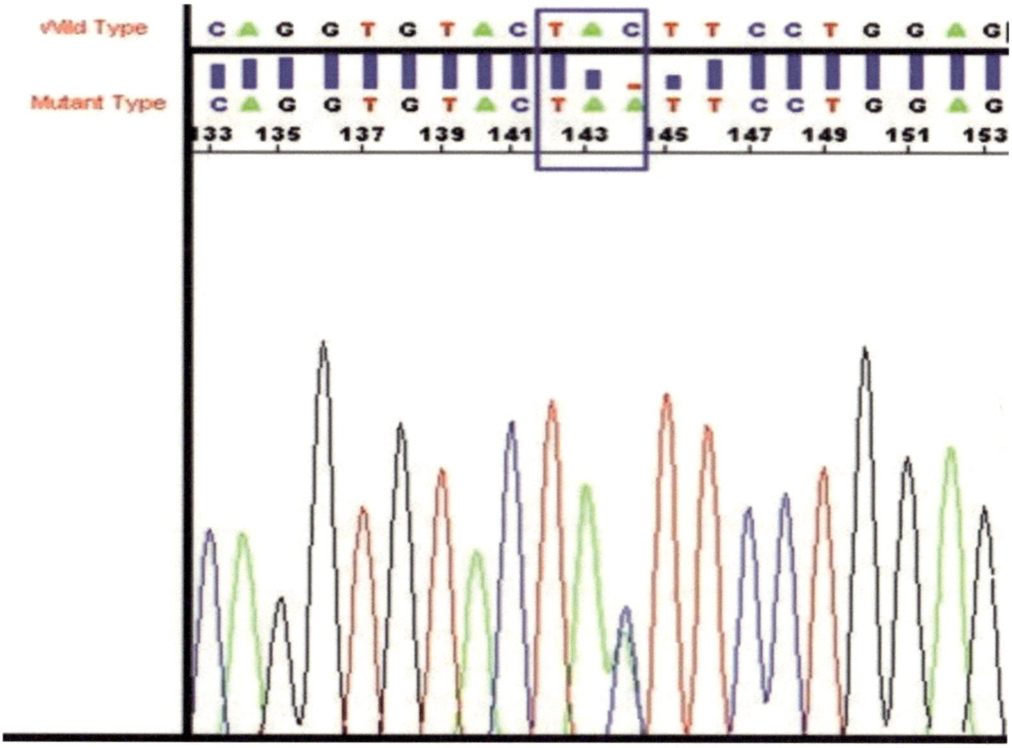

Figure 1. Electropherogram of the p.Y471X nonsense mutation in the MEFV gene revealed by DNA Sequencing analysis in the Turkish patient.

The case presented here was one of the patients who had misdiagnosis in particularly during the childhood losing time by unnecessary processes and treatments. Therefore, certain diagnosis determined by detailed DNA sequence analysis is essential for suspicious and undefined cases, and for cases disestablished by other limited screening methods. In the molecular analysis of Mediterranean fever gene, c.1413C>A nucleotide change in exon 5 resulting in p.Tyr471X nonsense mutation was determined (Figure I). We also exploited the fact that the p.Y471X creates a novel recognition site for the Tsp509I restriction enzyme to develop a PCR-RFLP assay in order to screen the affected families and healthy controls for the mutation.

Y471X nonsense mutation in MEFV gene is the first noted in Turkish FMF patients (7), and the second nonsense mutation of FMF mutation database worldwide. Inherited missens mutations reported in the 5th exon of MEFV gene in FMF patients are very rare. Though the fifth exon of the gene could not called as a critical region carrying the mutational hotspots, the result could demonstrate there is still way to walk on the road through the hidden side of FMF. Novel Y471X mutation in exon 5 of the MEFV gene located in the coiled coil domain of pyrin protein is implicated in association with actin binding interacting selectively with monomeric or multimeric forms of actin. Since effects of nonsense mutations in the amino acids are known damaging and pathogenic, we did not use the PolyPhen software (32) in order to evaluate the potential pathogenicity of this newly found amino acid substitution which we carry out regularly in our laboratory. Nevertheless, expression studies will be required.

Due to the abundance of mutations in exon 10 and clinical heterogeneity of the disease, different screening methods have been developed. As long been known the majority of FMF patients in classically affected populations were screened by routine methods for only common mutations, which primarily targets only the most prevalent MEFV mutations in a specific population; thus, rare or novel mutations can be overlooked. The first nonsense mutation in FMF era, Y688X, was evaluated by Touitou I. (5), and was suggested to have a location between two well-known hotspots for FMF mutations (codons 680 and 694) in exon 10. This finding contributed to the critical role of exon 10 for the MEFV function as an hotspot. Here, it is discussed that, the newly found Y471X nonsense mutation has a great significance in screening asymptomatic individuals since it was not found in one of the hot-spots of MEFV gene.

Autoinflammatory diseases are heterogeneous group of disorders, thus FMF like phenotypes and related genes most likely exists (33-36). In some cases, the causal genes may not only be the unique causes of the diseases. It is well known that Mendelian disorders caused by the dysfunction of a single gene have a wide heterogeneity of disease phenotypes (37). FMF has both genetic and phenotypic heterogeneity and mutations within a single gene are known to cause different clinical phenotypes in Turkey. Thus, all MEFV gene sequence variations found in symptomatic cases should not be considered as causative pathogenic disease mutations. In particular, FMF related Turkish patients with no MEFV mutation or with only single MEFV mutations may not actually reflect the phenotype seen in FMF.

Another point is subclinical inflammation concerning asymptomatic heterozygous patients without a second mutation mostly continues with the typical disease characteristics possibly due to the presence of other modifier genes and/or environmental factors. Therefore, factors other than casual MEFV gene and other pyrin-dependent effects should be contributing to the sustainable systemic inflammation that is sufficient for the occurrence of the symptomatic FMF related phenotype. Previously, MICA, TLR2 and SAA loci were shown as modifying alleles in FMF (5, 38). Synonimous or non-synonimous sequence variations of MEFV relevant genes involving SAA and TLR2 were previously considered as critical factors for the course of the disease. Both SAA1 locus and Arg753Gln TLR2 polymorphism were implied as genetic susceptible loci for a risk factor of developing secondary amyloidosis in different ethnic populations of FMF patients (26, 27, 30). Against the traditionally considered monogenic inheritance pattern, compound heterozygotes of 2 autoinflammatory disease genes were also reported describing patients who were found to have 2 or more reduced penetrance mutations, involving E148Q in MEFV, R92Q or P46L in

TNFRSF1A, V377I in MVK, and V198M in CIAS1 (29, 34, 35). For the purpose of screening mutations in other known autoinflammatory genes for typical FMF patients carrying 1 single heterozygous MEFV mutation, Booty et al screened 6 candidate genes that encode proteins known to interact with pyrin or genes functioning in IL-1B pathway involving ASC/PYCARD, SIVA, CASP1, PSTPIP1, POP1, and POP2 (6). A novel PSTPIP1 nucleotide mutation, two novel substitutions in ASC/PYCARD and SIVA genes were identified while Casp1, POP1, and POP2 were mutation negative. In a Jewish patient with FMF, novel W171X (513G>A) mutation was identified which is presumed as a stop codon, to remove the last 2 of the 6 helices in the CARD domain of ASC/PYCARD. In FMF patients with only 1 MEFV mutation, including milder FMF-associated mutations, 1 Turkish patient was identified as a carrier of W171X (6). To date, SNPs in ASC/PYCARD gene were identified in 5′/3′ region, exon 1, intron 1, exon 3 coding region involving rs79351176, rs8056505, rs11648861, rs79464842, rs73532217, rs75471387, rs11867108, rs61086377, rs76878620, and rs75216100. In the ASC/PYCARD protein, the conserved PyD domain is 91 aa in lenght (1-91) and CARD domain is 89 aa in lenght (107-195). The previously reported W171X (513G>A) mutation (31) corresponds to the exon 3 coding region of the ASC/PYCARD gene and results with a stop codon. Thus, in our sequencing analysis, we also searched the presence of mutations in the ASC/PYCARD gene in our entire patients group. However, this sequence was not mutated, and we have neither identified the above substitutions along the entire coding regions and flanking segments of ASC/PYCARD gene (unpublished data).

For investigating of mutations in other periodic fever disease genes, in a study of our group, a total of 75 Turkish patients and 25 ethnically matched healthy control individuals diagnosed with periodic fever was molecularly diagnosed for having mutations in causative disease genes (apart from the present patients group; unpublished data). Mutation screening of coding and noncoding regions of MVK, TNFRSF1A, and NLRP3/CIAS1 genes were carried out for different group of patients according to their clinical implications.

MVK gene transcript variant 1 (12q24; NM_000431.2→NP_000422.1) was fully sequenced in 25 periodic fever patients. Molecular diagnosis revealed the following results: p.Ser52Asn missense mutation was identified in 6 patients. In addition, p.Asp170Asp and p.Ser135Ser synonimous aminoacid mutations and IVS6-18 A>G, homozygous IVS9+24 G>A, and IVS 4+8 C/T intronic nucleotide substitutions were observed in the remaining patients group.

NLRP3 gene (CIAS1; 1q44; NM_004895.4→NP_004886.3) NACHT, LRR and PYD domains-containing protein 3 isoform a was fully sequenced in 25 periodic fever patients. Molecular diagnosis revealed the following nucleotide substitutions in the screened gene region: K608fsX611 frameshift mutation, p.Ser726Gly and p.Gln703Lys missense mutations, together with Ser34Ser, Ala242Ala, Arg260Arg, Thr219Thr ve Leu411Leu synonimous aminoacid mutations.

TNFRSF1A gene (12p13.2; NM_001065.3→NP_001056.1) tumor necrosis factor receptor superfamily member 1A precursor form was fully sequenced in 25 periodic fever patients. Molecular diagnosis revealed the following nucleotide substitutions in the screened gene region: p. Arg92Gln and p. Ala301Thr missense mutations with IVS6+10 A>G and IVS8-23 T>C intronic nucleotide substitutions.

Intronic nucleotide substitutions and synonimous aminoacid mutations of all the screened gene regions were also observed in the 25 ethnically matched healthy control individuals. Mutation frequency was 4% (1/25), 32% (8/25), and 40% (n:10/25) in TRAPS, HIDS, and CAPS patients.

Nonetheless, finding of symptomatic rare MEFV mutations in particular for at-risk populations and the individuals who have been asymptomatic and negative for common mutations makes detailed mutation screening critically important in FMF. It has been previously evidenced that there have been a number of patients who have typical FMF phenotype or FMF related symptoms with only one MEFV heterozygous mutation and/or even without any MEFV mutations (6, 7).

The majority of FMF patients in classically affected populations are screened by routine methods that are limited to the detection of common mutations. These tests primarily target the most prevalent MEFV mutations to rule out asymptomatic cases in at-risk populations. Therefore, while searching for the common mutations that underlie typical FMF symptoms, we should primarily consider the entire coding sequence of the MEFV gene before analyzing other recurrent fever genes. Patients with no mutation or with only single pyrin mutations may not actually reflect the phenotype seen in FMF. Compound heterozygotes of 2 autoinflammatory disease genes involving MEFV, TNFRSF1A, CIAS1, and MVK were reported (29, 34, 35). Thus, screening of other autoinflammatory disease genes, e.g. CIAS, were considered for the MEFV gene mutation/SNP negative FMF patients. In conclusion, by using sequencing analysis, we can prevent less common, population-restricted, novel sequence variants from being overlooked. This has implications for the characterization of typical and atypical FMF; screening for the most common mutations by routine methods is sufficient for the initial laboratory diagnosis of FMF in Turkish patients; however, the results should be confirmed by specific DNA sequencing of all coding exons and exon-intron flanking regions.

4. Conclusions

Among the newly identified mutations in this comprehensive study, Y471X, R151S, L709R, and K695N were observed as pathogenic reflecting the typical FMF character involving abdominal pain, fever, thoracic pain, myalgia, arthritis, and erysipelas like erythema. Rare mutations and SNPs have great importance for FMF pathogenesis. For this periodic fever disorder, heterogeneity is present in phases of allelic, frequency and critical locations of mutant alleles, and clinical appearance. Therefore, in particular for the suspicious cases; possible presence of other autoinflammatory disease gene mutations as we outlined above and rare mutations and SNP variations in the MEFV gene, molecular techniques, sample sizes, ethnic origins, and regions in the ancestral countries should be regarded as critical and determinative keys in FMF clinical and molecular diagnosis.

Sequencing analysis not only the common major mutations but also the detection of rare mutations can be carried out which have great importance in particular for at-risk populations. By means of sequencing analysis, we could prevent the missing of less common rare variants that might be restricted to the populations by routine techniques. The majority of FMF patients in classically affected populations are screened by routine methods that are limited to the detection of common mutations. These tests primarily target the most prevalent MEFV mutations to rule out asymptomatic cases in at-risk populations. Therefore, while searching for the common mutations that underlie typical FMF symptoms, we should primarily consider the entire coding sequence of the MEFV gene before analyzing other recurrent fever genes. In conclusion, by using sequencing analysis, we can prevent less common, population-restricted, novel sequence variants from being overlooked. This has implications for the characterization of typical and atypical FMF; screening for the most common mutations by routine methods is sufficient for the initial laboratory diagnosis of FMF in Turkish patients; however, the results should be confirmed by specific DNA sequencing of all coding exons and exon-intron flanking regions. We should consider gene mutation screening in early diagnosis and the follow-up of the clinical course in particular for the asymptomatic cases. Early determination of the disease causing mutation will be favorable in order to prevent abundant treatments in newly diagnosed patients.

Author details

Afig Berdeli and Sinem Nalbantoglu
Ege University, School of Medicine, Children's Hospital, Molecular Medicine Laboratory, Bornova, Izmir, Turkey

Acknowledgement

We would like to thank patients and clinicians for their participation and contribution in our study.

5. References

[1] Touitou I. The spectrum of Familial Mediterranean Fever (FMF) mutations. Eur J Hum Genet, 2001; 9(7):473-83.
[2] Schwabe AD, Peters RS. Familial Mediterranean fever in Armenians: analysis of 100 cases. Medicine (Baltimore), 1974; 53:453–62.
[3] Tufan A, Babaoglu MO, Akdogan A, Yasar U, Calguneri M, Kalyoncu U, Karadag O, Hayran M, Ertenli AI, Bozkurt A, Kiraz S. Association of drug transporter gene ABCB1 (MDR1) 3435C to T polymorphism with colchicine response in familial Mediterranean fever. J Rheumatol, 2007; 34(7):1540-4.
[4] Özçakar B., Yalçınkaya F., Yüksel S., Ekim M. The expanded clinical spectrum of familial Mediterranean fever. Clin Rheumatol, 2007; 26:1557–1560.

[5] Touitou I., The spectrum of Familial Mediterranean Fever (FMF) mutations, Eur J Hum Genet. 9(7) (2001) 473-83.

[6] Booty M., Chae J., Masters S., Remmers E., Barham B., Le JM., Barron KS., Holland SM., Kastner DL., Aksentijevich A. F amilial Mediterranean Fever With a Single MEFV Mutation. Where Is the Second Hit? Arthritis & Rheumatism, 2009; 60 (6): 1851–1861.

[7] Berdeli A, Mir S, Nalbantoglu S, Kutukculer N, Sozeri B, Kabasakal Y, Cam S, Solak M. Comprehensive analysis of a large-scale screen for MEFV gene mutations: do they truly provide a "heterozygote advantage" in Turkey? Genet Test Mol Biomarkers. 2011 Jul-Aug;15(7-8):475-82. Epub 2011 Mar 17.

[8] French FMF Consortium. (1997) A candidate gene for familial Mediterranean fever. Nat Genet, 17(1):25-31.

[9] The International FMF consortium. (1997) Ancient missensemutations in a new member of the RoRet gene family are likely to cause familial Mediterranean fever. Cell, 90: 797-807.

[10] Yu JW, Wu J, Zhang Z, Datta P, Ibrahimi I, Taniguchi S, Sagara J, Fernandes-Alnemri T, Alnemri ES., Cryopyrin and pyrin activate caspase-1, but not NF-kappaB, via ASC oligomerization, Cell Death Differ. 2006; 13(2):236-49.

[11] Chae, J.J. Komarow HD, Cheng J, Wood G, Raben N, Liu PP, et al. Targeted disruption of pyrin, the FMF protein, causes heightened sensitivity to endotoxin and a defect in macrophage apoptosis. Mol. Cell 2003; 11, 591–604.

[12] Diaz, A., Hu, C., Kastner, D. L., et al. Arthritis Rheum, 2004, 50: 3679–3689.

[13] Centola M, Wood G, Frucht DM, et al. The gene for familial Mediterranean fever, MEFV, is expressed in early leukocyte development and is regulated in response to inflammatory mediators. Blood, 2000, 95:3223–31.

[14] Gumucio DL, Diaz A, Schaner P, et al. Fire and ICE: the role of pyrin domain-containing proteins in inflammation and apoptosis. Clin Exp Rheumatol, 2002, 26:S45-53.

[15] Masumoto J, Dowds TA, Schaner P, et al. ASC is an activating adaptor for NF-kappa B and caspase-8-dependent apoptosis. Biochem Biophys Res Commun, 2003,303(1):69-73.

[16] Marek-Yagel D, Berkun Y, Padeh S, Abu A, Reznik-Wolf H, Livneh A, Pras M, Pras E. Clinical disease among patients heterozygous for familial Mediterranean fever. Arthritis Rheum. 2009 Jun;60(6):1862-6.

[17] Shoham, N.G. et al. Pyrin binds the PSTPIP1/CD2BP1 protein, defining familial Mediterranean fever and PAPA syndrome as disorders in the same pathway. Proc. Natl. Acad. Sci, 2003, 100:13501–13506.

[18] Jeru I, Papin S, L'Hoste S, et al. Interaction of pyrin with 14.3.3 in an isoform-specific and phosphorylation-dependent manner regulates its translocation to the nucleus. Arthritis Rheum, 2005, 52:1848–1857.

[19] Chae, J.J. et al. The B30.2 domain of pyrin, the familial Mediterranean fever protein, interacts directly with caspase-1 to modulate IL-1b production. Proc. Natl. Acad. Sci, 2006, 103: 9982–9987.

[20] Richards N, Schaner P, Diaz A, et al. Interaction between pyrin and the apoptotic speck protein (ASC) modulates ASC-induced apoptosis. J Biol Chem, 2001,276(42):39320–9.

[21] Balci-Peynircioglu B, Waite AL, Hu C, et al. Pyrin, product of the MEFV locus, interacts with the proapoptotic protein, Siva. J Cell Physiol, 2008.

[22] http://fmf.igh.cnrs.fr/ISSAID/infevers/

[23] Shohat M, Magal N, Shohat T, Chen X, Dagan T, Mimouni A, Danon Y, Lotan R, Ogur G, Sirin A, Schlezinger M, Halpern GJ, Schwabe A, Kastner D, Rotter JI, Fischel-Ghodsian N. Phenotype-genotype correlation in familial Mediterranean fever: evidence for an association between Met694Val and amyloidosis. Eur J Hum Genet. 1999 Apr;7(3):287-92.

[24] Yalçinkaya F, Tekin M, Cakar N, Akar E, Akar N, Tümer N. Familial Mediterranean fever and systemic amyloidosis in untreated Turkish patients. QJM. 2000 Oct;93(10):681-4.

[25] Papadopoulos V, Mitroulis I, Giaglis S. MEFV heterogeneity in Turkish Familial Mediterranean Fever patients. Mol Biol Rep. 2010 Jan;37(1):355-8.

[26] Cazeneuve C, Papin S, Jéru I, et al. Subcellular localisation of marenostrin/pyrin isoforms carrying the most common mutations involved in familial Mediterranean fever in the presence or absence of its binding partner ASC. J Med Genet, 2004, 41(3):e24.

[27] Gershoni-Baruch R, Brik R, Shinawi M, et al. The differential contribution of MEFV mutant alleles to the clinical profile of familial Mediterranean fever. Eur J Hum Genet, 2002,10:145–9.

[28] Livneh A, Langevitz P, Zemer D, et al. Criteria for the diagnosis of FMF. Arthritis Rheum, 1997, 40(10):1879-85.

[29] Singh-Grewal D, Chaitow J, Aksentijevich I, et al. Coexistent MEFV and CIAS1 mutations manifesting as familial Mediterranean fever plus deafness [letter]. Ann Rheum Dis, 2007, 66:1541.

[30] Ozen S, Berdeli A, Türel B, et al. Arg753Gln TLR-2 polymorphism in familial mediterranean fever: linking the environment to the phenotype in a monogenic inflammatory disease. J Rheumatol, 2006, 33(12):2498-500. Epub 2006 Oct 1.

[31] Samuels J, Ozen S. Familial Mediterranean fever and the other autoinflammatory syndromes: evaluation of the patient with recurrent fever. Curr Opin Rheumatol 2006;18:108–17.

[32] http://coot.embl.de/PolyPhen.

[33] Kastner DL, Aksentijevich I. Intermittent and periodic arthritis syndromes. In: Koopman WJ, Moreland LW, editors. Arthritis and allied conditions: a textbook of rheumatology. 15th ed. Philadelphia: Lippincott Williams & Wilkins; 2005. p. 1411–61.

[34] Stojanov S, Kastner DL. Familial autoinflammatory diseases: genetics, pathogenesis and treatment. Curr Opin Rheumatol, 2005, 17:586–99.

[35] Touitou I, Perez C, Dumont B, et al. Refractory auto-inflammatory syndrome associated with digenic transmission of low-penetrance tumour necrosis factor receptor-associated periodic syndrome and cryopyrin-associated periodic syndrome mutations. Ann Rheum Dis, 2006, 65:1530–1.

[36] Helen J Lachmann and Philip N Hawkins. Developments in the scientific and clinical understanding of autoinflammatory disorders. 2009.

[37] Bell J. Predicting disease using genomics. Nature, 2004, 429:453–6.
[38] Shaw PJ, Lukens JR, Burns S, et al. Cutting Edge: critical role for PYCARD/ASC in the development of experimental autoimmune encephalomyelitis. J Immunol, 2010, 184:4610–4.

Chapter 8

Pathophysiological Roles of Mutations in the Electrogenic Na^+-HCO_3^- Cotransporter NBCe1

George Seki, Shoko Horita, Masashi Suzuki,
Osamu Yamazaki and Hideomi Yamada

Additional information is available at the end of the chapter

http://dx.doi.org/10.5772/39225

1. Introduction

The electrogenic Na^+-HCO_3^- cotransporter NBCe1, belonging to the solute carrier 4 (SLC4) family, plays essential roles in the regulation of extracellular and intracellular pH [1,2]. Consistent with an essential role of NBCe1 in bicarbonate absorption from renal proximal tubules, homozygous mutations in NBCe1 cause proximal renal tubular acidosis (pRTA) [3-11]. These pRTA patients with NBCe1 mutations invariably present with ocular abnormalities such as band keratopathy, cataract, and glaucoma, indicating that NBCe1 also plays important roles in the maintenance of ocular homeostasis [12,13]. Some pRTA patients also have migraine, suggesting that NBCe1 may also contribute to the pH regulation in the brain [10]. In addition, mice models for NBCe1 deficiency have been developed [11,14].

In this review, we try to summarize the recent data about the pathophysiological roles of NBCe1 mutations.

2. Physiological roles of NBCe1 in kidney and pancreas

There are at least five mammalian NBCe1 variants, NBCe1A through NBCe1E as shown in Figure 1 [15,16]. NBCe1B differs from NBCe1A at the N-terminus, where the first 85 amino acids of NBCe1B replace the first 41 amino acids of NBCe1A [17]. NBCe1C differs from NBCe1B at the C-terminus, where the last 61 amino acids of NBCe1C replace the last 46 amino acids of NBCe1B [18]. NBCe1D and NBCe1E, identified from mouse reproductive tract tissues, contain a deletion of 9 amino acids in exon 6 of NBCe1A and NBCe1B, respectively [16].

Among these variants, NBCe1C is predominantly expressed in brain, but its physiological roles remain speculative [18]. NBCe1B is widely expressed in several tissues including pancreatic ducts, intestinal tracts, ocular tissues, and brain [2,12,13,19-22]. In the basolateral membranes of pancreatic ducts NBCe1B is thought to mediate bicarbonate uptake into cells, which may be essential for the bicarbonate secretion from pancreas [23-25]. Consistent with this view, some pRTA patients with NBCe1 mutations presented with an elevated serum amylase level [3,7]. However, none of these patients presented with a distinct form of pancreatitis. Probably, other acid/base transporters such as Na^+/H^+ exchanger 1 (NHE1) or H^+-ATPase in the basolateral membranes of pancreatic duct cells could at least partially compensate for the NBCe1 inactivation [26].

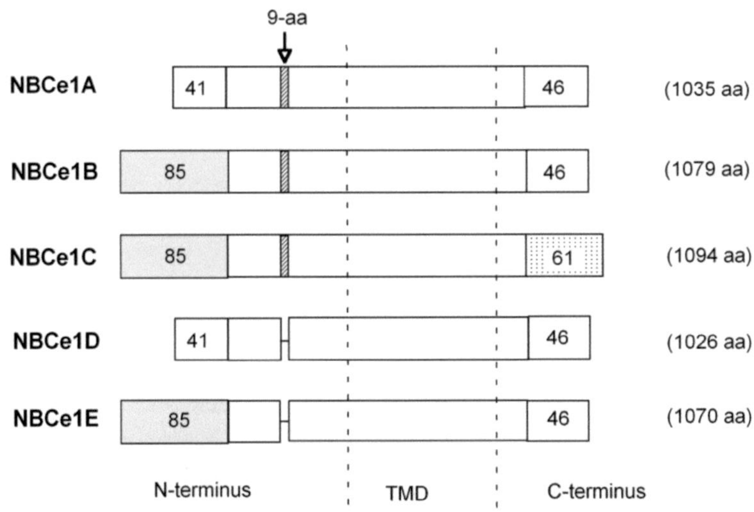

Figure 1. Structures of NBCe1 variants. Numbers of boxes indicate numbers of amino acids in N- or C-terminus. Note that NBCe1D and NBCe1E lack 9 amino acids (9-aa) in exon 6 of NBCe1A and NBCe1B, respectively. TMD: transmembrane domain.

NBCe1A is predominantly expressed in the basolateral membranes of renal proximal tubules, where it mediates bicarbonate exit from cells [2,27]. The opposite transport directions between NBCe1A in kidney and NBCe1B in pancreas may be related to the different stoichiometric ratios. Thus, NBCe1A in *in vivo* renal proximal tubules functions with $1Na^+$ to $3HCO_3^-$ stoichiometry, whereas NBCe1B in pancreatic ducts may function with $1Na^+$ to $2HCO_3^-$ stoichiometry [23,28]. However, these differences in transport stoichiometry may not be due to the intrinsic properties of NBCe1 variants, but rather reflect the environmental factors such as incubation conditions or cell types. Indeed, NBCe1A in isolated renal proximal tubules can function with either $1Na^+$ to $2HCO_3^-$ or $1Na^+$ to $3HCO_3$-stoichiometry depending on the incubation conditions [29-31]. Such changes in transport stoichiometry of NBCe1A can be also induced in *Xenopus* oocytes [32]. Moreover, NBCe1B may function with $1Na^+$ to $2HCO_3^-$ stoichiometry in cultured pancreatic duct cells, but may function with $1Na^+$ to $3HCO_3^-$ stoichiometry when expressed in cultured renal proximal tubular cells [33]. Regarding the electrogenicity of NBCe1A, recent work by Chen and Boron suggests that the predicted fourth extracellular loop corresponding to amino acids 704 to 735 may have an important role [34]. They found that replacing these residues with the corresponding residues of electroneutral Na^+-HCO_3^- cotransporter NBCn1-A creates an electroneutral NBC.

Although the basolateral membranes of renal proximal tubules are known to contain several bicarbonate transporters such as Na^+-dependent and Na^+-independent Cl^-/HCO_3^- exchangers [35,36], NBCe1A seems to play an essential role in bicarbonate absorption in this nephron segment. Consistent with this view, the homozygous inactivating mutations in NBCe1A cause severe pRTA with the blood bicarbonate concentration often less than 10 mM [3-11]. Functional deletion of NBCe1 in mice produces even more severe acidemia with the blood bicarbonate concentration around 5 mM [11,14]. By contrast, functional deletion of Cl^-/HCO_3^- exchanger AE1, which is responsible for a majority of basolateral bicarbonate exit from α-intercalated duct cells, produces only moderate acidemia in mice with the blood bicarbonate concentration around 17 mM [37]. This may probably reflect much higher bicarbonate absorbing capacity of renal proximal tubules than that of renal distal tubules.

3. NBCe1 mutations and pRTA

Until now, 12 homozygous mutations in NBCe1 have been identified in pRTA patients associated with ocular abnormalities as shown in Figure 2 [3-11].

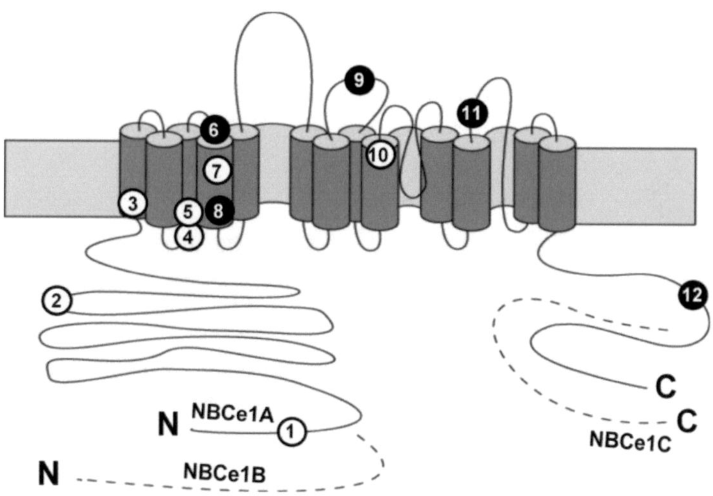

Figure 2. NBCe1 topology and pRTA-related mutations. Numbers in circles correspond to Q29X, R298S, S427L, T485S, G486R, R510H, W516X, L522P, N721TfsX29, A799V, R881C, and S982NfsX4. White numbers in black circles indicate mutations associated with migraine.

They include eight missense mutations R298S, S427L, T485S, G486R, R510H, L522P, A799V, and R881C, two nonsense mutations Q29X and W516X, and two frame shift mutations N721TfsX29 and S982NfsX4. Except the NBCe1A-specific mutation Q29X, which is expected to yield non-functional NBCe1A but leave both NBCe1B and NBCe1C intact [4], all the other mutations lie in the common regions of NBCe1 variants. The C-terminal mutant S982NfsX4 is expected to introduce a frameshift in exon 23 and a premature stop codon for both

NBCe1A (S982NfsX4) and NBCe1B (S1026NfsX4), yielding the mutant proteins with 51 fewer amino acids than the wild-type proteins. On the other hand, this mutation abolishes the translation of NBCe1C, the C-terminal variant skipping exon 24 [10,18].

Topological analysis using the substituted cysteine accessibility method suggests that most of these mutations are buried in the protein complex/lipid bilayer where they perform important structural roles [38]. In particular, the amino acid substitution analysis revealed that Thr^{485} might reside in a special position, which seems to require the OH group side chain to maintain a normal conformation of NBCe1A. Based on homology modeling to the crystallized cytoplasmic domain structure of AE1, Arg^{298} in the C-terminal cytoplasmic domain of NBCe1A was also predicted to reside in a solvent-inaccessible subsurface pocket and to associate with Glu^{91} or Glu^{295} via H-bonding and charge-charge interactions [39]. This unusual continuous chain of interconnected polar residues may be essential for HCO_3^- transporting ability of SLC4 proteins. Parker *et al.* recently found that in addition to a per-molecule transport defect as previous reported [7], the NBCe1 A799V mutant has an unusual HCO_3^--independent conductance that, if associated with mutant NBCe1 in muscle cells, could contribute to the occurrence of hypokalemic paralysis in the affected individual [40,41].

Functional analyses using different expression systems indicate that at least 50% reduction in NBCe1A activity would be required to induce severe pRTA [3,7,9]. However, no tight relationship between the degree of NBCe1A inactivation and the severity of acidemia exits, suggesting the involvement of other factors in the etiology of pRTA. Indeed, several mutants are found to display abnormal trafficking in mammalian cells [10,42,43]. As will be discussed later, defective membrane expression of NBCe1B in astrocytes may be responsible for the occurrence of migraine [10].

4. Physiological roles of NBCe1 in ocular homeostasis

The presence of NBCe1-like activity has been reported in several ocular tissues. Among these tissues, the physiological role of NBCe1 is established in the corneal endothelium. Thus, the corneal endothelium is known to mediate the electrogenic transport of sodium and bicarbonate into the aqueous humor, and this process is considered to be essential for corneal hydration and transparency [44]. Several lines of evidence suggest that NBCe1 is responsible for a majority of this transport. For example, Jentsch *et al.* found an electrogenic sodium-coupled bicarbonate cotransport activity compatible with NBCe1 in cultured bovine corneal endothelial cells [45]. Usui *et al.* later found the functional and molecular evidence for NBCe1 in cultured human corneal endothelial cells [46]. Immunohistological analysis confirmed the expression of NBCe1 in rat, human, and bovine corneal endothelium [12,13,47]. Furthermore, most of the pRTA patients with NBCe1 mutations presented with band keratopathy. The reduction of bicarbonate efflux by NBCe1 mutations may increase the local pH within the corneal stroma, which may facilitate local Ca^{2+} deposition resulting in band keratopathy [13].

Immunohistological analysis also detected the expression of NBCe1 in rat and human lens epithelium [12,13]. Functional analysis in cultured human lens epithelial cells revealed the presence of Cl^--independent, electrogenic Na^+-HCO_3^- cotransporter activity. This transport activity was largely suppressed by adenovirus-mediated transfer of a specific hammerhead ribozyme against NBCe1, consistent with a major role of NBCe1 in overall bicarbonate transport by the lens epithelium [13]. The lens is an avasuclar tissue, and the transport by lens epithelium may be essential for the maintenance of lens homeostasis and integrity [48]. A study in lens epithelial cell layers indeed detected an active fluid transport from their anterior to posterior sides against a hydrostatic pressure [49]. Probably, the transport activity of NBCe1 in lens epithelium may be essential for the lens homeostasis and transparency. Indeed, the pRTA patients with NBCe1 mutations often presented with cataracts.

Most of the pRTA patients with NBCe1 mutations also presented with glaucoma. Immunohistological analysis detected the expression of NBCe1 in human trabecular meshwork cells [13]. The electrogenic transport activity compatible with NBCe1 was also reported in human trabecular meshwork cells [50]. Because trabecular meshwork is the main site for aqueous outflow in the human eye [51], the inactivation of NBCe1 in trabecular meshwork cells may be responsible for the occurrence of high-tension glaucoma usually observed in the pRTA patients with homozygous NBCe1 mutations [10]. On the other hand, the NBCe1 expression was also detected in retina [12,52]. Interestingly, some of the family members carrying the heterozygous NBCe1 S982NfsX4 mutation, which has a dominant negative effect as will be discussed later, presented with normal-tension glaucoma without pRTA [10]. This type of glaucoma may be caused by dysregulation of extracellular pH in retina, because NBCe1 in retinal Müller cells may protect the excessive synaptic activities by counteracting the light-induced extracellular alkalosis [12,52,53].

NBCe1 was also found in human and rat pigmented and nonpigmented ciliary epithelial cells [12,13]. In addition to Na^+/H^+ and anion exchangers [54], NBCe1 may be also involved in influx and efflux of bicarbonate into/from these tissues, thereby contributing to the initial step of aqueous humor formation [55].

Regarding the NBCe1 variants expressed in ocular tissues, several studies suggest that NBCe1B is the predominant variant [12,47]. However, both NBCe1A and NBCe1B are indeed expressed in several ocular tissues [13,46]. Consistent with the latter view, the pRTA patient carrying the homozygous Q29X mutation, which inactivates NBCe1A but leaves NBCe1B and NBCe1C intact, presented with bilateral high-tension glaucoma [4]. She did not have band keratopathy or cataract.

5. NBCe1 mutations and migraine

It has been known that pH in the brain shows rapid changes in response to electrical activity. These changes in local pH may have an important influence on neurobiological responses by modifying numerous enzymes, ion channels, transporters, and receptors [19].

Among several acid/base transporters expressed in the brain, NBCe1 is intensively expressed in olfactory bulb, hippocampal dentate gyrus, and cerebellum, localizing in both glial cells and neurons [56]. Although a large number of transporters may be involved in the pH homeostasis of the brain interstitial space, acid secretion by glial cells via inward electrogenic Na^+-HCO_3^- cotransporter NBCe1B may have a significant role in the prevention of excessive neural activities. In fact, alkalosis in extracellular spaces is generally associated with enhanced neuronal excitability, while acidosis is known to suppress neural activity [19]. A recent study using NBCe1 knockout (KO) mice confirmed that NBCe1 mediates a depolarization-induced alkalinization (DIA) response in astrocytes [57]. This study revealed that NBCe1 also contributes partially to a DIA response in hippocampal neurons [57]. Bevensee *et al.* initially reported that the expression of NBCe1B is more abundant in astrocytes than in neuron, while NBCe1C show the reverse pattern of expression [18]. However, the expression of NBCe1C was also found in rat astrocytes [22]. Despite the intensive expression of NBCe1 in brain and the potential contribution of NBCe1 to the extracellular pH regulation in brain, the physiological significance of NBCe1 in brain had still remained speculative. However, recent work revealed an unrecognized association of migraine with NBCe1 mutations [10].

Migraine is a common, disabling, multifactorial disorder, affecting more than 10% of the population with women more affected than men [58]. Although genetic factor plays a substantial role in ordinary migraine, the genetic basis has been established only in familial hemiplegic migraine (FHM), a rare autosomal dominant subtype of migraine with aura. In addition to a similar headache phase as found in ordinarily migraine, FHM patients experience prolonged hemiparesis [59]. Thus far, three genes have been identified as the genetic basis for FHM: *CACNA1A* encoding the α1 subunit of voltage-gated neuronal Cav2.1 calcium channels [60], *ATP1A2* encoding the α2 subunit of Na^+/K^+ ATPase [61], and *SCN1A* encoding the neuronal voltage-gated sodium channel Nav1.1 [62]. These mutations are thought to cause migraine by enhancing neuronal excitability [63].

We recently identified two sisters with pRTA, ocular abnormalities and hemiplegic migraine. Genetic analysis excluded pathological mutation in *CACNA1A*, *ATP1A2*, and *SCN1A*, but identified the homozygous S982NfsX4 mutation in the C-terminus of NBCe1 [10]. Several heterozygous members of the family also presented with glaucoma and migraine with or without aura. This mutant showed a normal electrogenic activity in *Xenopus* oocytes. When expressed in mammalian cells, however, the S982NfsX4 mutant showed almost no transport activity due to a predominant retention in the endoplasmic reticulum (ER). Several mutant proteins that are retained in the ER are known to exert a dominant negative effect by forming hetero-oligomer complexes with wild-type proteins [64], and NBCe1 can also form the oligomer complexes [65]. Indeed, co-expression analysis uncovered a dominant negative effect of the mutant through hetero-oligomer formation with wild-type NBCe1, which may be responsible for the occurrence of migraine and glaucoma in the heterozygous family members. To further substantiate NBCe1 mutations as a cause of migraine, we re-investigated the other pRTA pedigrees with distinct NBCe1 mutations, and found 4 additional homozygous patients with migraine: hemiplegic migraine with episodic ataxia in L522P [8], migraine with aura in N721TfsX29 [6], and migraine without aura in R510H and R881C [3,7]. Transient expression of GFP-tagged NBCe1B constructs carrying these mutations in C6 glioma cells revealed a remarkable coincidence between the apparent lack of membrane expression and the occurrence of migraine. From these and other results, we concluded that the near total loss of

NBCe1B activity in astrocytes can cause migraine potentially through dysregulation of synaptic pH [10]. We cannot exclude a possibility that the inactivation of NBCe1C is also involved in the pathogenesis of migraine.

Cerebral cortical hyperexcitability causing cortical spreading depression (CSD) seems to be the underlying pathophysiological mechanism of migraine aura [63]. In general, neuronal firing may lead to a rise in extracellular K^+ concentration and further depolarization, but uptake of K^+ into astrocytes can counteract this process. Therefore, enhanced neurotransmitter release by *CACNA1*A mutations, excessive neuronal firing by *SCN1A* mutations, or impaired clearance of K^+ and/or glutamate by *ATP1A2* mutations can all induce CSD [63].Neuronal excitation may also elicit an initial extracellular alkalosis, probably mediated by Ca^{2+}/H^+ exchange [19]. Upon depolarization, however, glial cells secret acid via inward electrogenic Na^+-HCO_3^- cotransport NBCe1, i.e. DIA, overwhelming the initial extracellular alkalosis. Under normal condition, the net extracellular acidosis due to DIA makes surrounding neuronal cells less excitable, because protons suppress excitatory NMDA receptors, with a steep sensitivity in the physiological range of extracellular [19]. Absence of DIA due to defective membrane expression of NBCe1 in astrocytes may cause a positive feedback loop of increased neuronal activity leading to further NMDA-mediated neuronal hyperactivity, causing complete depolarization of a sizable population of brain cells, i.e. CSD. We therefore think that migraine associated with NBCe1 mutations represents a primary headache most likely caused by dysfunctional local pH regulation in the brain as shown in Figure 3.

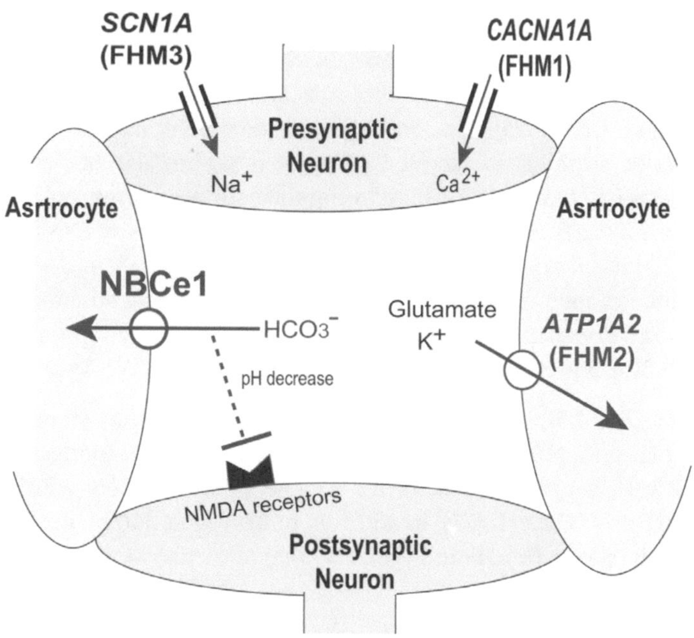

Figure 3. Migraine-associated transporters. While *SCN1A* and *CACNA1A* may directly regulate neuron excitation, *ATP1A2* may regulate neuron excitation indirectly via uptake of K^+ and/or glutamate into astrocytes. On the other hand, NBCe1-mediated uptake of HCO_3^- into astrocytes may also regulate neuron excitation by affecting pH-sensitive NMDA receptors.

6. Roles of N-terminal sequences in NBCe1 functions

When expressed in *Xenopus* oocytes, NBCe1B and NBCe1C showed much lower activities than that of NBCe1A [66-68]. The deletion from of the cytoplasmic N-terminus of an 87-amino acid sequence markedly enhanced the activities of both NBCe1B and NBCe1C by more than 3-fold, indicating that this sequence contains an autoinhibitory domain [66,68]. On the other hand, this sequence also contains a binding domain for inositol 1,4,5-triphosphate receptors (IP_3R) binding protein released with IP_3 (IRBIT). IRBIT is dissociated from IP_3R in the presence of physiological concentrations of IP_3, the process of which has an important role in the regulation of IP_3R functions [69,70].

We and others found that IRBIT binds to and activates NBCe1B and NBCe1C expressed in *Xenopus* oocytes [67,71]. Because this binding requires the cytoplasmic sequence of a 62-amino acid sequence in the N-terminus of NBCe1B and NBCe1C, IRBIT does not bind to NBCe1A that lacks this sequence [67]. Co-expression of IRBIT markedly activates the NBCe1B activity by several-fold. Because this stimulation is not associated with the significant changes in the amount of NBCe1B expressed in the plasma membranes of *Xenopus* oocytes, IRBIT may induce the stimulation of per-molecule activity of NBCe1B [67,68]. Interestingly, Lee et al. found that a mutant IRBIT lacking a protein phophatase-1 (PP-1) binding site stimulates NBCe1B to a 50% greater than can be achieved by the removal of autoinhibitory domain [68]. These results suggest that the stimulatory mechanism of IRBIT may involve not only the neutralization of autoinhibitory domain but also other factors.

The stimulation of NBCe1B by IRBIT has been also confirmed in pancreatic ducts *in vivo* [25]. Thus in secretory epithelia such as pancreatic ducts, IRBIT has a central role in fluid and bicarbonate secretion by activating both NBCe1B and the cystic fibrosis transmembrane conductance regulator CFTR [25]. The subsequent study revealed that the with-no-lysine (WNK) kinases act as scaffolds to recruit Ste20-related proline/alanine-rich kinase (SPAK), which phosphorylates CFTR and NBCe1B, reducing their surface expression. In addition to the direct activation of NBCe1B and CFTR, IRBIT opposed the effects of WNKs and SPAK by recruiting PP-1 to dephosphorylate CFTR and NBCe1B, restoring their surface expression [72]. In contrast to these complex modes of IRBIT-mediated transport stimulation in secretory epithelia, the dephosphorylation of IRBIT by PP-1 may rather partially suppress the stimulatory effect of IRBIT on NBCe1B in *Xenopus* oocytes, which do not express WNKs or SPAK [68,73].

The injection of inositol 4,5-bisphoshate (PIP_2) into *Xenopus* oocytes stimulated the whole currents of NBCe1B and NBCe1C [74]. IRBIT reduced the PIP_2-induced stimulation of NBCe1B and NBCe1C, suggesting that IRBIT and PIP_2 may compete with one another in stimulating NBCe1B and NBCe1C [71]. In addition to the regulation by the binding of IRBIT or PIP_2, the N-terminus of NBCe1B and NBCe1C may also play a role in the inhibition by intracellular Mg^{2+} [75].

7. Phenotypes of NBCe1-deficient mice

Two types of NBCe1-deficient mice, NBCe1 KO and W516X knockin (KI) mice, have been produced [11,14]. Both types of mice show severe acidosis and early lethality. Thus, NBCe1

KO mice exhibited severe metabolic acidosis (blood HCO_3^- concentration of 5.3 mM), growth retardation, hyperaldosteronism, anemia and splenomegaly, abnormal enamel mineralization, intestinal obstruction, and early death before weaning. Splenomegaly might be due to hemolytic anemia due to severe acidemia. The white pulp and the red pulp were severely disrupted in spleen of KO mice. A significant reduction in the cAMP-stimulated short circuit current was detected in colon of KO mice in the presence of a carbonic anhydrase inhibitor acetazolamide, which might reduce the availability of HCO_3^-.

A homozygous NBCe1 W516X mutation was identified in a girl with severe pRTA (blood HCO_3^- concentration of 10 mM), growth retardation, and the typical ocular abnormalities including band keratopathy, cataracts, and glaucoma [11]. Homozygous W516X KI mice also presented with severe metabolic acidosis (blood HCO_3^- concentration of 3.9 mM), growth retardation, hyperaldosteronism, anemia and splenomegaly, and early death before weaning [11]. Due to the process of nonsense-mediated decay, the expression of NBCe1 mRNA was halved in the heterozygous and virtually absent in the homozygous W516X KI mice. The NBCe1 activity in isolated renal proximal tubules from the homozygous KI mice was severely reduced to less than 20% of the activity in tubules from wild-type mice. The rate of bicarbonate absorption in the homozygous KI mice was also markedly reduced to less than 20% of that in wild-type mice, confirming the indispensable role of NBCe1 in bicarbonate absorption from renal proximal tubules. Alkali therapy was effective in prolonging the survival, and partially improving growth retardation and bone abnormalities of the homozygous KI mice. The prolonged survival time by alkali therapy uncovered the development of corneal opacities due to corneal edema in the homozygous KI mice. These results confirmed that the normal NBCe1 activity in corneal endothelium is essential for the maintenance of corneal transparency not only in humans but also in mice [11].

Unlike NBCe1 KO and W516X KI mice, NHE3 KO mice showed only a mild acidemia with blood HCO_3^- level of around 21 mM [76]. In the apical membranes of renal proximal tubules, Na^+/H^+ exchanger type 3 (NHE3) has been considered to mediate a majority of proton secretion into lumen [77]. However, functional analysis using isolated renal proximal tubules from NHE3 KO mice revealed the residual amiloride-sensitive NHE activity, which corresponded to approximately 50% of the wild-type activity [78]. This residual NHE activity, which could represent NHE8 [79], might be able to at least partially compensate for the loss of NHE3 activity. In contrast to such an effective compensation mechanism in the apical membranes, Na^+-dependent and Na^+-independent Cl^-/HCO_3^- exchangers in the basolateral membranes of renal proximal tubules [35,36] may be unable to compensate for the loss of NBCe1A activity.

Author details

George Seki, Shoko Horita, Masashi Suzuki, Osamu Yamazaki and Hideomi Yamada
Department of Internal Medicine, Faculty of Medicine, University of Tokyo, Japan

8. References

[1] Romero MF, Hediger MA, Boulpaep EL, Boron WF. Expression cloning and characterization of a renal electrogenic Na^+/HCO_3^- cotransporter. Nature 1997; 387: 409-413.

[2] Romero MF, Boron WF. Electrogenic Na^+/HCO_3^- cotransporters: cloning and physiology. Annu Rev Physiol 1999; 61: 699-723.

[3] Igarashi T, Inatomi J, Sekine T, *et al.* Mutations in SLC4A4 cause permanent isolated proximal renal tubular acidosis with ocular abnormalities. Nat Genet 1999; 23: 264-266.

[4] Igarashi T, Inatomi J, Sekine T, *et al.* Novel nonsense mutation in the Na^+/HCO_3^- cotransporter gene (SLC4A4) in a patient with permanent isolated proximal renal tubular acidosis and bilateral glaucoma. J Am Soc Nephrol 2001; 12: 713-718.

[5] Dinour D, Chang MH, Satoh J, *et al.* A novel missense mutation in the sodium bicarbonate cotransporter (NBCe1/SLC4A4) causes proximal tubular acidosis and glaucoma through ion transport defects. J Biol Chem 2004; 279: 52238-52246.

[6] Inatomi J, Horita S, Braverman N, *et al.* Mutational and functional analysis of SLC4A4 in a patient with proximal renal tubular acidosis. Pflugers Arch 2004; 448: 438-444.

[7] Horita S, Yamada H, Inatomi J, *et al.* Functional analysis of NBC1 mutants associated with proximal renal tubular acidosis and ocular abnormalities. J Am Soc Nephrol 2005; 16: 2270-2278.

[8] Demirci FY, Chang MH, Mah TS, Romero MF, Gorin MB. Proximal renal tubular acidosis and ocular pathology: a novel missense mutation in the gene (SLC4A4) for sodium bicarbonate cotransporter protein (NBCe1). Mol Vis 2006; 12: 324-330.

[9] Suzuki M, Vaisbich MH, Yamada H, *et al.* Functional analysis of a novel missense NBC1 mutation and of other mutations causing proximal renal tubular acidosis. Pflugers Arch 2008; 455: 583-593.

[10] Suzuki M, Van Paesschen W, Stalmans I, *et al.* Defective membrane expression of the Na^+-HCO_3^- cotransporter NBCe1 is associated with familial migraine. Proc Natl Acad Sci U S A 2010; 107: 15963-15968.

[11] Lo YF, Yang SS, Seki G, *et al.* Severe metabolic acidosis causes early lethality in NBC1 W516X knock-in mice as a model of human isolated proximal renal tubular acidosis. Kidney Int 2011; 79: 730-741.

[12] Bok D, Schibler MJ, Pushkin A, *et al.* Immunolocalization of electrogenic sodium-bicarbonate cotransporters pNBC1 and kNBC1 in the rat eye. Am J Physiol Renal Physiol 2001; 281: F920-F935.

[13] Usui T, Hara M, Satoh H, *et al.* Molecular basis of ocular abnormalities associated with proximal renal tubular acidosis. J Clin Invest 2001; 108: 107-115.

[14] Gawenis LR, Bradford EM, Prasad V, *et al.* Colonic anion secretory defects and metabolic acidosis in mice lacking the NBC1 Na^+/HCO_3^- cotransporter. J Biol Chem 2007; 282: 9042-9052.

[15] Boron WF, Chen L, Parker MD. Modular structure of sodium-coupled bicarbonate transporters. J Exp Biol 2009; 212: 1697-1706.

[16] Liu Y, Xu JY, Wang DK, Wang L, Chen LM. Cloning and identification of two novel NBCe1 splice variants from mouse reproductive tract tissues: a comparative study of NCBT genes. Genomics 2011; 98: 112-119.

[17] Abuladze N, Song M, Pushkin A, *et al.* Structural organization of the human NBC1 gene: kNBC1 is transcribed from an alternative promoter in intron 3. Gene 2000; 251: 109-122.

[18] Bevensee MO, Schmitt BM, Choi I, Romero MF, Boron WF. An electrogenic Na^+-HCO_3^- cotransporter (NBC) with a novel COOH-terminus, cloned from rat brain. Am J Physiol Cell Physiol 2000; 278: C1200-C1211.

[19] Chesler M. Regulation and modulation of pH in the brain. Physiol Rev 2003; 83: 1183-1221.

[20] Marino CR, Jeanes V, Boron WF, Schmitt BM. Expression and distribution of the Na^+-HCO_3^- cotransporter in human pancreas. Am J Physiol 1999; 277: G487-G494.

[21] Satoh H, Moriyama N, Hara C, *et al.* Localization of Na^+-HCO_3^- cotransporter (NBC-1) variants in rat and human pancreas. Am J Physiol Cell Physiol 2003; 284: C729-C737.

[22] Majumdar D, Maunsbach AB, Shacka JJ, *et al.* Localization of electrogenic Na/bicarbonate cotransporter NBCe1 variants in rat brain. Neuroscience 2008; 155: 818-832.

[23] Ishiguro H, Steward MC, Lindsay AR, Case RM. Accumulation of intracellular HCO_3^- by Na^+-HCO_3^- cotransport in interlobular ducts from guinea-pig pancreas. J Physiol 1996; 495 (Pt 1): 169-178.

[24] Ishiguro H, Steward MC, Wilson RW, Case RM. Bicarbonate secretion in interlobular ducts from guinea-pig pancreas. J Physiol 1996; 495 (Pt 1): 179-191.

[25] Yang D, Shcheynikov N, Zeng W, *et al.* IRBIT coordinates epithelial fluid and HCO_3^- secretion by stimulating the transporters pNBC1 and CFTR in the murine pancreatic duct. J Clin Invest 2009; 119: 193-202.

[26] Steward MC, Ishiguro H, Case RM. Mechanisms of bicarbonate secretion in the pancreatic duct. Annu Rev Physiol 2005; 67: 377-409.

[27] Boron WF. Acid-base transport by the renal proximal tubule. J Am Soc Nephrol 2006; 17: 2368-2382.

[28] Yoshitomi K, Burckhardt BC, Fromter E. Rheogenic sodium-bicarbonate cotransport in the peritubular cell membrane of rat renal proximal tubule. Pflugers Arch 1985; 405: 360-366.

[29] Seki G, Coppola S, Fromter E. The Na^+-HCO_3^- cotransporter operates with a coupling ratio of 2 HCO_3^- to 1 Na^+ in isolated rabbit renal proximal tubule. Pflugers Arch 1993; 425: 409-416.

[30] Seki G, Coppola S, Yoshitomi K, *et al.* On the mechanism of bicarbonate exit from renal proximal tubular cells. Kidney Int 1996; 49: 1671-1677.

[31] Muller-Berger S, Nesterov VV, Fromter E. Partial recovery of in vivo function by improved incubation conditions of isolated renal proximal tubule. II. Change of Na-HCO_3 cotransport stoichiometry and of response to acetazolamide. Pflugers Arch 1997; 434: 383-391.

[32] Muller-Berger S, Ducoudret O, Diakov A, Fromter E. The renal Na-HCO_3-cotransporter expressed in Xenopus laevis oocytes: change in stoichiometry in response to elevation of cytosolic Ca^{2+} concentration. Pflugers Arch 2001; 442: 718-728.

[33] Gross E, Hawkins K, Abuladze N, *et al.* The stoichiometry of the electrogenic sodium bicarbonate cotransporter NBC1 is cell-type dependent. J Physiol 2001; 531: 597-603.

[34] Chen LM, Liu Y, Boron WF. Role of an extracellular loop in determining the stoichiometry of Na^+-HCO_3 cotransporters. J Physiol 2011; 589: 877-890.

[35] Preisig PA, Alpern RJ. Basolateral membrane H-OH-HCO_3 transport in the proximal tubule. Am J Physiol 1989; 256: F751-F765.

[36] Seki G, Fromter E. Acetazolamide inhibition of basolateral base exit in rabbit renal proximal tubule S2 segment. Pflugers Arch 1992; 422: 60-65.

[37] Stehberger PA, Shmukler BE, Stuart-Tilley AK, Peters LL, Alper SL, Wagner CA. Distal renal tubular acidosis in mice lacking the AE1 (band3) Cl^-/HCO_3^- exchanger (slc4a1). J Am Soc Nephrol 2007; 18: 1408-1418.

[38] Zhu Q, Kao L, Azimov R, *et al.* Topological location and structural importance of the NBCe1-A residues mutated in proximal renal tubular acidosis. J Biol Chem 2010; 285: 13416-13426.

[39] Chang MH, DiPiero J, Sonnichsen FD, Romero MF. Entry to "formula tunnel" revealed by SLC4A4 human mutation and structural model. J Biol Chem 2008; 283: 18402-18410.

[40] Deda G, Ekim M, Guven A, Karagol U, Tumer N. Hypopotassemic paralysis: a rare presentation of proximal renal tubular acidosis. J Child Neurol 2001; 16: 770-771.

[41] Parker MD, Qin X, Williamson RC, Toye AM, Boron WF. HCO_3^--independent conductance with a mutant Na/HCO_3 cotransporter (SLC4A4) in a case of proximal renal tubular acidosis with hypokalemic paralysis. J Physiol 2012: (in press) doi: 10.1113/jphysiol.2011.224733

[42] Li HC, Szigligeti P, Worrell RT, Matthews JB, Conforti L, Soleimani M. Missense mutations in Na^+:HCO_3^- cotransporter NBC1 show abnormal trafficking in polarized kidney cells: a basis of proximal renal tubular acidosis. Am J Physiol Renal Physiol 2005; 289: F61-F71.

[43] Toye AM, Parker MD, Daly CM, *et al.* The human NBCe1-A mutant R881C, associated with proximal renal tubular acidosis, retains function but is mistargeted in polarized renal epithelia. Am J Physiol Cell Physiol 2006; 291: C788-C801.

[44] Hodson S, Miller F. The bicarbonate ion pump in the endothelium which regulates the hydration of rabbit cornea. J Physiol 1976; 263: 563-577.

[45] Jentsch TJ, Keller SK, Koch M, Wiederholt M. Evidence for coupled transport of bicarbonate and sodium in cultured bovine corneal endothelial cells. J Membr Biol 1984; 81: 189-204.

[46] Usui T, Seki G, Amano S, *et al.* Functional and molecular evidence for Na^+-HCO_3^- cotransporter in human corneal endothelial cells. Pflugers Arch 1999; 438: 458-462.

[47] Sun XC, Bonanno JA, Jelamskii S, Xie Q. Expression and localization of Na^+-HCO_3^- cotransporter in bovine corneal endothelium. Am J Physiol Cell Physiol 2000; 279: C1648-C1655.

[48] Mathias RT, Rae JL, Baldo GJ. Physiological properties of the normal lens. Physiol Rev 1997; 77: 21-50.

[49] Fischbarg J, Diecke FP, Kuang K, *et al.* Transport of fluid by lens epithelium. Am J Physiol 1999; 276: C548-C557.

[50] Lepple-Wienhues A, Rauch R, Clark AF, Grassmann A, Berweck S, Wiederholt M. Electrophysiological properties of cultured human trabecular meshwork cells. Exp Eye Res 1994; 59: 305-311.

[51] Bill A. Blood circulation and fluid dynamics in the eye. Physiol Rev 1975; 55: 383-417.

[52] Newman EA. Sodium-bicarbonate cotransport in retinal astrocytes and Muller cells of the rat. Glia 1999; 26: 302-308.

[53] Borgula GA, Karwoski CJ, Steinberg RH. Light-evoked changes in extracellular pH in frog retina. Vision Res 1989; 29: 1069-1077.

[54] Counillon L, Touret N, Bidet M, *et al.* Na^+/H^+ and Cl^-/HCO_3^- antiporters of bovine pigmented ciliary epithelial cells. Pflugers Arch 2000; 440: 667-678.

[55] Shahidullah M, To CH, Pelis RM, Delamere NA. Studies on bicarbonate transporters and carbonic anhydrase in porcine nonpigmented ciliary epithelium. Invest Ophthalmol Vis Sci 2009; 50: 1791-1800.

[56] Schmitt BM, Berger UV, Douglas RM, *et al.* Na/HCO_3 cotransporters in rat brain: expression in glia, neurons, and choroid plexus. J Neurosci 2000; 20: 6839-6848.

[57] Svichar N, Esquenazi S, Chen HY, Chesler M. Preemptive regulation of intracellular pH in hippocampal neurons by a dual mechanism of depolarization-induced alkalinization. J Neurosci 2011; 31: 6997-7004.

[58] Lipton RB, Scher AI, Kolodner K, Liberman J, Steiner TJ, Stewart WF. Migraine in the United States: epidemiology and patterns of health care use. Neurology 2002; 58: 885-894.

[59] The International Classification of Headache Disorders: 2nd edition. Cephalalgia 2004; 24 Suppl 1: 9-160.

[60] Ophoff RA, Terwindt GM, Vergouwe MN, *et al.* Familial hemiplegic migraine and episodic ataxia type-2 are caused by mutations in the Ca^{2+} channel gene CACNL1A4. Cell 1996; 87: 543-552.

[61] De Fusco M, Marconi R, Silvestri L, *et al.* Haploinsufficiency of ATP1A2 encoding the Na^+/K^+ pump alpha2 subunit associated with familial hemiplegic migraine type 2. Nat Genet 2003; 33: 192-196.

[62] Dichgans M, Freilinger T, Eckstein G, *et al.* Mutation in the neuronal voltage-gated sodium channel SCN1A in familial hemiplegic migraine. Lancet 2005; 366: 371-377.

[63] Goadsby PJ. Recent advances in understanding migraine mechanisms, molecules and therapeutics. Trends Mol Med 2007; 13: 39-44.

[64] Alper SL. Genetic diseases of acid-base transporters. Annu Rev Physiol 2002; 64: 899-923.

[65] Kao L, Sassani P, Azimov R, *et al.* Oligomeric structure and minimal functional unit of the electrogenic sodium bicarbonate cotransporter NBCe1-A. J Biol Chem 2008; 283: 26782-26794.

[66] McAlear SD, Liu X, Williams JB, McNicholas-Bevensee CM, Bevensee MO. Electrogenic Na/HCO_3 cotransporter (NBCe1) variants expressed in Xenopus oocytes: functional comparison and roles of the amino and carboxy termini. J Gen Physiol 2006; 127: 639-658.

[67] Shirakabe K, Priori G, Yamada H, *et al.* IRBIT, an inositol 1,4,5-trisphosphate receptor-binding protein, specifically binds to and activates pancreas-type Na^+/HCO_3^- cotransporter 1 (pNBC1). Proc Natl Acad Sci U S A 2006; 103: 9542-9547.

[68] Lee SK, Boron WF, Parker MD. Relief of autoinhibition of the electrogenic Na-HCO_3 cotransporter NBCe1-B: role of IRBIT vs. amino-terminal truncation. Am J Physiol Cell Physiol 2012; 302: C518-C526.

[69] Ando H, Mizutani A, Matsu-ura T, Mikoshiba K. IRBIT, a novel inositol 1,4,5-trisphosphate (IP3) receptor-binding protein, is released from the IP3 receptor upon IP3 binding to the receptor. J Biol Chem 2003; 278: 10602-10612.

[70] Ando H, Mizutani A, Kiefer H, Tsuzurugi D, Michikawa T, Mikoshiba K. IRBIT suppresses IP_3 receptor activity by competing with IP_3 for the common binding site on the IP_3 receptor. Mol Cell 2006; 22: 795-806.

[71] Thornell IM, Wu J, Bevensee MO. The IP_3 receptor-binding protein IRBIT reduces phosphatidylinositol 4,5-bisphosphate (PIP_2) stimulationon of Na/bicarbonate cotransporter NBCe1 variants expressed in Xenopus laevis oocytes (Abstract). FASEB J 2010; 24: 815.816.

[72] Yang D, Li Q, So I, *et al.* IRBIT governs epithelial secretion in mice by antagonizing the WNK/SPAK kinase pathway. J Clin Invest 2011; 121: 956-965.

[73] Devogelaere B, Beullens M, Sammels E, *et al.* Protein phosphatase-1 is a novel regulator of the interaction between IRBIT and the inositol 1,4,5-trisphosphate receptor. Biochem J 2007; 407: 303-311.

[74] Wu J, McNicholas CM, Bevensee MO. Phosphatidylinositol 4,5-bisphosphate (PIP_2) stimulates the electrogenic Na/HCO_3 cotransporter NBCe1-A expressed in Xenopus oocytes. Proc Natl Acad Sci U S A 2009; 106: 14150-14155.

[75] Yamaguchi S, Ishikawa T. The electrogenic Na^+-HCO_3^- cotransporter NBCe1-B is regulated by intracellular Mg^{2+}. Biochem Biophys Res Commun 2008; 376: 100-104.

[76] Schultheis PJ, Clarke LL, Meneton P, *et al.* Renal and intestinal absorptive defects in mice lacking the NHE3 Na^+/H^+ exchanger. Nat Genet 1998; 19: 282-285.

[77] Alpern RJ. Cell mechanisms of proximal tubule acidification. Physiol Rev 1990; 70: 79-114.

[78] Choi JY, Shah M, Lee MG, *et al.* Novel amiloride-sensitive sodium-dependent proton secretion in the mouse proximal convoluted tubule. J Clin Invest 2000; 105: 1141-1146.

[79] Goyal S, Vanden Heuvel G, Aronson PS. Renal expression of novel Na^+/H^+ exchanger isoform NHE8. Am J Physiol Renal Physiol 2003; 284: F467-F473.

Chapter 9

The Mutations and Their Relationships with the Genome and Epigenome, RNAs Editing and Evolution in Eukaryotes

Daniel Frías-Lasserre

Additional information is available at the end of the chapter

http://dx.doi.org/10.5772/49968

"Mutations have been crucial for geneticists, as day and night for astronomers. Whithout the successions of days and night we would not know about stars. Whithout mutations we would know very little about inheritance and the existence of genes."
Gustavo Hoecker Salas
(December 5, 1915- March 19, 2008)
National Prize of Science of Chile in 1989

1. Introduction

The idea of variation in nature is very old, in Heraclitus of Ephesus (504-500 BC) we find the first ideas of changes when he stated: "we never bathed in the same river". However in the field of biology, the Greeks considered that the species were immutables. This concept changes with the first scientific ideas of organic evolutions and heredity. Lamarck proposed the first evolutionary theory where the organisms evolved from simple forms. Also he proposed an hereditary model in which the environmental influences are very important as an agents of evolutionary change and proposed the Theory of acquired characters. With the Mendelism advent, Lamarcks's Theory was left behind and all the mutations in the living organisms were attributed to Mendelian "factors". However in recent years with the development of epigenesis, genomic imprinting and the horizontal transferences of the genes, Lamarck's ideas have resurfaced.

The concept of mutation was coined by Hugo De Vries in 1901, whom worked with plants species of the genus Oenothera where he discovered some phenotypic hereditary characteristics that he coined as "mutations" and "mutants" to those individuals that have these phenotypic alterations. In opinion of De Vries, these mutations give origin to a new species that he named "elementary species" [1], [2]. Thus, this gave birth to the saltacionist Theory of Evolution that he described in his book entitled " Mutations". The harmony between Mutation Theory and Mendel model of heredity, the simplicity of the experimental method and the vast accumulation of supporting data, explain the big impact in the biological world [3]. Also, De Vries ventured with a hipothesis: " With the knowledge of the principles of the mutations will be possible in the future to induce mutations artificially" [4]. Wilhelm Johannsen argued that evolution consisted of discontinuous changes between "pure lines" and carried out their classic experiments in the beans *Phaseolus vulgaris*, through which coined the concepts of phenotype, genotype and gene [5] Other important step in the advances of the genetics as an experimental discipline, was the stablishment of relationships between mutations and genes discovered by Thomas Hunt Morgan in 1939 using *Drosophila* as biological material. Later Timoféeff- Ressovsky distinguished mutations at gene level and chromosomal aberrations. Morgan named mutations to these changes in individuals genes with variable effects [6] . Year later Morgan perfected the gene concepts as " the hereditary unit indivisible by recombination, located in the loci in a homologous chromosomal pair that can spontaneously mutate and belong to the linkage unit" [7]. In the framework of this concept the genes are located in a fixed position, specifically in a locus, concept coined by Morgan in 1915, and could change of position only by structural chromosomal reorganization [6]. This concept was accepted by the great majority of the scientific community of this time, prevailing until the discovery of transposable genetic elements in the second half of last century. However it is necessary to refer to some exceptions to the classic concept of the gene. Richard Goldschmidt in his book Theoretical Genetics denied the existence of an corpuscular gene; according to his opinion, in the chromosome only there is a definite pattern of changes that corresponds with the mutation and: "the mutation create the gene" [8].

Mutations have been historically the cornerstone of biological disciplines: in basic science, to understand biodiversity and evolution of species, in medicine to explain phenotypic variation and diseases, in education to justify the individual differences found between the students within a classroom and also in agriculture and veterinary in the improvement of plants and animals useful to man. Thus, Mutations have allowed the explosive growth of genetics as an experimental science. In multicellular organisms the cell differentiation requires a series of genetic and epigenetic changes. The mutations (epimutations) can occurs also post transcriptionally in the different type of RNAs that constitute the epigenome. This article explores this theme, in the framework of the adaptation, phenotypic plasticity and evolution of eukaryotes.

2. Mutations at genome level

At the beginning of the genetics as an experimental discipline, mutations have been associated to the classic Mendelian genes and, with the advent of molecular genetics these genetic changes are produced in the coding area of the DNA. A gene occupied a definite place in the chromosome that was associated with a well determined phenotype,thus the gene was simultaneously a unit of mutation and function and were indivisible by recombination [7]. Archivald Garrod in 1909 was interested in to explain the origins and inheritance of human diseases. Also he was the first proposing the concept that a gene is in direct relationship with the production of a specific protein and that establishes the genetic control of some inborn error of the metabolism. He showed that an alteration in an enzyme was linked to amino acid metabolism. In 1941 Beadle and Tatum postulated the hypothesis "one gene-one enzyme". Thus, each gene control the production, function and specificity of a particular enzyme. Studies conducted in differents organisms proves that the capacity to synthetize the appropriate amino acid is caused by the modification or loss of a single enzyme. This concept was changed by Vernon Ingram who postulated the hypotesis "one gene-one polypeptide" in base to the sickle cell anemia disease in humans . Also Ingram postulated that this disease is caused by a single gene mutation which is letal in homozygous with severe sickle cell anemia, and is semiletal in heterozygous that show an attenuated sickle cell anemia. Normal homocigotes individuals are normal for the form of their blood cells and their hemoglobin in an electrophoretic analysis migrated differently in comparation to those heterozygotous individuals. The fingerprint show that the differences between normal and diseased individuals was only a single amino acids substitution in one of the beta chain of polypeptide. The glutamic acid in normal individuals is replaced by valina in individuals with sickle cell anemia. The difference between valina and glutamic acids is only one base in the codon. Moreove, the amino acid changes in one chain is independent of changes in the other chain, suggesting that the gene determining the alpha and beta chain are located in different loci. Thus one gene codes for one polypeptide and several polypeptides may be necessary for a functional enzyme of the organism. In 1961, Seysmour Benzer studing the fine structure of genes by using mutants in the phage T4 of E.coli, use for first time the concept of cistron. Inside of a gene, there are differents cistrons or "functional units". Benzer demostrated the hypotesis of Ingram, the cistron corresponds to a sequence of nucleotides that code for a polypeptidic chain [9, 10]

The ideas about the genetic action and its mutability were complemented by Goldschmidt in1940 [11] who defined the gene on the basis of its physiological action. With the first DNA sequencing by Frederick Sanger , it was clearly demostrated by C. Yanofsky that the gene is a nucleotide sequence that encodes for proteins. Thus, within the genes there are information for the amino acid sequence of the primary structure of protein. [12] Any mutation at nucleotides of a gene may cause an alteration in the primary structure of the protein. Depending on the phenotypic effect causing these mutations can be lethal, semiletal, deletereos or innocuous (silent mutation). Many researchers were interested in inducing mutations with differents agents in plants and animals such as Hermann Muller in *Drosophila* ,Milislav Demerec in bacteria, Áke Gustafsson in barley, George Snell in mice, G.W. Beadle, E.L. Tatum in *Neurospora* ,Lederberg and Tatum in *E.coli* [13].

An important step in the process of regulation of gene expression were the Jacob and Monod experiments in *E. coli*. Using mutations were able to establish the first model of expression and gene silencing in prokaryotes. Based in pioneering works of Calvin Bridges and Goldschmidt on the effects of homeotic mutation on development in *Drosophila*, García-

Bellido and Lewis proposed a model of gene regulation of development in eukaryotes [14, 15]. The homeotic mutations have been fundamentals to explain the genetic basis of development, adaptation and evolution in eukaryote organisms. However, in recent years have found that in regions of DNA does not code for proteins are transcribed an enormous amount of non-coding RNA (ncRNAs), which together with proteins, regulate gene expression. These RNA, including the rRNA and tRNA, together with the mRNA and chromatin are part of epigenome. The mutation at the level of the epigenome have been called epimutations and also cause phenotypic changes, including diseases but also evolutionary novelties that even can be inherited through a non-Mendelian pattern of inheritance.Then will delve into this important topic .

3. Epimutations at epigenome level

The concept of epigenome is a recent concept in genetics that arises with epigenesis concept. The epigenome involved the chemical changes at DNA level such as methylation and also histones acetylation, chromatin remodeling and phenotypic changes that originate by ncRNAs [16]. The epigenesis is a old concept that was coined in 1942 by Conrrad H. Waddington to explain as an adults can be formed from a cygote by cell differentiation and gene regulation. In a multicellular organism each cell has an epigenotype that is determined by which genes are functioning in that particular cell. The differentiation of multicellular organisms is controlled by epigenetic markers and are transmitted through cell division. However, have been demonstrated that epigenetic changes in germ cell line could be hereditable transgenerationally. Epigenesis is a heritable changes in the expression of genes that not involve a change in the nucleotide structure of DNA but only changes in the chromatin. These changes alter the capacity of genes to respond to external signals [17]. Epigenetic changes allows heritable or transgenerational modifications in the expression of genes without the need of mutations at DNA level and not necessarily following the Mendelian model of heredity. In classical model of Mendelian heredity a gene's effects were assumed to be independent of its parental origin, but is know that some genes have differents effects depending if gene was inherited via a sperm or an egg. This process is know as genomic imprinting. At present there is a lot of evidence that genomic imprinting inclusive may influence human behavior. Is know that children who inherit a chromosomal deletion of 15q11-q13 from their father have behavior different of children who inherit a similar deletion from their mother [18, 19, 20]. Also, experimental animal models in mouse shows that in utero or early life environmental exposures produce effects that can be inherited transgenerationally and are accompanied by epigenetic alterations [21]. These changes in the epigenome have been named as "epimutations". In humans there are just a few reports that have been used to suggest inheritance of epimutations and the search of these epigenetic inheritance is under way [18]. Some evidences have been described in colorectal cancer [22, 23, 24, 25].

Epigenesis and epimutation concepts also extend to ncRNAs that have different functions and in human genome constitute about of 60% of the total transcriptional output [26, 27, 28,

29, 30]. The ncRNAs are short single-stranded between 18 to 30nt length such as micro RNA(miRNAs) Small interfering RNA (siRNAs), small nuclear RNA (snRNAs), Small nucleolar RNAs(snoRNAs), piwi- interacting RNAs (piRNAs) and long nc RNA (lncRNA) 200-2800 nt length. All these ncRNAs are hairpin that are paired in some places similar to tRNAs. The homologies detected between the ncRNAs with endogenous viruses, tramposons and introns revealed that ncRNAs probably originates from RNA viruses [31]. In the eukaryote genome, the ncRNAs are located in the non coding areas of mRNAs, endogenous viruses, tramposons and also transcribed from non coding DNA areas. The ncRNAs not transcribed for proteins and are characterized for a great variety of processes that included genomic imprinting, as enhancers of transcriptional regulation, mRNA processing and modification, sex determination by dosage compensation, protein degradation, oncogenic, tumor-suppresive, neural and synaptic plasticity of learning and memory and cognitive capacity by regulating dendrite morphogenesis during early development and also viral and tramposons defense [28,29,30,32,33,34]. Most of the mRNA stability elements are considered to be located in the 5′- and 3′- untranslated regions (UTRs) of genes where are located ncRNAs [35, 36] In the following paragraphs are detailed the features and the functions of each ncRNAs in eukaryotes. Also describes the effects of the mutations in the origin of disease, and also in the adaptation and evolution of the species. In Table 1 are shows the principal hallmark characteristics of these smalls and long ncRNAs.

Name	Length in nucleotides (nt)	Principal functions	References
siRNAs	21-23 nt	mRNA cleavage	[41]
miRNAs	21-23 nt	Regulate developmental timing	[50-52]
piRNAs	29-30 nt	Tramposons silencing in gametes	[61]
snRNAs	90-216 nt	Efficiency of splicing, maintaining telomeres	[69-70]
snoRNAs	< 70 nt	Guide methylation of rRNAs,tRNAs and other snRNAs	[69,72]
lnc RNAs	200-2800 nt	X chromosome inactivation, human brain development	[76,77,94]_

Note: lncRNAs always act in Cis position in the chromosome and small ncRNAs in Trans position [76].

Table 1. Principal Hallmark characteristics of small and long non-coding RNAs

4. The mutations at non-coding RNAs level

4.1. Short interfering RNAs

The eukaryotic genome encode an ample amount of short interfering RNAs, in different cells and tissues principally miRNAs, siRNAs and piRNAs that have less than 200 nt length and are highly conserved. These short ncRNAs are engaged in specific gene regulation and modulate the development of several eukaryote organisms including mammals and are involved in gene silencing in higher eukaryotes [27,37]. They act by binding to complementary sites on targets mRNAs to induce cleavage or repression of transcription in a specific manner. Thus these ncRNAs could participate in the degradation of some specific sequence of mRNA. Also, a mutation in proteins required for miRNAS function or biogenesis can affect animal development [37, 38, 39,40]. Generally the target genes and the mechanism of target suppression are unknown, the reason for this is that miRNAs have a very short sequence of nucleotides, and also the interaction of base pairs with target mRNAs may be affected by a protein complex [38]. Unlike miRNAs of animals, miRNA target of plants are more easily identified because of near-perfect complementarity to their target sequences and act as siRNAs and destroy its target mRNA [41]. In plants, the miRNAs target sites are generally found into the protein–coding segment of the target mRNAs but in animals are found in untranslated region 3'UTR [40, 41]. MiRNAs and siRNAs are processed from a double-stranded RNA precursors about 70 nt by a specific ribonuclease, DICER that excises long RNA into short duplexes of 21-23 nucleotides called siRNAs and miRNAs. Only one type of DICER is found *in C. elegans* and humans indicating that the same DICER is acting on both miRNAs and siRNAs precursors [42,43]. However, two mutants, Dicer 1 and Dicer 2, have been discovery in *Drosophila* . Dicer 1 block the production of miRNA precursors. In a different way, Dicer 2 block the processing of siRNA precursors [44]. The excised short RNAs are associated with an ARGONAUTE proteins and constitute an RNA-inducing silencing complex (RISC) that is able to target near- perfect complementary RNAs for their degradation or for the control of translation [38, 45]. In contrast to DICER , studies in *C.elegans* and *in Drosophila* embryos suggest that the maturation and function of siRNAs and miRNas have differents requirements for argonaute proteins [45]. Mutations in these proteins required for miRNAs function or biogenesis impair animal development [46]. Micro RNAs are highly conserved across a wide range of species, for this reason it is not uncommon that homologies have been described in miRNA binding sites [38, 47]. It was shown that a large subset of *Drosophila* miRNAs with homologs in the human genome is perfectly complementary to several classes of sequence motifs previously demonstrated to mediate in negative posttranscription regulation [48,49]. The functions of miRNAs began to be studied in the founding members of miRNAs was in lin-4 and let-7, genes that regulate developmental timing, were discovery from molecular analysis on *Caenorhabditis elegans* [50, 51,]. Both are 21-22 nt RNAs associated with apparent precursor RNAs with stem-loop structure, and both mediate post-transcriptional regulation of target mRNAs via imperfectly complementary sites in their 3' UTRs [37]. MiRNAs play significant regulatory roles in physiological aspect of development and pathologies in plants, flies, fishes, and mammals [52]. In *C.elegans* miRNAs involves to lys mi RNAs that regulates left-right asymmetry in the nervous system [34], and in *Drosophila* bantam miRNA control tissue growth and apoptosis [39]; miR-14 *in Drosophila* suppresses cell death and is required for normal fat metabolism control [53]. In *Bombix mori* has been discovered that miRNAs are relates with the molting stages and, based on the analysis of target genes, have been hypothesized that miRNAs regulate development on complex stages [54].In mouse miR-375 is involved in the pancreatic- islet-specific that regulates insulin secretion[55] and miR-181 is important in hematopoietic differentiation [56].In the sheep, the variety Texel, was identified the myostatin GDF8 gene in chromosome 2 . This gene has direct relation with a major effect on muscle mass. Also have been discovery that this gene has relation with the coding of a miRNA which is highly expressed in the skeletal muscle. A transition of G to A in 3' UTR occurs in an allele of the gene GDF8. This mutation inhibits the production of myostatin causing muscular hypertrophy [57]. MiRNAs also have a role in a normal development and function of heart muscle in vertebrates. In mouse embryos, overexpression of miRNAmiR-1 in the heart, during mid-embryogenesis originated lethality due to cardiomyocyte deficiency and heart failure [58].There are many evidences that mutations in miRNAs cause disease in humans. For example, karyotyping showing that chronic lymphocytic leukemia (CLL) has a genetic basis consisting in a deletion located in 13q14 chromosome. These deletion is associated to other diseases such as mantle cell lymphoma, multiple myeloma and prostate cancers [59].In humans, has been demonstrated that the hemizygous and/or homozygous loss at 13q14 constitute the most frequent chromosomal abnormality in CLL. Also has been demonstrate that two mutation in miRNAs : miR15 and miR16 are located into a 30-kb deletion area in CLL. Both genes are deleted or down-regulated in the majority of CLL [42]. In plants many mRNA target encode transcription factors that are important in morphogenesis regulation and, due to the high complementarity with mRNA targets act as siRNAs guiding the destruction of their mRNA target. In plants, miRNA target sites are principally found within the protein-coding segment of the target mRNA, but in animals miRNA act in 3′ untraslated region (3′UTR) [40,41,60].A set of 3′ UTR motifs, such as the Brd-box (AGCUUUA), the K-box (CUGUGAUA) and the GY-box(GUCUUCC), were characterized as motifs involved in negative post-transcriptional regulation of genes in the enhancer of split and, Brd gene complexes of *Drosophila* the 5′ends of miRNAs may be important for target recognition [37]

5. Mutations in Piwi interacting non-coding RNAs

PiRNAs are other class of small ncRNAs molecules that have 29-30 nt lenght and form the piRNA-induced silencing complex (piRISC) protein in the germ line of many animal species. Piwi proteins bind to piRNAs, which map to transposons. PiRNAs are important regulators of gametogenesis and have been proposed to play roles in transposon silencing [61].

PiRNAs are produced by the primary processing of single-stranded transcripts of heterochromatic master loci [62] The piRISC complex protects the integrity of the genome from invasion of transposable elements and other genetic elements as viruses and silencing them. They express only in gonads, specially during the spermatogenesis regulating the meiosis.[63,64] but also has been described during de ovogenesis [61]. As a result of the loss of piRNAs silencing, in *Drosophila* piwi mutations lead to transposable element over expression and cause a transposition burst. PiRNAs mutants in females exhibit two types of abnormalities, over expression of transposons and severely underdeveloped ovaries [62,65].

Piwi proteins and piRNAs have conserved functions in transposon silencing in the embryonic male germ line. Piwi proteins are proposed to be piRNAs-guided endonucleases that initiate secondary piRNA biogenesis.The biogenesis and piRNA amplification is fundamental for the silencing of LINE1 transposons. Experimental data in mice in base to mutations in Mili and Miwi 2 alleles revealed that the defective piRNAs results in spermatogenic failure and sterility. [66].The relevance of the non-coding genome in human disease has mainly been studied in the context of the widespread disruption of miRNAs expression and function that is seen in human cancer. At present we are only beginning to understand the nature and extent of the piRNAs, snoRNAs, transcribed ultraconserved regions (T-UCRs) and large intergenic non-coding RNAs (lincRNAs) are emerging as key elements of cellular homeostasis [67]. Genomic imprinting causes parental origin–specific monoallelic gene expression through differential DNA methylation established in the parental germ line. However, the mechanisms underlying how specific sequences are selectively methylated are not fully understood. Has been found that the components of the piRNAs pathway are required for de novo methylation of the differentially methylated region (DMR) of the imprinted mouse Rasgrf1 locus, but not other paternally imprinted loci. A retrotransposon sequence within a ncRNAs spanning the DMR was targeted by piRNAs generated from a different locus. A direct repeat in the DMR, which is required for the methylation and imprinting of Rasgrf1, served as a promoter for this RNA. Has been proposed a model in which piRNAs and a target RNA direct the sequence-specific methylation of Rasgrf1.[68]

6. Mutations in small nuclear ncRNAs

SnRNAs are short molecules of RNA that are located within the nucleus of cells and participate in a variety of processes such as RNA splicing, regulation of transcription factors (7SK RNA) or RNA polimerase II (B2 RNA) and maintaining the telomeres [69]. RNA-RNA interactions between snRNAs or between snRNAs and the pre-mRNAs play critical roles in the accuracy and efficiency of the splicing. The snRNAs also are combined with the protein factors, they make an RNA-protein complex called small nucleoriboprotein (snRNP).The presence of dynamic RNA-RNA interactions within a ribonucleoprotein (RNP) complex like the spliceosome suggests that the snRNAs themselves may need to adopt more than one RNA conformation in order to execute their functions during splicing. Not all of these interactions are established simultaneously, nor do they persist once established. Rather, interactions are formed, modified, disrupted, and replaced during spliceosome assembly and splicing. [70]. The complex structure of spliceosome and the varied interactions between their protein subunits make than any mutations in the nucleotide structure of the snRNAs cause alterations in some of its interactions and functions. Thus, it has been demostrate that in yeast alternative RNA folding can cause cold sensitive function of RNA and that in the case of U2 snRNA, for which the potential to form the alternative structure is conserved, disrupting the alternative folding relieves the cold sensitive defect. This finding suggests that alternative RNA folding may provide a general explanation for the common occurrence of cold-sensitive mutations in RNA and RNA binding proteins [70]. In the yeast *Schizosaccharomyces pombe* there are pre-mRNA processing (prp) mutants that are temperature sensitive or cold sensitive for growth. Some these mutants accumulated the U6 snRNAs precursor at the nonpermissive temperature [71]. Small snoRNAs, are ancient ncRNA that guide the methylation of rRNAs, tRNAs and other snRNAs. These snoRNAs are less than 70 nt in length including 10-20 nucleotides of antisense elements for base pairing rRNA processing involves a number of snoRNAs [69,72]. These activities involve direct base-pairing of the snoRNA with pre-rRNA using different domains. A mutation consisting of single nucleotide insertion in the guide domain shifts modification to an adjacent uridine in rRNA, and severely impairs both processing and cell growth [73].Have been described that U3 and U14 snoRNAs have been implicated in processing steps leading to 18S rRNA formation in eukaryotes. In addition, 18S rRNA formation in vertebrates requires U22 snoRNAs ,and in yeast it requires snR10 and snR30 snoRNAs.The role of snoRNAs in rRNA processing is distinct from the function of the majority of snoRNAs that serve as guide RNAs for rRNA modification. Mutations in U3 snoRNAs of Xenopus were tested for function in oocytes. The results show that U3 mutagenesis uncoupled cleavage at sites 1 and 2, flanking the 5′ and 3′ ends of 18S rRNA, and generated novel intermediates: 19S and 18.5S pre-rRNAs [74] This study reveals that budding yeast snoRNAs gene promoters are typically demarcated by a single, precisely positioned binding site for the telomere-associated protein Tbf1, which is required for full snoRNAs expression. Tbf1 is known to bind to subtelomeric regions of *S. cerevisiae* chromosomes, where it contributes to the maintenance of telomere length and the regulation of telomeric gene silencing. The subtelomeric binding protein Tbf1 is a global transcriptional activator in budding yeast, where it activates snoRNA genes [75]

7. Mutations in macro or long non-coding RNAs

Macro or long coding RNAs are conserved and unlike the short RNA, always act in Cis position in the chromosomes and can be up to several hundred thousand nucleotides long , about 200-2800 nt. In the eukaryotic genome and, specially in mammals there are thousands of lncRNAs that are expressed in different cell lines and tissue and exhibit tissue-specific expression patterns. At moment there are a small amount of lncRNA in which are know in its function and stability, althought has been assumed that they are generally unstable. Reciently an genome-wide analysis in the mouse neuroblastoma cells, using a custom ncRNAs array has been determined that lncRNA show a similar range of half-lives to proteins-coding transcripts, suggesting that lncRNAs are not unstable and also that the stability of lncRNAs is a regulated process and depend of where are located in the genome these lncRNAs. Thus, the intergenic RNAs show more stability that those originated from introns of mRNA [76]. Also it is know that in mammals these lncRNAs have different regulatory functions , principally X chromosome inactivation by heterochromatinization (Xist gene) and coats the inactive X chromosome from which it is transcribed. This represents part of the mechanism by which transcriptional silencing is achieved [77]. The lncRNAs roX in flies plays a role in dosage compensation in sex determination similar to XIST gene in mammals [78]. Also the lncRNAs are involves in the regulation of transcriptional and post transcriptional pathway programming, regulation of mRNA splicing, epigenetic gene activation in the regulation of Hox genes that regulate development and also in genomic imprinting and as enhacers of gene expression and in the length of telomere in the chromosomes [79,80,81,82,83,84,85,86,87,88,89,90].

In addition, several lncRNAs have been shown to be mis regulated in various diseases including cancer and neurological disorders [83,91]. One such alterations in an lncRNA, is Malat1 RNA (metastasis-associated lung adenocarcinoma transcript). Malat1 also is highly abundant in neurons and It is enriched only when RNA polymerase II-dependent transcription is active. Knock-down studies revealed that Malat1 modulates the recruitment of SR family pre-mRNA-splicing factors to the transcription site of a transgene array. Malat1 controls the expression of genes involved not only in nuclear processes, but also in the function of the synapse. In cultured hippocampal neurons, knock-down of Malat1 decreases synaptic density, whereas its over-expression results in a cell-autonomous increase in synaptic density. These results suggest that Malat1 regulates synapse formation by modulating the expression of genes involved in synapse formation. [91]. lncRNAs are present not only in animals but also in plants where they are involved in gene silencing and in the phenotypic plasticity [92]. In mouse a lncRNAs that has been coined as Rubie (RNA upstream of BMP4 expressed in inner ear) originate malformation in the vestibular apparatus. The Mutation is expressed in developing semicircular canals. However, was discovered that the SWR/J allele of Rubie is disrupted by an intronic endogenous retrovirus that causes anormal splicing and premature polyadenylation of the transcript. Rubie lies in the conserved gene desert upstream of Bmp4, within a region previously shown to be important for inner ear expression of Bmp4 [93]. Also in vertebrates and specifically in humans has been described mutations in transposables elements that are related to neurodegerative diseases. The mutation was located in a degenerated long interspersed elements (LINES). This mutation expressed in the brain and causes lethal infantil encephalopathy suggesting that these repetitive elements are important in human brain development [94].

8. The RNA editing

The epimutations at ncRNAs are very important for the adaptation of organism and could be also heritable. Traditionally has been considered that mutations are nucleotide changes that occur at the DNA level and also that are the only new source of genetic variation. However, an special epigenetic regulatory mechanism was discovered from the mitochondria of protozoa *Trypanosome* where a number of genes are expressed in a unconventional manner, the nucleotide sequence of primary transcripts is modified post-transcriptionally through the insertion or deletion of Uridine. These nucleotide alteration was coined as RNA editing [95,96] and also should be considered as "post-transcriptional epimutations". The RNA editing has been detected in unicellular and multicellular eukaryotes but not in prokaryotes. After this discovery, it was thought that this process affects only mRNAs, but now is known that also the editing occur in tRNAs, rRNAs and miRNAs [73,97,98,99]. In humans RNA editing is a change of adenosine to inosine mediated by the enzyme adenosine deaminase, acting on double – stranded RNA, where the inosine acts as guanosine [73,98]. In mammals also has been described another kind of RNA editing consisting in a change of cytosine to uridine [100]. This unexpected epigenetic mechanism that occurs only in eukaryotes, changes the function of mutations at DNA level and their importance in the evolution of prokaryotes and eukaryotes. Thus the epimutations in ncRNAs also are very important in the adaptation of eukaryotes, specially in reaction norm and phenotypic plasticity.

9. The post-transcriptional nc RNAs epimutations and their role in the norm of reaction and phenotypic plasticity

Until recently it was thought that in eukaryotes the mutations important for the organism were located into the areas of DNA that code for proteins. Under this framework, protein were the only molecules that regulate the action of genes and, a mutation into the a structural gene could cause a change in the primary structure of proteins. A single amino acid change could cause a serious disease. With the advances in molecular genetics and the discovery of ncRNAs, now we know that In the ncRNAs also occurs epimutations that can also cause phenotypic changes and diseases. These epimutations are more difficult to interpret at a molecular level because they do not affect the protein sequence. Generally the epimutation in ncRNAs alter the RNA structural ensamble between ncRNAs and mRNAs and, alter the message of genetic information in the cells [101,102]. Similar to proteins, the epimutations produced in the ncRNAs into cells that belonging to differents organs and tissues within the body in eukaryotes can cause a great variety of illness.

The non-coding region of DNA previously thought was garbage, we now know it is not. An exception to this rule is the contribution of by the transposable elements described in maize by Barbara McClintock in 1947, dubbed as controlling elements. The merit of her discovery was the realization that the genome is not static and there are genes that are unstable in terms of location in the genome and could promote its own transposition. Now we know that these transposable elements are found in unicellular and multicellular organisms and have a viral origin [31]. Also the discovery of transposable elements and horizontal transferences of genes had led to the understanding that the genome is a "fluid mosaic of genetic information" from different origins, where the horizontal transfer mediated by virus, tramposons and viruses play an important role in the genic flow between the organisms, not necessarily related genetically [31]. Reciently, in prokaryotes and eukaryotes there are many evidences in that another class of molecular interaction occurs in the regulation of gene action and cellular processes, principally manifested by small ncRNAs that base pairs with mRNAs and regulate the gene expression postranscriptional [101,103]. NcRNAs are a very good tool for the inactivation of specific messages, for example some classes of these ncRNAs such as siRNAs and miRNAs have been found in the regulation of of development and cell death. The nc RNAs act also in prokaryotes, in the replication and maintenance of extrachromosomal elements they have an epistatic effect to any transcriptional signals for their specific mRNAs.Thus, a single ncRNA can regulate multiple genes and have profound effects on cell physiology[104].

10. Conclusions

The mutations not only occur in the structural genes but also in those areas that code for ncRNAs, in the mRNA messenger (RNA editing) and also in the introns and in both ends of mRNA, specifically in the 3'UTR and 5'UTR regions where as well are located ncRNAs. Thus mRNA is not only an intermediary between DNA and protein, as is expressed in the classic Crick's Central Dogme of Molecular Biology, but also correspond to a relevant producer of miRNAs and siRNAs. In addition the transcription of all eukaryotic genome generates a large amount of differents ncRNAs which together with proteins regulating the expression of genes. The experimental evidences show that ncRNAs do not occur randomly in all cells but there are an enrichment of a particular ncRNAs depending of their function and cell where they act. There is now evidences that the environmental and developmental influences have effects on the phenotype. The epigenetic changes at DNA and RNA level such as DNA methylation, acetylation of histones, epimutation and RNA editing have an importance in the Darwinian fitness and could be adaptative [105]. Also many of these changes are inherited in a different way that the classic Mendelian model of heredity. One of the assumptions of population genetics is that genes are vertically transmitted to the progeny according to the laws of Mendelian inheritance. In this context, and based on Weissmann's barriers between somatic and germinal cells, only genetic changes that take place within gametes are inherited by the next generation. However at present there are evidences about a non-Mendelian model of heredity which has a close proximity to a neo-Lamackian inheritance model.

This model is based on epigenetic changes induced by the environment, in the epimutations at ncRNAs level, in the mRNA editing and also in horizontal gene transfers. Thus epimutations could be heritable. In this type of heredity there must be no barriers that prevent the changes in somatic cells could be integrated into the genomic information that resides in the nucleus of germ cells. The transposable elements, viruses and ncRNAs can be vectors incorporating somatic mutations within the genome and epigenome of the germ cells. Thus could be evade the Weissman's barriers between somatic and germ cells through retrovirus [106]. Also a mutation in piRNAs which block the action of a virus or transposable element of somatic origin could facilitate the negative impact of mobile elements in germ cells and this change may be inherited.

In humans has been postulated that cardiovascular and metabolic function and that elements of the heritable or familial component of susceptibility to cardiovascular disease, obesity and other non-communicable diseases (NCD) can be transmitted across generations by non-genomic means. Placenta's inaccurate nutritional cues,increases the risk of NCD. Endocrine or nutritional interventions during early postnatal life can reverse epigenetic and phenotypic changes induced, for example, by unbalanced maternal diet during pregnancy. Elucidation of epigenetic processes may permit perinatal identification of individuals most at risk of later NCD and enable early intervention strategies to reduce such risk [105].

Unlike prokaryontes,the eukaryote genome expresses numerous types of ncRNAs that play a fundamental role in the regulation and gene expression. Those small molecules have the possibility of interact with differents kinds of proteins generating a homeostatic system that can respond quickly to environmental changes. Both class of molecules, protein and ncRNAs, are the manifestation of a great amount of information accumulated within the genetic and epigenetic programs. The epigenetic plasticity protects individuals from environmental changes and explain the classic concepts of reaction norm and phenotypic plasticity that previously had been poorly explained on its genetic basis. But now we know that if there is an epigenetic control for these phenotypic changes. Also, these ncRNAs contribute to the processing of information in at least two form: a) Saving a lot of information on their small molecules with a minimal of energy cost.b) Rapid acquisition of information from environmental with a rapid response and adaptation. Further ncRNAs appear to facilitates the acceleration of the evolution of an organism's information contained and functional computanional system. This new picture provides a new dimensions about information processing in the brain [70] and in other cells belonging to other tissues where the ncRNAs can mitigate the negative effects of the environment, increasing adaptability and acceleration in the organic evolution.

Author details

Daniel Frías-Lasserre
Institute of Entomology, Universidad Metropolitana de Ciencias de la Educación, Santiago, Chile

Acknowledgements

Financed by the project code B-12-1, Direction of Extension of the Metropolitan University of Educational Sciences, Santiago, Chile

11. References

[1] Blakeslee AF (1933) The work of Professor Hugo De Vries. Scientific Monthly 36: 378-380.
[2] Blakeslee AF (1935) Hugo De Vries 1848-1935. Science 81: 581-582.
[3] Shull GH (1933) Hugo De Vries at eighty-five. Journal of Heredity 24 (1):3-6.
[4] Gustafsson A (1963) Mutations and the Concept of Variability: 89-104. Recent Plant Breeding Research. Almquist ,Wiksell / John Willey, Sons.
[5] Sarkar S (1999) From the Reaktionsnorm to the Adaptative Norm : The Norm of Reaction, 1909-1960. Biological Philosophy 14 : 235-252.
[6] Timoféef- Ressovsky NW (1939) Les mechanisms des mutations et la structure du gene. Actualités Scientifiques et Industrialles, 812. Genétique. Exposés publies sous la direction de B Ephrusi, Institut Biologie Physico-Chemique, Paris. Hermans and Cie, Editeurs.

[7] Mogan HT (1934) La relación de la genética con la Medicina y la Fisiología. Conferencia Nobel presentada en Estocolmo el 4 de Junio de 1934. Genetica Suplement. 2: 627-631.
[8] Lima-de-Faria (1957) Goldschmidt's interpretation of the gene concept and the problem of chromosome organization. Hereditas 43:462-465.
[9] Benzer S.(1955) Fine structure of a genetic region in bacteriophage. Science 41:344-354.
[10] Benzer S (1959) On the topology of the genetic fine structure. Proceedings of the National Academy of Sciences, 45: 1607-1620.
[11] Goldschmidt RB (1940) Chromosomes and genes. American Association for the Advancement of Science, 14: 56-66
[12] Yanofsky C (1967) Gene structure and protein structure. Scientifican American, 216: 80-94.
[13] Bonner DM (1948) Genes as determiners of cellular biochemestry. Science 108: 735-739.
[14] García- Bellido A (1977) Homeotic and atavic mutation in insects. American Zoology 1:613-629
[15] Lewis EB (1978) A gene complex controlling segmentation in *Drosophila.* Nature 276: 565-570.
[16] Ahmad A, Zhang Y, Cao XF (2010) Decoding the epigenetic language of plant development . Molecular. Plant 3: 719-728.
[17] Koerner MV, Pauler FM, Huang R ,Barlow DP (2009) The function of non-coding RNAs in genomic imprinting. Development, 136: 1771-1783.
[18] Haig D. (2000) Genomic imprinting, Sex-Biased Dispersal, and Social Behavior, 907:149-163.
[19] Hulten M., Amstrong S, Challinor P, Gould C, Hardy G, Leedham P, Lee T, McKeown C. (1991) Genomic imprinting in an Angelman and Prader- Willi translocation family. Lancet 338: 638-639.
[20] SkuseDH, James RS, Bishop DV, Coppin B, Dalton P, Aamondt-Leeper G, Bacarese-Hamilton M, Creswell C, McGurk R, Jacobs PA. (1997)Evidence from Turne's síndrome o fan imprinted X-linked locus affecting cognitive function. Nature 387 (6634): 705-708).
[21] Nilsson E, Larsen G, Manikkam M, Guerrero-Bosagna C, Savenkova MI, Skinner MK. (2012) Environmentally Induced Epigenetic Transgenerational Inheritance of Ovarian Disease.PloS ONE 7(5):e36129.doi:10.1371/journal.pone.0036129
[22] Chan TI,Yuen ST, Kong CK, Chan YW, Chan ASY (2006) Heritable germline epimutation of MSH2 in a family with hereditary nonpolyposis colorectal cancer. Nature Genetics 38: 1178-1183.
[23] Hitchins MP, Wong JJ, Suthers G, Suter CM, Martin DI, Hawkins NJ, Ward RL (2007) Inheritance of a cancer associated MLH1 germ-line epimutation. New England Journal of Medicine 356: 697-705.
[24] Mercer TR, Dinger ME, Mattick JS (2009) Long non-coding RNAs: Insights into functions. Nature Review of Genetics. 10:155-159.

[25] Eddy, S. R. Non-coding RNA genes and the modern RNA world (2001) Nature Review of Genetics12: 919-929.

[26] Mattick, J.S.; Makunin, I.V. Non-coding RNA.(2006) Human Molecular. Genetics. 1: 17-29.

[27] Stort, G. 2002. An expanding universe of noncoding RNAs. Science 296:1260-1263.

[28] Ryan, J.; Taft, R. J.; Pang, K.C.; Mercer, T.R. Dinger, M.; Mattick, J. S. 2002. Non-coding RNAs: regulators of disease. Journal of Pathoogy. 220: 126-139.

[29] Taft, R.J.; Pang, K. C.; Mercer, T. R.; Dinger, M.; Mattick, J.S.2010. Non-coding RNAs: regulators of disease. Journal of Pathology. 220:126-139

[30] Sánchez L(2008).Sex determining mechanism in insects. International Journal of Devevelopment Biology 52: 837-956

[31] Frias-Lasserre DA. (2012) Non Coding RNAs and Viruses in the Framework of the Phylogeny of the Genes, Epigenesis and Heredity. International Journal of Molecular Science 2012, *13*(1), 477-490

[32] Azzalin CM, Reichenbach P, Khoriauli L, Giulotto E, Lingner J. (2007) Telomeric repeat containing RNA and RNA surveillance factors at mammalian chromosome ends. Science 318: 798-801.

[33] Orom UA, Shiekhattar R.(2011) Long non coding RNAs and enhancers. Current Opinion in Genetics & Development 21:194-199.

[34] Johnston RJ, Horbert O (2003) A microRNA controlling left/right neuronal asymmetry in *Caenorhabditis elegans* Nature 426: 845-849.

[35] Holcik M, Liebhaber, S A. (1997). Four highly stable eukaryotic mRNAs assemble 3'untranslated region RNA-protein complexes sharing cis and trans componenets.Proceedings of National Academy of Science 94 (6): 2410-2414.

[36] Mazumder B, Seshadri V , Fox, P. 2003.Translational control by the 3'-UTR: the ends specify the means. Trends in Biochemical Sciences 28: 91-98.

[37] Lai EC (2003). MicroRNAs: Runts of Genome Assert Themselves. Current Biology 13:R925-R936.

[38] Enright, AJ, John B, Gaul U, Tuschl T, Sander Ch, Marks D S, (2003) MicroRNA targets in *Drosophila* Genome Biology 5: R1- R1-14.

[39] Brennecke J, Hipfner DR, Stark A, Russell RB, Cohen SM (2003) *bantam* encodes a developmentally regulates microRNA that controls cell proliferation and regulates the pro-apoctotic genes hid in *Drosophila.* Cell 113: 25-36.

[40] Lee RC, Feinbaum RL, Ambros V. (1993) The *C.elegans* heterochronic gene lin-4 encodes small RNAs with antisense complementarity to lin-14. Cell 75: 843-854.

[41] Rhoades MW, Reinhart BJ, Lim LP,Burge CB, Bartel DP. Prediction of plant microRNA targets. (2002) Cell, 110: 513-520.

[42] Calin G A, Calin Dan Dumitru, Masayoshi Shimizu,Roberta Bichi, Simona Zupo,Evan Noch, Hansjuerg Aldler, Sashi Rattan, Michael Keating, Kanti Rai,Laura Rassenti, Thomas Kipps, Massimo Negrini, Florencia Bullrich, and Carlo M. Croce . (2002) Frequent deletions and down-regulation of micro- RNA genes *miR15* and *miR16* at

13q14 in chronic lymphocytic leukemia. Proceedings of National Academy of Science U S A. November 26; 99(24): 15524–15529.

[43] Grishok, A., Pasquinelli, A.E., Conte, D., Li, N., Parrish, S., Ha,I., Baillie, D.L., Fire, A., Ruvkun, G., and Mello, C.C. (2001).Genes and mechanisms related to RNA interference regulate expression of the small temporal RNAs that control *C. elegans* developmental timing. Cell 106: 23–34.

[44] Lee YS, Nakahara K, Phan JW, Kim,K, HeZ, SontheIMER EJ, Carthew RW. (2004).Distinct roles for *Drosophila* Dicer-1 and Dicer-2 in the siRNA/miRNA silencing pathways. Cell 117: 69-81.

[45] Okamura K, Ishizuka A, Siomi H, Siomi M. (2004) Distinct roles for Argonaute proteins in small RNA- directed RNA cleavage pathways.Genes & Development 18: 1655-1666.Hamilton A.J, Baulcombe D.C. (1999). A specie of small antisence RNA in posttranscriptional gene silencing in plants. Science 286: 950-952.

[46] Ketting RF, Fischer SE, Bernstein E, Sijen T, Hannon GJ, Plasterk RHA. (2001) Dicer functions in RNA interference and in synthesis of small RNA involved in developmental timing in *C. elegans*. Genes and Development 15: 2654–2659

[47] Moss E.G, Tang L (2003) Conservation of the heterochronic regulator Lin-28, its developmental expression and microRNA complementary sites. Development Biology 258: 432-442.

[48] Lagos-Quintana M, Rauhut R, Meyer J, Borkhardt, Tuschl.(2003) New micro RNAs from mouse and human. RNA 9:175-179.

[49] Landtthaler, Yalcin A,Tuschi T. 2004. The human DiGeorge Syndrome critical region gene 8 and its *D.melanogaster* homolog are required for miRNA biogenesis. Current Biology 14:2162-2167.

[50] Chalfie M, Horvitz Ch M, Sulston JE (1981) Mutations that lead to reiteration in the cell lineages of *C.elegans*. Cell 24: 59-69.

[51] Ambros, V., and Horvitz, H.R. (1984). Heterochronic mutants of the nematode *Caenorhabditis elegans*. Science *226*, 409–416.

[52] Carrington JC, Ambros V (2003) Role of microRNAs in plant and animal development. Science 301: 336–338.

[53] Xu P,Vernooy SY, Guo M, Hay BA (2003). The *Drosophila* micro RNA Mir-14suppresses cell death and is required for normal fat metabolism. Current Biology 13: 790-795.

[54] Yu X, Zhou Q, Li S-C, Luo Q, Cai Y, et al. (2008) The Silkworm (*Bombyx mori*) microRNAs and Their Expressions in Multiple Developmental Stages. PLoS ONE 3(8): e2997. doi: 10.1371/journal.pone.0002997.

[55] Poy MN, Eliason L, Krutzfeldt J, Kuwajima S, Ma X , MacDonald P. E., Pfeffer, S. Tuschl T., Rajewsky N., Rorsman, P. Stoffel, M. (2004) A pancratic islet-specific microRNA Regulates insulin secretion.Nature 432:226-230.

[56] Chen CZ, Li L. Lodish HF,Bartel DP (2004) MicroRNAs modulate hematopoietic lineage differentiation. Science 303:83-86.

[57] Clop A, Marcq F, Takeda H, Pirottin D, Tordoi X, Bibe B, Bouix J, Caiment F, Elsen JM, Eychenne F, Larzul C, Laville E, Meish F, Milenkovic D, Tobin J, Charlier C, George M. (2006). Nature Genetics 38: 813-818.

[58] Zhao, Y., Ransom, J. F., Li, A., Vedantham, V., von Drehle, M., Muth, A. N., Tsuchihashi, T., McManus, M. T., Schwartz, R. J. and Srivastava, D. (2007). Dysregulation of cardiogenesis, cardiac conduction, and cell cycle in mice lacking miRNA-1. Cell 129, 303–317

[59] Dong JT, Boyd JC, Frierson HF JR. (2001)Loss of heterozygosity at 13q14 and 13q21 in high grade, high stage prostate cancer. Prostate 49:166-171.

[60] Xie Z, Kasschau KD, Carrington JC (2003) Negative feedback regulation of dicer-like1 in *Arabidopsis* by microRNA-guide mRNA degradation. Current Biology 13: 784-789.

[61] Wilcznska A, Minshall N, Armisen J, Miska E A, Standart N (2009) Two Piwi proteins, Xiwi and Xili, are expressed in the Xenopus female germline. RNA 15:337–345.

[62] Malone CD, Brennecke J, Dus M, SDtark A, McCombie R, Sachidanandam R, Hannon J H (2009) Specialized piRNA pathways act in germline and somatic tissues of the Drosophila ovary. Cell 137:522–535.

[63] Kim V. N, 2006. Small RNAs just got bigger, Piwi-interacting RNAs (piRNAs) in mammalian testes, Gene and Development., 20:1993-1997.

[64] Mikiko C. Siomi, Sato K, Pezic D, Aravin AA. 2011.PIWI-interacting small RNAs: the vanguard of genome defence. Nature Reviews Molecular Cell Biology 12, 246-258.

[65] Sarot E, Payen-Groschêne G, Bucheton A, Pélisson A (2004) Evidence for a piwidependent RNA silencing of the gypsy endogenous retrovirus by the Drosophila melanogaster flamenco gene. Genetics 166:1313–1321.

[66] De Fazio, S., Bartonicek, N., Di Giacomo, M., Abreu-Goodger, C., Sankar, A., Funaya, C., Antony, C., Moreira, P.N., Enright, A.J. & O'Carroll, 2011.The endonuclease activity of Mili fuels piRNA amplification that silences LINE1 elements D. Nature. 2011 Oct 23. doi: 10.1038/nature10547.

[67] Esteller M.2011.Non-coding RNAs in human disease. Nature Reviews Genetics 12, 861-874

[68] Watanabe T, Tomizawa S ,Mitsuya K, Totoki Y, Yukamoto, Y, Kuramochi-Miyagawa S, Lida N, Hoki Y, Murphy P J, Toyoda A, Gotoh K, Hiura H, Arima T, Fujiyama A, Sado T, Shibata T, Nakano T, Lin H, Ichiyanagi K, Soloway P, Sasaki H. 2011. Role for piRNAs and Noncoding RNA in de Novo DNA Methylation of the Imprinted Mouse *Rasgrf1* Locus. Science 332: 848-852.

[69] Laurent GS, Wahlestedt C (2007). Noncoding RNAs:couplers of analog and digital information in nervous system function?. Trends in Neurosciences 30:612-621.

[70] Zavanelli MI, Britton JS, Igel A H, Ares M. 1994. Mutations in an Essential U2 Small Nuclear RNA Structure Cause Cold-Sensitive U2 Small Nuclear Ribonucleoprotein Function by Favoring Competing Alternative U2 RNA Structures. Molecular and Cellular Biology 14: 1689-1697.

[71] Urushiyama S, Tani T Ohshima Y. 1996. Isolation of novel pre-mRNA splicing mutants of *Schizosaccharomyces pombe.* Molecular and General Genetics MGG 253: 118-127

[72] Kiss T.(2002) Small nucleolar RNAs: an abundant group of noncoding RNAs with diverse cellular functions. Cell. 109: 145-148.

[73] Liang H,Landweber LF (2007) Hypothesis: RNA editing of microRNA target sites in human?. RNA 13:463-467.

[74] Borovjagin A, Gerbi SA. (2001). *Xenopus* U3 snoRNA GAC-Box A9 and Box A Sequence Play Dictinct Functional Roles in rRNA Processing. Molecular and Cellular Biology 21: 6210-6221.

[75] Preti M, Ribeyre C,Pcali CH, BDieci G.(2010) The Telomere-Binding Protein Tbf1 Demarcates snoRNA Gene Promoters in Saccharomyces cerevisiae. Molecular Cell 38, 614–620.

[76] Clark MB, Johnston RL, Inostroza-Ponta M, Fox AH, Fortini E, Moscato P. Dinger ME, Mattick JS (2012). Genome-wide analysis of long noncoding RNA stability. Genome Research. http://www.genome.org/cgi/doi/10.1101/gr.131037.111.

[77] Tian D, Sun S, Lee JT.(2010) The long non-coding RNA,JPX, is a molecular switch for chromosome inactivation. Cell 143:390-403.

[78] Deng X., Meller V.H. (2006). Non-coding RNA in fly dosage compensation. Trends in Biochemical Sciences 31: 526-532.

[79] Koerner, M.V.; Pauler, F.M.; Huang, R.; Barlow, D.P. (2009) The function of non-coding RNAs in genomic imprinting. Development, 136, 1771–1783.

[80] Satterlee, J.S.; Barbee, S.; Jin, P.; Krichevsky, A.; Salama, S.; Schratt, G.; Wu, D.Y. (2007) Noncoding RNAs in the brain. Journal of Neurosciences., *27*, 11856–11859.

[81] Dinger, M.E.; Amaral, P.P.; Mercer, T.R.; Pang, K.C.; Bruce, S.J.; Gardiner, B.B.; Askarian-Amiri, M.E.; Ru, K.; Soldà, G.; Simons, C.Simons C, Sunkin SM, Crowe ML, Grimmond SM, Perkins AC, Mattick JS. (2008) Long noncoding RNAs in mouse embryonic stem cell pluripotency and differentiation. Genome Research., *18*, 1433–1445

[82] Dinger ME, Pang KC, Mercer TR, Crowe ML, Grimmond SM, Mattick JS (2009). NRED: a database of long noncoding RNA expression. Nucleic Acid Research 37: D122-126.

[83] Taft, R.J.; Pang, K.C.; Mercer, T.R.; Dinger, M.; Mattick, J.S.(2010) Non-coding RNAs: Regulators of disease. Journal of Pathology, *220*, 126–139.

[84] Thakur, N.; Tiwari, V.K.; Thomassin, H.; Pandey, R.R.; Kanduri, M.; Gondor, A.; Grange, T.; Ohlsson, R.; Kanduri, C. (2004) An antisense RNA regulates the bidirectional silencing property of the Kcnq1 imprinting control region. Molecular Cell Biology, *24*, 7855–7862.

[85] Kurakawa R.(2011) Long non-coding RNAs as a regulator for transcription. Program of Molecular Biology 51:29-41

[86] Raman, R.P.; Kanduri, C. (2011).Transcriptional and post transcriptional programming by long noncoding RNAs. Program of Molecular Subcellular Biology, 51, 1–27.

[87] Azzalin, C.M.; Reichenbach, P.; Khoriauli, L.; Giulotto, E.; Lingner, J. (2007) Telomeric repeat containing RNA and RNA surveillance factors at mammalian chromosome ends. Science, 318, 798–801.

[88] Schoeftner, S.; Blasco, M.A. (2007) Developmentally regulated transcription of mammalian telomeres by DNA dependent RNA polymerase II. Natural Cell Biology, 10, 228–236.

[89] Arora, R.; Brun, C.M.C.; Azzalin, C.M. Terra. (2011) Long noncoding RNAs at eukaryotic telomeres. Program of Molecular Subcellular Biology, *51*, 65–94.

[90] Orom, U.A.; Shiekhattar, R. (2011) Long non-coding RNAs and enhancers. Current. Opinion in Genetics Development, 21: 194–198.

[91] Bernard D, Prasanth KV, Tripathi V, Colasse S, Nakamura T, Xuan Z, Zhang MQ, Sedel F, Jourdren L, Coulpier F, Triller A, Spector DL, Bessis A (2010) A long nuclear-retained non-coding RNA regulates synaptogenesis by modulating gene expression. The EMBO Journal (2010) 29: 3082 – 3093.

[92] De Lucia F, Dean C. (2011) Long non-coding RNAs and chromatin regulation. 14:168-173. Epub 2010

[93] Roberts KA, Abraira VE,Tucker AF, Goodrich LV, Andrews NC (2012) Mutation of *Rubie*, a novel Long Coding RNA Located Upstream of *Bmp4*, Causes Vestibular Malformation in Mice. PLoS ONE 7(1): e29495.doi:10.1371/journal.pone.0029495.
Cartault F, Munier P Benko, E, Desguerre I , Hanein S, Boddaert N, Bandiera S, Vellayoudoma J, Krejbich-Trototf P, Bintnerg M, Hoarauf JJ,Girardb M, Géninh E, de Lonlayb P, Fourmaintrauxa A, Navillej M, Rodriguezk D, Feingold J, Renouil M, Arnold Munnich A, Westhofm E, Fähling M, Lyonnetb S,Henrion-Caude A. (2012) Mutation in a primate-conserved retrotransposon reveals a noncoding RNA as a mediator of infantile encephalopathy. www.pnas.org/cgi/doi/10.1073/pnas.111159610.

[94] Benne R. (1992) RNA editing in trypanosomes.Molecular Biology Report 16: 217-227.

[95] Benne R. Van der Burg J,BrakenhoffJPJ, Sloof P, Van Boom JH, Tromp MC, (1986) Major transcript of the frameshifted coxll gene from *Trypanosome* mitochondria contains four nucleotides that are not incoded in the DNA.Cell 46:819-826.

[96] Rubio MAT,Pastar I, Gaston KW, Ragone FL, Janzen ChJ, Cross GAM, Papavasiliou,FN,Alfonso JD.(2007) An adenosine-to inosine tRNA editing enzyme that can perform C-to-U deamination of DNA. PNA 104: 7821-7826.

[97] Luciano DJ, Mirsky H, Vendetti NJ,Maas S, (2004) RNA editing of miRNA precursor. RNA 10:1174-1177.

[98] Gott, J.M.; Emerson, R.B. (2000). Functions and mechanisms of RNA editing. Annual Review of Genetics 34, 499-531. Syndrome of an imprintedX-linked locus affecting cognitive function. Nature: 387: 705-708.

[99] Blanc V, Davidson NO (2003) C-to-U RNA Editing: Mechanisms Leading to Genetic Diversity. The Journal of Biological Chemestry 278: 1395-1398.

[100] Shimoni Y, Friedlander G, Hertzroni G, Niv G, Altuvia S, Biham O, Margalit H. (2007) Regulation of gene expression by small non-coding RNAs: a quantitative view. Molecular Systems Biology 3:138.

[101] Halvorsen M., Martin JS, Broadaway S, Laederach A. (2010) Disease-Associated Mutations that alter the RNA structural ensamble.Plos Genetics 6 (8): e1001074.doi: 10.1371/journal.pgen.1001074.

[102] Storz G, Altuvia S, Wassarmann KM (2005) An abundance of RNA regulators Annual Review of Bichemical 74:199-217.

[103] Gottesman S. (2005). Micros for microbes: non-coding regulatory RNAs in bacteria. Trends in Genetics 21:7399-404.

[104] Hanson M, Godfrey KM, Lillycrop KA, Burdge GC, Gluckman PD.(2011) Developmental plasticity and developmental origins of non-communicable disease: theoretical considerations and epigenetic mechanisms. Progress in Biophysic and Molecular Biology. 106:272-80.

[105] Steele EJ, EJ, Lindle RA, Blanden RV (1998) Lamarck's signature. Allen and Unwin, Sydney, Australia, 286 pp.

Chapter 10

Screening of Gene Mutations in Lung Cancer for Qualification to Molecularly Targeted Therapies

Paweł Krawczyk, Tomasz Kucharczyk and Kamila Wojas-Krawczyk

Additional information is available at the end of the chapter

http://dx.doi.org/10.5772/48689

1. Introduction

In many developed countries non-small-cell lung cancer (NSCLC), which accounts for approximately 85% of lung cancers, is the first cause of death in patients with malignant neoplasms. Depending on patients' medical status, surgical resection is possible in early stages of NSCLC. Regrettably, only 15-30% of newly diagnosed NSCLC cases can be qualified for operation. Therefore, chemotherapy and radiotherapy plays the dominant role in the multidisciplinary treatment of patients with NSCLC and small-cell lung cancer (SCLC). Unfortunately, both options of treatment in locally advanced and metastatic lung cancer have limited efficacy [1]. Molecularly targeted therapies offer new possibilities of lung cancer treatment in genetically predisposed patients. Within the next few years, personalised therapy of whole lung cancer population based on screening of different gene mutations will become a fact.

The development of cancer usually depends on strong carcinogenic effect of substances found in cigarette smoke on bronchial epithelial cells. Those carcinogens lead to genetic disorders that cause appearance of preinvasive changes: squamous dysplasia preceding carcinoma *in situ* and squamous cell carcinoma as well as atypical adenomatous hyperplasia (AAH) preceding development of adenocarcinoma. The preinvasive cells as well as cancer cells are characterised with large genome changes. Comparative genomic hybridisation (CGH) studies have identified chromosomal aberrations, particularly amplifications and deletions, in lung cancer cells. Cancer cells exhibit deletions of chromosome 17 short arm, with loss of *p53* gene (deletion of 17(p12-13) and chromosome 9 short arm, with loss of *p16* gene (*CDKN2A*) (deletion of 9(p21-22). Both mentioned genes are suppressor genes and lack of their protein products allows aneuploid cancer cells to survive and accumulate serious chromosomal aberrations like deletions 3(p14-21), 8(p21-23), 13(q14), 13(q22-24) and allelic losses at 9(p21), 13(q24) as well as gains at 1(q21-31), 3(q21-22), 3(q25-27), 5(p13-14), 8(q23-

24), 7(p12). The presence of deletions generates abnormal expression or impaired function of tumour suppressor genes such as *RB1, FHIT, RASSF1A, SEMA3B* and *PTEN*. However, the gain of chromosomal region including oncogenes is associated with overexpression or increased activity of *MYC, KRAS, EGFR, CCDN1, MCM2, RUVBL1, SOX2* and *BCL2* genes [2, 3]. Moreover, cell subclones with new genetic abnormalities may become dominant within metastases or within persistent or recurrent cancer deposits through selective pressures exerted by chemotherapy or molecularly targeted therapy [4].

Deletion of chromosome 17 short arm, with loss of *p53* gene, is the most frequent disturbance in lung cancer (50-70%). Squamous cell carcinoma (SCC) of lung exhibits higher frequencies of deletions at chromosomal regions 3(p14-21), 8(p21-23), 17(p13) (*p53* gene), 13(q14) (*RB1* gene), 9(p21) (*CDKN2A* gene) and amplification of 3(q21-22) (*SOX2* gene) when compared with adenocarcinoma (AC). Amplification of 7(p11) and 14(q13) causing increased gene dosage and protein expression of thyroid transcriptional factor-1/NK2 homeobox-1 (TITF-1/NKX2-1) and of epidermal growth factor receptor (EGFR) are prevalent in lung adenocarcinoma [2, 3].

2. Genetic mutations in lung cancer cells

Apart of chromosomal aberrations single gene mutations can appear in lung cancer cells. These mutations can be revealed with molecular biology techniques. Mentioned mutations do not often appear simultaneously in one cancer cell (less than 3% of tumour cells). They concern genes important for correct proliferation, differentiation and cell growth such as oncogenes and genes for signal proteins involved in a complicated network of intracellular signal transmission (predominantly genes for tyrosine and threonine-serine kinases).

The most important kind of genetic disturbances observed in NSCLC cells are point mutations (single nucleotide substitutions), small (few to a few dozen base pairs) deletions or insertions and formation of fusion genes as a result of translocation of gene fragments, usually within a single chromosome. Some of these alterations change the structure of proteins (sense mutations) which play an important role in oncogenesis, others shift the expression of oncogenes and suppressor genes, while some remain silent. Such processes lead to protein malfunction: they can increase or decrease protein expression or cause differences in normal enzyme activity.

Accumulation of driver mutations in different genes is detected depending on history of tumour exposure to carcinogens. Failure of DNA repair and progressive genetic instability leads to appearance of mutation that drives cancer development, its growth and metastases [4]. Molecular type of lung cancer is partially consistent with histological type of tumour. Although frequency of occurrence of some driver mutations is extremely rare, in only 20% of NSCLC tumours important mutations are not detected. Small cell lung cancer is less characterised in terms of incidence of genetic mutations. Until 2011, 1738 mutated genes and tens of thousands of different types of mutations were identified in NSCLC [2, 5, 6, 7]. Figure 1 shows the percentage of tumours with identified mutations in all histological types of NSCLC.

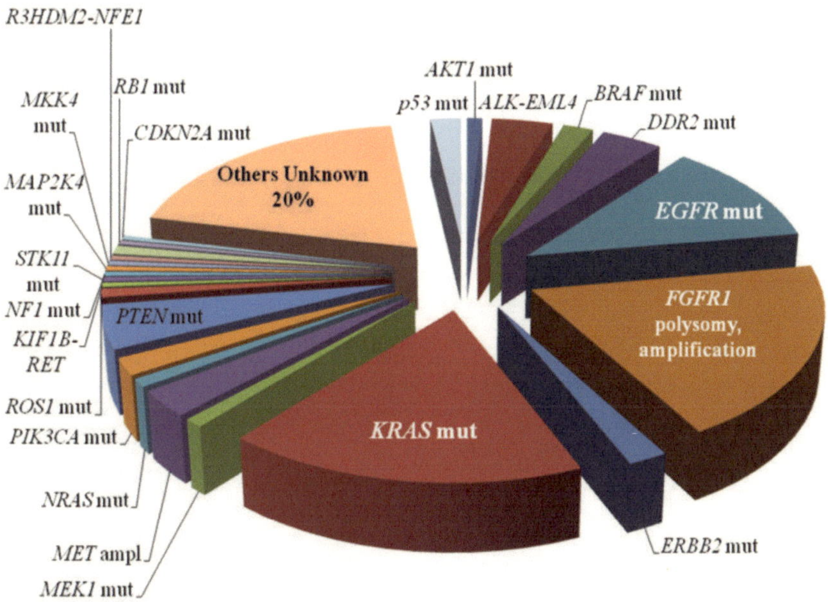

Figure 1. The percentage of NSCLC tumours with identified mutations in different genes (*EGFR* gene amplification and polysomy, as well as *p53* gene abnormalities which are common in NSCLC tumours have not been included on the graph).

NSCLC is a heterogeneous aggregate of histological subtypes, which traditionally have been grouped together because of similarities of treatment outcome. Ideally, a tumour classification system should include morphologic and genetic distinctions between tumour types, which will help to define specific subset of patients responsive to certain molecularly targeted treatment. In terms of genetic mutations squamous cell carcinomas are the least described. Mutations have not been detected in over 50% of already screened tumours (Fig. 2). On the other hand adenocarcinoma cases are definitely better described and in only 20% of tumours screening fails to describe any mutations. Among 10-15% of non-smokers (but also light-smokers and former smokers) adenocarcinoma might develop regardless of tobacco smoking. In these cases in almost all tumours different genetic mutations have been found, mostly in epidermal growth factor receptor (*EGFR*) and *KRAS* genes as well as presence of *EML4-ALK* fusion gene (Fig. 3). Accumulated evidence suggested that lung cancer in ever smokers and never smokers follow distinct molecular pathways and may therefore respond to distinct therapy. One could speculate than non-small cell lung cancer in ever and never smokers are two distinct disorders regarding their molecular level and the manner of treatment planning [5, 6, 7, 8, 9, 10, 11, 12].

The most frequent irregularity found among squamous cell carcinoma patients is an amplification of gene for fibroblast growth factor receptor type 1 (FGFR) and *p53* gene abnormalities. These disturbances could overlap with other mutations. In SCC it is extremely rare to detect *EGFR, PTEN, ERBB2 (HER2), PIK3CA, DDR2* or *BRAF* mutations, which are more typical for adenocarcinoma [5, 6, 7].

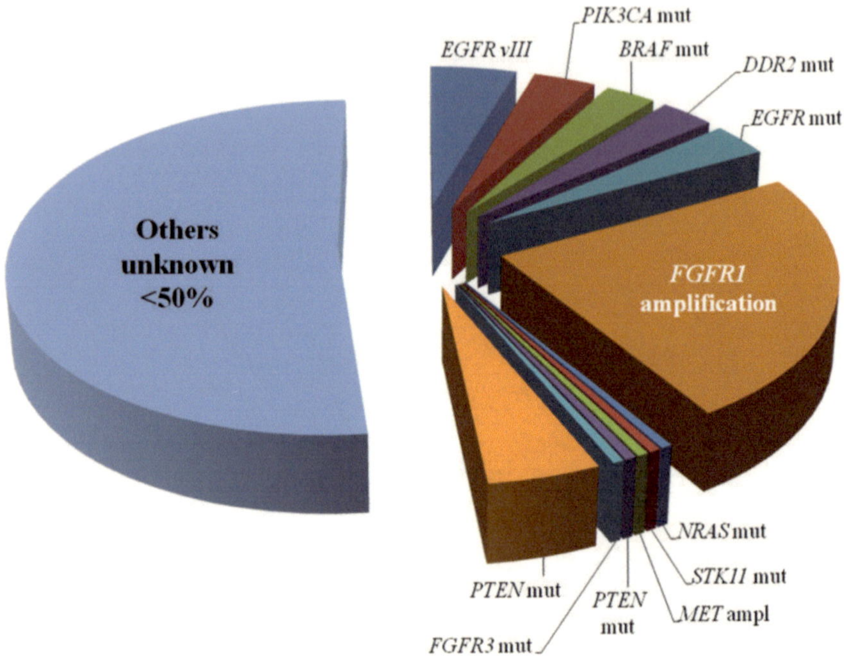

Figure 2. The percentage of SCC tumours with identified mutations in different genes (*p53* gene abnormalities which are common in SCC tumours have not been included on the graph)

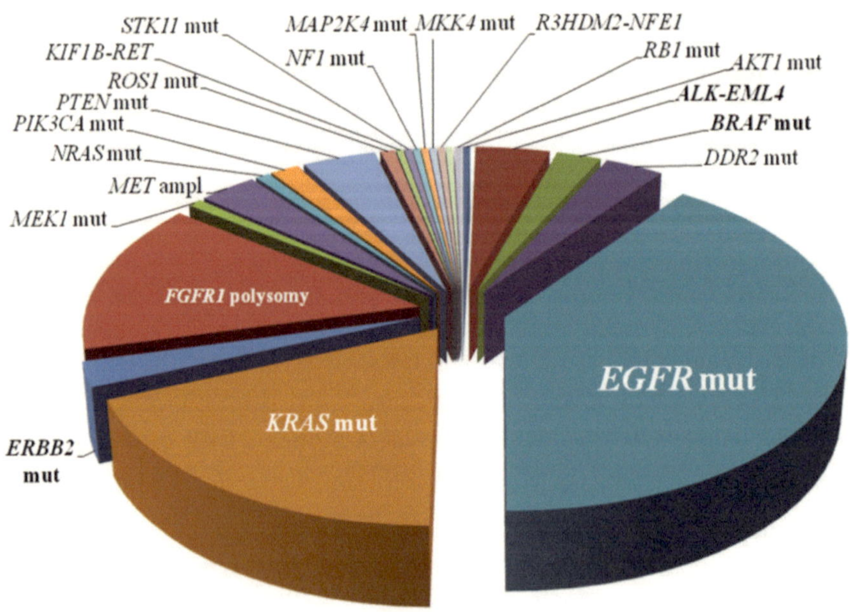

Figure 3. The percentage of AC tumours with identified mutations in different genes (*EGFR* gene amplification and polysomy have not been included on the graph).

Among patients with adenocarcinoma the most often detected irregularities are in *EGFR* gene, Kirsten rat sarcoma viral oncogene homolog (*KRAS*) gene and *p53* gene. In non-smoking Caucasian population activating mutations in *EGFR* gene appear with frequency of over 50%. The most common mutations in this gene are: small (9-21 base pair) deletions in exon 19 (48% of detected mutations) and missense mutations in exon 21 (L858R, 41% of detected mutations). Substitutions in exon 18-21 or insertions and duplications in exon 20 are rare but they also appear [2, 9, 13].

Mutations in exon 18-21 of *EGFR* gene concern tyrosine kinase domain of the EGF receptor. Overexpression of EGFRs' tyrosine kinase function leads to hyperphosphorylation of intracellular signalling proteins of Pi3K/Akt or RAS/RAF/MAPK pathways without having to activate the receptor with its specific ligand – the EGF. The activation of Pi3K/Akt pathway results in stimulation of transcription factors such as STAT or excessive proliferation of cancer cells. Mutations in *EGFR* gene are most common in papillary AC, less frequent in adenocarcinoma with „lepidic predominant" growth and least frequent in solid AC [2, 13].

Mutations in *KRAS* gene are also common and are detected in 15-25% of adenocarcinoma cases. *KRAS* gene, which is coding a low molecular weight guanosine triphosphatase (GTPase) is considered to be the most frequently mutated oncogene in lung AC arising in patients with history of smoking. Most *KRAS* mutations involve replacing glycine with other amino acids such as valine, aspartic acid and glutamic acid in codon 12. Less frequent mutations consider codon 13 and 61. The emergence of the mutation causes the reduction of GDPase activity with subsequent potent activation of mitogenic and proliferative signalling through the RAF/MEK/ERK/MAPK cascade. Mutations in *KRAS* gene are most common in solid mucinous adenocarcinoma and in acinar adenocarcinoma [2, 5, 6, 7].

Among other mutations detected in more than 2% of adenocarcinomas are *EML4-ALK* fusion gene, substitution V600E in *BRAF* oncogene, substitutions in codon 542, 545 and 1047 of *PIK3CA* oncogene, insertion in exon 20 of *ERBB2* gene, polysomy of *FGFR1* gene and amplification of *cMET* gene. Both anaplastic large cell lymphoma kinase (*ALK*) and echinoderm microtubule associated protein 4 (*EML4*) genes are located in chromosome 2p and fusion of both involves small inversions within this region. *EML4-ALK* fusion results in constitutive activation of ALK kinase. *EML4-ALK* fusion gene is prevalent in lung adenocarcinoma (2-4%), especially in signet ring cell carcinoma (<15%), in younger patients and in never- or light smokers. *EML4-ALK* fusion gene is mutually exclusive with *EGFR* and *KRAS* gene mutations. Recently, new fusion genes have been discovered in lung adenocarcinomas, including fusion of kinesis family member 5B (*KIF5B*) with ret proto-oncogene (*RET*) and fusion of coiled-coil domain containing protein 6 (*CCDC6*) with *RET* as well as fusions of *ALK* with c-ros oncogene 1 receptor tyrosine kinase (*ROS1*) [2, 5, 6, 7, 14, 15].

Information about the mutations mentioned above come from large databases such as *Catalogue of Somatic Mutations in Cancer* (COSMIC), *My Cancer Genome*, *The Cancer Genome*

Atlas and the results obtained by the American *Lung Cancer Mutation Consortium* (LCMC) [5, 6, 7, 16].

3. Molecular biology methods in lung cancer diagnostics

Mutation testing has become an essential determinant in clinical practice in decision of treatment options for patients with non-small-cell lung carcinomas. Unfortunately NSCLC tumours, in which the molecular diagnostics is carried out, are highly heterogeneous and the cytological and histological material is often insufficient to complete the analysis (small percentage of cancer cells or DNA fragmentation in the process of paraffin embedding). Direct sequencing is still a frequently used method despite having low sensitivity and being time-consuming and labour-intensive. However, direct sequencing and particularly next generation sequencing (technology based on reversible dye terminators, sequencing by ligation and pirosequencing) are the methods of high-throughput screening for unknown mutations. Microarrays containing oligonucleotide mutation probes are emerging as useful platforms for the diagnosis of multiple genetic abnormalities in cancer cells [17, 18].

The multiplex SNaPshot PCR (minisequencing) technique is a PCR (polymerase chain reaction)-based assay for detection of known mutations. Specific primer which anneals immediately adjacent to the mutated region is extended by one base using a fluorescently labeled ddNTPs, which are detected in capillary electrophoresis. No further extension is possible because of the ddNTP binding. This kind of reaction is being used more and more frequently because of its fast and sensitive detection of many known mutations in a single assay [19].

Recent advances in molecular techniques have enabled the design of sensitive detection assays based on quantitative real-time PCR, but usually with limited degree of mutation coverage. Allele-specific PCR (ASP-PCR), amplification refractory mutation system PCR (ARMS-PCR), clamp PCR and mutant-enriched PCR (ME-PCR) are among these techniques. The most frequently used is the ARMS–PCR method that can detect a known SNP (single nucleotide polymorphism). It consists of two complementary reactions: one containing an ARMS primer specific for the normal DNA sequence that cannot amplify mutant DNA at a given locus and the other one containing a mutant-specific primer that cannot amplify normal DNA. High resolution melting (HRM) real-time PCR is also a technique that might allow fast screening for mutations. The real-time PCR technology itself is highly flexible and many alternative instruments and fluorescent probe systems have been developed recently [17, 18].

For detecting polysomy, gene amplifications and the presence of fusion genes molecular probes labelled with different fluorochromes and fluorescence *in situ* hybridisation (FISH) technique are being used. Techniques related to FISH, but allowing to label only one gene fragment, are silver *in situ* hybridisation (SISH) and chromogenic *in situ* hybridisation (CISH). The FISH technique requires an assessment of signal quantity from labelled genes and chromosome fragments with fluorescence microscopy whereas SISH or CISH staining can be analysed in light microscope [17, 18].

Routine genetic testing for somatic mutations in lung cancer biopsies is becoming the standard for providing optimal patients care. However, it is unclear whether this testing should be routine for all lung cancer patients, because the prevalence of the most common mutations is very low especially in heavy smokers with squamous cell carcinoma. Moreover, great number of molecular biology methods and variety of biological material acquired from patients create a critical need for robust, well-validated diagnostic tests and equipment that are both sensitive and specific for mutations. An *In Vitro* Diagnostic Medical Device (IVD) is defined in Directive 98/79/EC of European Parliament and of the Council. IVD is described as any medical device which is a reagent, calibrator, control material, kit, equipment or system, whether used alone or in combination, intended by the manufacturer to be used *in vitro* for the examination of specimens, including blood and tissue donations, derived from the human body for the purpose of providing information concerning pathological state and congenital abnormalities of patients as well as to monitor therapeutic effect. IVD equipment is labelled by CE marking according to European Product Safety Regulations [20].

4. Molecularly targeted therapies in lung cancer

Molecularly targeted drugs are directed against abnormal proteins and other molecules, specific for cancer cells, participating in metabolic pathways. Excess activation of those pathways is essential for growth and unrestrained proliferation of cancer cells. Blocking these pathways results in inhibition of cell division and in cell apoptosis. Therefore, molecularly targeted drugs show high efficacy in two groups of patients:

1. if the mutation of the gene encoding a signalling pathway protein results in excessive activity while changing its structure, what allows more effective binding of the drug (e.g. activating mutations in *EGFR* gene and the efficacy of tyrosine kinase inhibitors of EGFR),
2. if the mutation of the gene encoding a signalling pathway protein results in excessive activity of the pathway and its blocking, regardless of the matching of the drug to the target protein, impairs tumour cell proliferation, which can be achieved at two levels:
   a. direct blocking of abnormal protein
   b. blocking of subsequent signalling pathway proteins stimulated by the abnormal protein [21].

Therefore, many of the therapies currently under development target several signalling proteins, especially tyrosine kinase receptors (e.g. EGFR, HER2, HER3, IGF-1R, cMET) or proteins in downstream signalling pathway (RAS/RAF/MAPK/mTOR and Pi3K/AKT) [19, 21].

Excessive stimulation of epidermal growth factor receptor increases proliferation of cancer cells in different kinds of tumours, i.a. in non-small-cell lung cancer. Cell growth signal is transmitted from EGFR (HER1), after its heterodimerisation with other member of HER family (ERBB2 – HER2, HER3 or HER4), through phosphorylation of Pi3K/AKT and

RAS/RAF/MAPK/mTOR pathway. The phosphorylation takes place due to EGFR tyrosine kinase activity, which performs hydrolysis of ATP to ADP and free phosphate. Tyrosine kinases are a part of EGFR but also other cell receptors and signalling proteins. Phosphorylation disorder initiated by EGFR tyrosine kinase is associated with the development of NSCLC that is independent from tobacco smoke carcinogens. Blocking of EGFR function may be achieved by using small molecule tyrosine kinase inhibitors (TKI) or monoclonal antibodies (such as cetuximab), which bind to extracellular domain of EGFR. Inhibition of tyrosine kinase function by TKI-EGFR is much more effective if the amino acid structure of the enzyme is disrupted by activating mutations in *EGFR* gene (described in the previous section). Cetuximab on the other hand demonstrates better effectiveness when high expression of EGFR is present on cancer cell surface [2, 9, 11, 12, 21, 22].

At the moment, two reversible EGFR TKIs are in use: gefitinib and erlotinib. Phase III study IPASS, carried out among Asian patients (up to 40% of *EGFR* gene mutation NSCLC carriers), has proven higher efficacy of gefitinib (71,2% response rate, longer progression free survival (PFS) up to 12 months and significant improvement in quality of life, but without overall survival (OS) prolongation) in compare to chemotherapy consisting of carboplatin and paclitaxel in patients with activating *EGFR* gene mutations. However, among patients with wild type *EGFR* gene, first line chemotherapy of advanced NSCLC with gefitinib was ineffective. The study included more than 1 200 adenocarcinoma patients, with a retrospective biomarker analysis performed on specimens from 437 tumour samples with evaluable *EGFR* gene mutation data. Mutations in *EGFR* gene were identified in 261 (59,7%) of these patients. Later studies comparing efficacy of erlotinib or gefitinib and standard chemotherapy had proven that EGFR TKIs are effective in first line of treatment (NEJ 002, WJTOG 3405, OPTIMAL, EURTAC studies) but only in patients with activating mutations in *EGFR* gene (Table 1). Moreover, OPTIMAL study showed that patients with deletion in exon 19 had longer median PFS than those with substitution L858R in exon 21 of *EGFR* gene. However, IPASS and WJTOG 3405 studies have not proven these observations [2, 11, 12, 21, 22, 23].

The BR.21 study concerned the effectiveness of erlotinib monotherapy in second or third line therapy in patients with advanced NSCLC. Erlotinib has prolonged PFS and improved quality of life when compared to best supportive care in the whole patients group, but an objective response was achieved in only 10% of patients. Patients with *EGFR* gene amplification, detected with FISH technique, responded more frequently to therapy with erlotinib. 61 (38,4%) of 159 tumours analysed in BR.21 study were positive for an increased *EGFR* gene copy number. Response rates were 21% and 5% in patients who were FISH-positive and FISH-negative, respectively. This benefit seemed to extend to survival (HR=0,43; p=0,004). It is not certain, if this result was related with underestimation of *EGFR* gene mutations in FISH-positive patients due to the use of sequencing method for *EGFR* gene mutation analysis. The INTEREST study confirmed this suggestion, demonstrating the superiority of gefitinib over docetaxel in second line of treatment in patients with activating mutation of *EGFR* gene. Application of reversible TKI-EGFR in II and III line of treatment in patients without activating mutations in *EGFR* gene is controversial [2, 11, 12, 21, 22, 23].

Study	**Patients with mutation**	**Treatment arms**	**Response rate**	**Median PFS**	**PFS (favouring TKI-EGFR)**
IPASS	216 Asian patients	gefitinib vs. paclitaxel/carboplatin	71% vs. 47%	9,5 vs. 6,3 months	HR=0,48 (95% CI: 0,36-0,64)
JP 0056 (NEJ 002)	200 North-East Japan patients	gefitinib vs. paclitaxel/carboplatin	74% vs. 31%	10,8 vs. 5,4 months	HR=0,31 (95% CI: 0,22-0,41)
WJTOG 3405	177 Asian patients	gefitinib vs. docetaxel/carboplatin	62% vs. 32%	9,2 vs. 6,3 months	HR=0,49 (95% CI: 0,34-0,71)
OPTIMAL	165 Asian patients	erlotinib vs. gemcitabine/carboplatin	83% vs. 36%	13,1 vs. 4,6 months	HR=0,16 (95% CI: 0,10-0,26)
EURTAC	170 Caucasian patients	erlotinib vs. platinum doublet	58% vs. 15%	9,7 vs. 5,2 months	HR=0,42 (95% CI: 0,27-0,64

Table 1. Prospective, randomised studies of efficacy of first-line TKI-EGFR and standard chemotherapy in patients with *EGFR* gene mutations [12].

The phase III SATURN study was designed to examine the effect of erlotinib in maintenance therapy dedicated to patients who had clinical benefit after 4 cycles of standard chemotherapy. PFS was significantly prolonged (HR=0,71; p<0,0001) and response rate (11,9% vs. 5,4%) was improved with erlotinib compared to best supportive care in all patients. However, significantly prolonged PFS was observed with erlotinib mainly in group of patients whose tumours had *EGFR* mutation (HR=0,10; p<0,0001) [2, 11, 12, 23].

Although controversial clinical trial results, National Comprehensive Cancer Network (NCCN) recognises that the presence of EGFR-activating mutations represents a "critical" biomarker for appropriate patients selection for TKI-EGFR therapy [24].

Some genetic irregularities may be responsible for occurrence of primary or secondary resistance to reversible TKI-EGFR and disease progression even after more than ten months of therapy. *EGFR* wild-type gene and *KRAS* gene mutations are associated with intrinsic TKI-EGFR resistance. Moreover mutations in *KRAS* and *EGFR* genes do not occur simultaneously in the same cancer cell. Patients with mutated *KRAS* gene experience better PFS with standard chemotherapy than with TKI-EGFR therapy. However, a subgroup of 90 patients from SATURN study who had *KRAS* mutation showed no significant difference in PFS in erlotinib-arm and placebo-arm. Although KRAS mutation has been associated with clinical outcomes with cetuximab in colorectal cancer, no association was reported from analyses of clinical studies of cetuximab in combination with chemotherapy in patients with NSCLC. Currently, *KRAS* mutation testing is not recommended in molecular diagnosis of NSCLC patients [11, 12].

The secondary resistance to reversible TKI-EGFR is connected with the inability to extend overall survival with erlotinib or gefitinib therapy. Underlying mechanism of resistance to reversible EGFR TKIs is an amplification of *IGF1R* and *MET* gene, but also mutations in exon 20 of *EGFR* and *HER2* genes. The presence of such abnormalities may have a pivotal role in qualification to novel therapies, currently in their last phase of clinical trials. Inhibitors of insulin-like growth factor receptor 1 (IGF1-R), both small molecule as well as monoclonal antibodies, and inhibitors of receptor for hepatocyte growth factor (cMET) (e.g. tivantinib – ARQ-197 or MetMab) may be used in some patients treated with reversible TKI-EGFR among whom a resistance for the therapy has occurred as an alternative way of Pi3K/AKT pathway stimulation created through overexpression of IGF1R and cMET (Figure 4) [25, 26, 27].

The occurrence of T790M mutation in exon 20 of *EGFR* gene and mutations in exon 20 of *HER2* gene may be important for the proper qualifications for the treatment with irreversible EGFR TKIs. Drugs like afatinib (BIBW-2992), PF-00299804 or neratinib (HKI-272) may be effective in case of resistance to reversible TKI-EGFR when a secondary mutation is present (e.g. T790M). The action of afatinib remains until the EGFR protein is removed from the cancer cell surface. Furthermore, afatinib also blocks HER2 and HER4 proteins which are preferential heterodimerisation partners for EGFR during stimulation by EGF. In LUX-Lung 1 study, afatinib efficacy (prolongation of PFS) was proven as a rescue treatment after failure of erlotinib or gefitinib if duration of second-line TKI-EGFR treatment exceeded 24 weeks (HR=0,38, p<0,0001). Irreversible TKI-EGFR may also be more effective than reversible TKI-EGFR in first-line of treatment of patients with activating mutations of *EGFR* gene. In the LUX-Lung 2 study, 129 patients with activating *EGFR* mutations and no previous TKI-EGFR treatment received afatinib as a single agent. Overall response rate was 60% with a promising PFS of 14 months. LUX-Lung 3 and LUX-Lung 6 studies are designed to compare effectiveness of afatinib and chemotherapy based on pemetrexed and cisplatin or gemcitabine and cisplatin in patients with *EGFR* mutations. As first-line treatment of patients with known *EGFR* mutation, PF-00299804 showed encouraging efficacy, which exceeded the erlotinib effectiveness. In patients with T790M and T854A mutations in *EGFR* gene, the combination of irreversible TKI-EGFR therapy with application of monoclonal antibody against EGFR (cetuximab) may be also reasonable [11, 12, 25, 26, 27].

Big hopes for the development of lung adenocarcinoma therapy are related to phase III studies over a novel, small molecule, molecularly targeted drug – crizotinib, an inhibitor of ALK, ROS1 and cMET. Crizotinib is particularly active in patients with *EML4-ALK* fusion gene, inducing disease control in up to 90% of such patients and prolonging their overall survival. In patients with *EML4-ALK* fusion gene, 64% of patients treated with crizotinib survived more than 2 years and 77% of patients survived more than 1 year. Newly defined kinase fusions (KIF5B with RET and ROS1 with ALK and with other fusion partners) may be also promising targets for molecular therapies [11, 12, 14, 15, 26, 27].

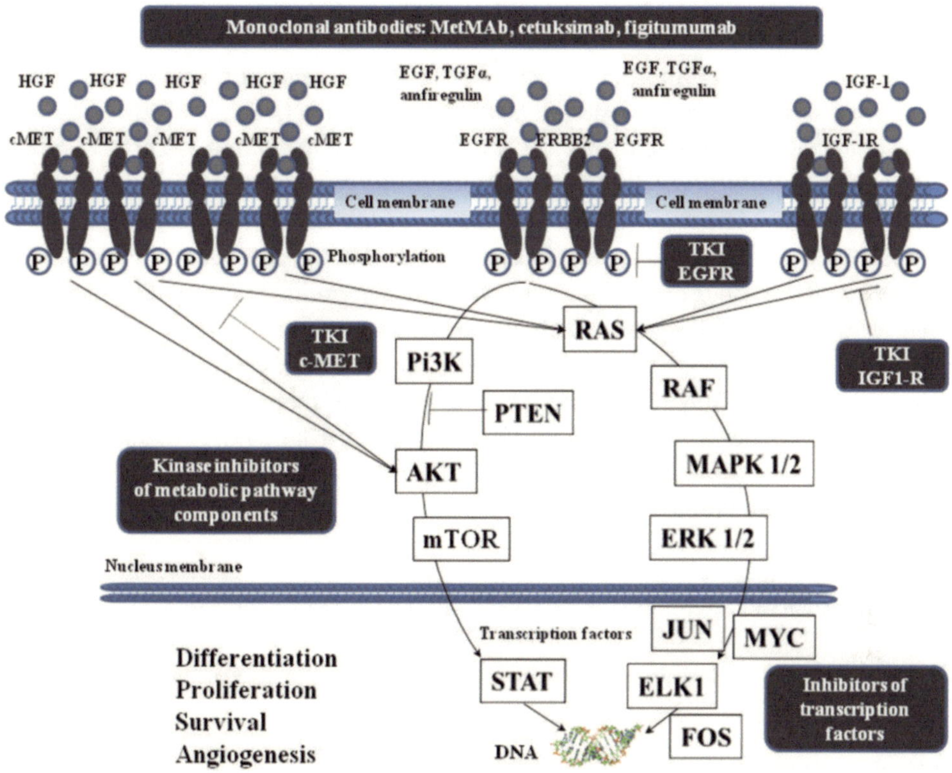

Figure 4. *EGFR* pathway components and possibility of new molecularly targeted therapies application in resistance to reversible TKI-EGFR.

Drugs inhibiting neoangiogenesis within the tumour have also found an application in molecularly targeted therapy of patients with NSCLC. These drugs are bevacizumab – a monoclonal antibody directed against vascular endothelial growth factor (VEGF) and small molecule drugs, inhibiting tyrosine kinase functions of VEGFR, PDGFR, FGFR, RET and c-Kit (vargatef, sunitinib) [26, 27]

American *Lung Cancer Mutation Consortium* (LCMC) had screened NSCLC tumour samples not only for *EGFR* and *ALK* mutations, but also for other known mutations such as *KRAS, EGFR, EML4-ALK, BRAF, HER2, PIK3CA, NRAS, MEK1, AKT1* and *MET* gene irregularities.

Mutations were found in 54% (280/516) of completely tested tumours, in 15 certified genetic laboratories. Mutation screening is not only for research purposes, but is also designed to determine patients who might benefit from molecularly targeted therapies. Molecular testing could definitely identify the mutations associated with response or resistance to targeted therapies [16]. Nowadays, we have an opportunity to match molecularly targeted therapies with the structure of proteins that are taking part in signalling pathways of neoplasm cells. The efficiency of tyrosine kinase inhibitors of EGFR (erlotinib, gefitinib) and ALK (crizotinib) in NSCLC patients bearing *EGFR* or *ALK* activating mutations is the example of such relationship. These observations create new possibilities for personalisation of known molecularly targeted therapies (registered and tested in clinical trails) in large population of NSCLC patients [16]. LCMC idea was used to describe potential capability of therapy of NSCLC patients, based on presence of mutations in cancer cells. Similarly, the BATTLE program at the M.D. Anderson Cancer Centre in Houston assessed biomarker-guided treatment in patients with previously treated, advanced NSCLC and biopsy-amenable disease. For this purpose, cancer gene databases should be created to determine what is known about germline and somatic gene variants as well as treatment options and their outcomes. According to recent cancer genomic knowledge, clinical trials of novel molecularly targeted drugs, could be offered to cancer patients who are unlikely to benefit from a standard therapy, with relatively poor prognosis and to patients who are more likely to benefit from a novel therapy due to the presence of tumour genetic abnormalities that predict sensitivity, lack of resistance or toxicity of a treatment (Table 2) [4, 16, 19, 26, 27].

Genetic abnormality	**Treatment**	**Mechanism of action**
activating mutation of *EGFR*	erlotinib or gefitinib	small molecule, reversible TKI-EGFR
activating mutation of *EGFR*	erlotinib + OSI-906 or MM-121 or MK-0646	small molecule, reversible TKI-EGFR + small molecule TKI IGF-1R or fully human monoclonal antibody against ErbB3
KRAS mutation; *MET* amplification	erlotinib + tivantinib (ARQ-197) or onartuzumab (MetMAb); JTP-74057 (GSK1120212);	small molecule TKI-EGFR + small molecule TKI cMET or monovalent (one-armed) monoclonal antibody against cMET; small molecule inhibitor of MEK 1/2 serine/threonine kinase;
fusion gene *EML4-ALK* and fusion genes with *ROS1* gene component; *ROS1* mutation	crizotinib, AP-26113, LDK-378, AF-802	small molecule TKI of ALK, ROS1 and cMET; small molecule TKI of ALK and EGFR; small molecule TKI of ALK

NRAS, MEK1 or *BRAF* mutation	GSK-1120212	small molecule inhibitor of MEK 1/2 serine/threonine kinase
BRAF, NRAS mutation	GSK-2118436; vemurafenib (PLX-4032)	small molecule inhibitor of BRAF serine/threonine kinase
mutation in exon 20 of *EGFR* (e.g. T790M); *HER2* mutation	Afatinib (BIBW2992), neratinib, PF299804, CI-1033, EKB-569, AV-412/MP-412, lapatinib	small molecule, irreversible TKI of pan-HER; small molecule, irreversible TKI of EGFR and HER2
PIK3CA mutation	BEZ-235, GDC-0491, SAR-245409, BKM-120, BYL-716, OSI-027, PX-866, MK-8669	small molecule inhibitor of mTOR and PI3K kinases; small molecule inhibitor of pan-PI3K; small molecule selective inhibitor of PI3Kα
MEK1 mutation	JTP-74057 (GSK-1120212); selumetinib (AZD-6244), GDC-0973, MEK-162, MSC-1936369B	small molecule inhibitor of MEK 1/2 serine/threonine kinase (MAPK/ERK kinase1/2 kinases);
DDR2 mutation (S768R)	erlotinib + dazatinib or nilotynib	small molecule inhibitor of BCR-ABL, SRC, c-Kit, EPH and PDGFRβ
FGFR amplification	PD-173074, ponatinib (AP24534), BGJ-398, FP-1039	small molecule TKI of FGFR and VEGFR; small molecule kinase inhibitor of native and mutated BCR-ABL, VEGFR2, FGFR1, PDGFRα, mutated FLT3 and LYN; small molecule TKI of FGFRs; monoclonal antibody against FGFR1
PDGFR amplification, *PDGFR* mutation, *c-Kit* mutation	MEDI-575, IMC-3G3, sunitinib, sorafenib, OSI-930, pazopanib (votrient)	Monoclonal antibody against PDGFR α; small molecule inhibitors of kinases of VEGFR1-3, RET, c-Kit, PDGFR α and β
FGFR and/or *PDGFR* amplification	intedanib (BIBF-1120), dovitinib (TKI258)	small molecule inhibitor of angiokinase (FGFR, PDGFR, VEGFR)
BRCA1 deficiency	olaparib + cisplatin	small molecule inhibitor of poly(ADP-ribose) polymerase (PARP)
AKT1 mutation	MK-2206, GSK-2110183	AKT inhibitors

Table 2. An example of qualification possibilities for molecularly targeted therapies based on NSCLC cell molecular signature (in most countries gefitinib, erlotinib and crizotinib are the only registered drugs in NSCLC therapy; other indications for therapy are hypothetical and are based only on the results of early clinical trials).

5. Summary

It is worth remembering that the presence of mutations may overlap with much more severe genetic abnormalities of lung cancer cells. These irregularities result in profound changes in cancer cells ability to proliferate and in effect it becoming invulnerable to selective molecularly targeted therapies. Therefore, at present only few above mentioned drugs may be used in lung cancer patients instead of standard chemotherapy. In most cases, molecularly targeted therapies will find an application in patients who have already exhausted all standard chemotherapy forms.

Multiple genetic alterations in lung cancer tumours and different targeted therapies based on appropriate molecular status of patients are still under investigation. However, the problems with proper obtaining and storage of tumour tissue for molecular testing as well as choosing adequate molecular methods for gene mutation screening is still open for discussion.

Author details

Paweł Krawczyk
Corresponding author
Department of Pneumonology, Oncology and Allergology,
Medical University of Lublin,
Lublin, Poland

Tomasz Kucharczyk and Kamila Wojas-Krawczyk
Department of Pneumonology, Oncology and Allergology,
Medical University of Lublin,
Lublin, Poland

6. References

[1] Jemal A, Bray F, Centem MM, Ferlay J, Ward E, Forman D (2011) Global cancer statistics. CA Cancer j. clin. 61: 69-90.
[2] Kadara H, Kabbout M, Wistuba II (2012) Pulmonary adenocarcinoma: a renewed entity in 2011. Respirology. 17: 50-65.
[3] Dehan E, Ben-Dor A, Liao W (2007) Chromosomal aberrations and gene expression profiles in non-small cell lung cancer. Lung cancer. 56: 175-184.
[4] Dancey JE, Bedard PL, Onetto N, Hudson TJ (2012) The genetic basis for cancer treatment decision. Cell. 148: 409-420.
[5] Catalogue of Somatic Mutations in Cancer – COSMIC. http://www.sanger.ac.uk/genetics/CGP/cosmic/
[6] My Cancer Genome. www.mycancergenome.org/
[7] The Cancer Genome Atlas. https://tcga-data.nci.nih.gov/tcga/

[8] Subramanian J, Govindan R (2007) Lung cancer in never smokers: a review. J. clin. oncol. 25(5): 561-570.

[9] Rudin CM, Avila-Tang E, Harris CC, Herman JG, Hirsch FR, Pao W, Schwartz AG, Vahakangas KH, Samet JM (2009) Lung cancer in never smokers: molecular profiles and therapeutic implications. Clin. cancer res. 15(18): 5646-5661.

[10] Begun S (2012) Molecular changes in smoking-related lung cancer. Expert rev. mol. diagn. 12: 93-106.

[11] Kulesza P, Ramchandran K, Patel JD (2011) Emerging concepts in pathology and molecular biology of advanced non-small cell lung cancer. Am j clin pathol. 136: 228-238.

[12] Dienstmann R, Martinez P, Felip E (2011) Personalizing therapy with targeted agents in non-small cell lung cancer. Oncotarget 2: 135-177.

[13] Yun CH, Boggon TJ, Li Y (2007) Structures of lung cancer-derived EGFR mutants and inhibitor complexes: Mechanism of activation and insights into differential inhibitor sensitivity. Cancer cell. 11: 217-227.

[14] Pao W, Hutchinson KE (2012) Summary of KIF5B-RET fusions in individuals with lung cancer. Nature med. 18: 349-351.

[15] Takeuchi K, Soda M, Togashi Y, Suzuki R, Sakata S, Hatano S, Asaka R, Hamanaka W, Ninomiya, Uehara H, Choi YL, Satoh Y, Okumura S, Nakagawa K, Mano H, Ishikawa Y (2012) RET, ROS1 and ALK fusions in lung cancer. Nature med. 18: 378-381.

[16] Lung Cancer Mutation Consortium. http://www.golcmc.com/

[17] Felip E, Gridelli C, Baas P (2011) Metastatic non-small-cell lung cancer: consensus on pathology and molecular tests, first-line, second-line, and third-line therapy. 1st ESMO Consensus Conference in Lung Cancer; Lugano 2010. Ann. oncol. doi:10.1093/annonc/mdr150

[18] Pirker R, Herth FJF, Kerr KM (2010) Consensus for EGFR mutation testing in non-small cell lung cancer. Results from a European Workshop. J. thorac. oncol. 5(10): 1706-1713.

[19] Heist RS, Engelman JA (2012) SnapShot: non-small cell lung cancer. Cancer cell. 21: 448-448.e2

[20] Eur-Lex Access to European Union law. http://eur-lex.europa.eu/LexUriServ/

[21] Salgia R, Hensing T, Campbell N (2011) Personalized treatment of lung cancer. Semin. oncol. 38: 274-283.

[22] Sun S, Schiller JH, Spinola M, Minna JD (2007) New molecularly targeted therapies for lung cancer. J. clin. invest. 117(10): 2740-2750.

[23] Janku F, Garrido-Laguna I, Petruzelka LB, Stewart DJ, Kurzrock R (2011) Novel therapeutic targets in non-small cell lung cancer. J. thorac. oncol. 6(9): 1601-1612.

[24] National Comprehensive Cancer Network. http://www.nccn.org/professionals/

[25] Doebele RC, Oton AB, Peled N, Camidge DR, Bunn PA (2010) New strategies to overcome limitations of reversible EGFR tyrosine kinase inhibitor therapy in non-small cell lung cancer. Lung cancer. 69: 1-12.

[26] ClinicalTrials. gov http://clinicaltrials.gov/

[27] National Cancer Institute. http://www.cancer.gov/clinicaltrials

Chapter 11

Clinical and Genetic Heterogeneity of Autism

Yu Wang and Nanbert Zhong

Additional information is available at the end of the chapter

http://dx.doi.org/10.5772/48700

1. Introduction

Autism (MIM 209850) comprises a heterogeneous group of disorders with a complex genetic etiology, characterized by impairments in reciprocal social communication and presence of restricted, repetitive and stereotyped patterns of behavior [1]. With an early onset prior to age 3 and prevalence as high as 0.9–2.6% [2,3], autism occurs predominantly in males, with a ratio of male: female of 4 to 1. It is one of the leading causes of childhood disability and inflicts serious suffering and burden for the family and society [4].

Diagnosis of autism is based on expert observation and assessment of behavior and cognition, not etiology or pathogenic mechanism. This is further emphasized by the current trend in the DSM-V, in which the category of Asperger syndrome is removed and the diagnostic criteria for autism are modified under the new heading of autism spectrum disorder (ASD). The change in diagnostic criteria is not based on known similarities or differences in causation between these clinically defined categories, but rather on the consensus of opinions of expert clinicians. For autism, several diagnostic instruments are available. Two are commonly used in autism research: the Autism Diagnostic Interview-Revised (ADI-R) that is a semi-structured parent interview [5], and the Autism Diagnostic Observation Schedule (ADOS) uses observation and interaction with the child(ren) [6]. The Childhood Autism Rating Scale (CARS) is used widely in clinical environments to assess severity of autism based on observation of children [7]. The M-CHAT was developed in the late 1990s as a first-stage screening tool for ASD in toddlers' age 18 to 24 months, with a sensitivity of 0.87 and a specificity of 0.99 in American children [8, 9].

2. Clinical heterogeneity of ASD

Autistic conditions are a spectrum of disorders, rather than a distinct clinical disorder, which means that the symptoms can be present in a variety of combinations with a range of severity. The disease has variable cognitive manifestations, ranging from a non-verbal child with mental retardation to a high-functioning college student with above average IQ with inadequate social skills [10]. Clinical heterogeneity of autism showed three major categories: idiopathic autism, autistic spectrum disorder (ASD), and syndromatic autistics that usually resulted from an identified syndrome with known genetic etiology. Traditionally, ASD includes autism, Asperger syndrome, where language appears normal, Rett syndrome and pervasive developmental disorder not otherwise specified (PDD-NOS), in which children meet some but not all criteria for autism. Rett syndrome (RTT), occurring almost exclusively in females, is characterized by developmental arrest between 5 and 18 months of age, followed by regression of acquired skills, loss of speech, stereotypic movements (classically of the hands), microcephaly, seizures, and intellectual difficulties. These disorders share deficits in social communication and show variability in language and repetitive behavior domains [1]. Autistic individuals may have symptoms that are independent of the diagnosis. Mental retardation is present in approximately 75% of cases of autism, seizures in 15 to 30% of cases, attention deficit hyperactivity disorder (ADHD) in 59-75% of cases, schizophrenia (SZ) in 5% of cases, obsessive-compulsive disorder (OCD) in about 60% of cases and electroencephalographic abnormalities in 20 to 50% of cases [11]. In addition, approximately 15 to 37% of cases of autism have a comorbid medical condition such as epilepsy, sensory abnormalities, motor abnormalities, sleep disturbances, and gastrointestinal symptoms. Five to 14% of cases had a known genetic disorder or chromosomal anomaly. The 4 most common conditions associated with autistic phenotypes are fragile X syndrome, tuberous sclerosis, 15q duplications, and untreated phenylketonuria. Other conditions associated with autistic phenotypes include Angelman syndrome, Cowden disease, Smith-Lemli-Opitz syndrome, cortical dysplasia-focal epilepsy (CDFE) syndrome, Neurofibromatosis, and X-linked mental retardation.

3. Autism is a complex genetic disorder

It is widely held that autism is largely genetic in origin; several dozen autism susceptibility genes have been identified in the past decade, collectively accounting for about 20% of autistic cases. There is strong evidence from twin and family studies for the importance of complex genetic factors in the development of autism [12, 13]. Family studies have shown that a recurrence rate of autism in siblings of affected proband is as high as 8–10% [12, 14]. Thus, the recurrence risk in siblings is roughly 100 times higher than that found in the general population. The substantial degree of familial clustering in ASD could reflect shared environmental factors, but twin studies strongly point to genetics. Several epidemiological studies among sex-matched twins have clearly demonstrated significant differences of concordance rates in the monozygotic (MZ) and dizygotic (DZ) twins. The largest of these studies [15] found that 60% of the MZ pairs were concordant for autism compared with none of the DZ pairs, suggesting a heritability estimate of >90% assuming a multifactorial threshold model. This is what is observed in every twin study in autism, and is overall consistent with heritability estimates of about 70–80% [15, 16]. One exception is a very recent study with a large sample of twins, which, despite showing a concordance of about 0.6 for MZ twins and 0.25 for DZ twins, comes to the conclusion that shared environment plays a larger role than genetic factors [17]. However, the question of how a shared environment would have a more major role than genetics is not clear. Moreover, studies in families show that first-degree relatives of an autistic proband have a markedly increased risk for autism relative to the population, consistent with a strong familial or genetic effect observed in twins [18]. This is not to dispute the role of the environment but to emphasize that genes play an important role. Similar to other common diseases with genetic contributions, autism was thought to fit a model in which multiple variants, each with small to moderate effect sizes, interact with each other and perhaps in some cases, environmental factors, to lead to autism; a situation referred to as complex genetics [13].

4. Genetic heterogeneity of autism

Although autism is highly heritable, the identification of candidate genes has been hindered by the heterogeneity of the disease. Autism genetics is highly complex, involving many genes/loci and different genetic variations, including translocation, deletion, single nucleotide polymorphism (SNP) and copy number variation (CNV) [13, 19, 20]. The most obvious general conclusion from all of the published genetic studies is the extraordinary etiological heterogeneity of autism. No specific gene accounts for the majority of autism; rather, even the most common genetic forms account for not more than 1–2% of cases [21]. Further, these genes, including those mentioned earlier, represent a diversity of molecular mechanisms that include cell adhesion, neurotransmission, synaptic structure, RNA processing/splicing, and activity-dependent protein translation. Genetic heterogeneity of autistic cases has been documented by identification of single gene mutations and genomic variations including CNV. The mutant genes identified from autistic patients are: *FMR1, MECP2, CNTNAP2, PTEN, DHCR7, CACNA1C, UBE3A, TSC2, NF1, ARX, NLGN3, NLGN4, NRXN1, FOXP1, FOXP2, GRIK2*, and *SHANK3* (Table 1). Genomic variation including copy number deletion or duplication at loci of 1q21.2, 1q42.2, 2q31.1, 3p25.3, 7q11.23, 7q22.1, 7q36.3, 11q13.3, 12q14.2, 15q11-13, 16p11.2, 16q13.3, 17q11.2, 17q12, 17q21.32, 22q13.33, or Xp22.11 may also associate with autism.

5. Genotype/phenotype correlation in ASD

The presence of genetic and phenotypic heterogeneity in autism with a number of underlying pathogenic mechanisms is highlighted in this current review. There are at least three phenotypic presentations with distinct genetic underpinnings: (1) autism with syndromic phenotype characterized by rare, single-gene defects (Table 2); (2) broad autistic phenotypes caused by genetic variations in single or multiple genes, each of these variations being common and distributed continually in the general population but resulting in variant clinical phenotypes when it reaches a certain threshold through complex gene-gene and gene-environment interactions; and (3) severe and specific phenotype caused by 'de-novo' mutations in the patient or transmitted through asymptomatic carriers of such mutations (Table 3) [48, 49]. Understanding the neurobiological processes by which genotypes lead to phenotypes, along with the advances in developmental neuroscience and neuronal networks at the cellular and molecular level, are paving the way for translational research involving targeted interventions of affected molecular pathways and early intervention programs that promote normal brain responses to stimuli and alter the developmental trajectory [50]. Recent genetic results have improved our knowledge of the genetic basis of autism. Nevertheless, identification of phenotypic markers remains challenging due to phenotypic and genotypic heterogeneity.

Gene	Genetic alteration	Location	Reference
FMR1	The number of CGG in *FMR1* alleles is classified as intermediate mutation (45 to 55), premutation (55 to 200), or full mutation (>200)	5′untranslated region	22-24
MECP2	T158M, T158A	Missense mutation	25
CNTNAP2	3709delG	Exon 22	26
	G731S, I869T R1119H, D1129H, I1253T, T1278I	Exon 14, 17 Exon 20, 21, 23, 24	27
	H275A	Exon 6	28
	CNV (microdeletion)	Promoter	29
PTEN	Deletion	Exon 2	30
CACNA1C	G406R	Missense mutation	31
UBE3A	D15S122	5' end of *UBE3A*	32, 33
TSC2	SNP	Intron 4, 9; exon 40	34
NF1	SNP	Intron 27	35
NLGN3	R451C	Missense mutation	36, 37
NLGN4	1186insT	Frameshift mutation	37
NRXN1	*De novo* 320-kb deletion	Promoter and initial coding exons	38, 39
	Missense structural variant	Neurexin1ß signal peptide region	40
FOXP1	*De novo* intragenic deletion	Exons 4-14	41
FOXP2	Del CAA;	Exon 5	42, 43
	Frequency of the TT allele	Intron 15	
GRIK2	SNP	M867I	44
SHANK3	*De novo* Q321R	Stop codon	45
	1-bp insertion	Exon 11	46
	De novo 7.9-Mb deletion	22q13.2-qter	47

Table 1. Genetic alteration identified from autism

Gene/loci	Chromosome	Phenotype (human/mouse)	Mechanism involved	Risk of autism	Reference
CNTNAP2	7q35-q36.1	Recessive EPI syndrome, ASD, ADHD, TS, OCD	Chromosomal rearrangements and large deletions, disruption of the transcription factor *FOXP2*, SNP	Not conclusive	51-54
CHD7	8q12.1	CHARGE	Mutations/deletions of gene *CHD7*, Chromatin remodeling; disruption of the transcription factor *FOXP2*; SNP;	15–50%	55, 56
TSC1	9q34.13	Tuberous Sclerosis type I.	Mutation in gene *TSC1* and subsequent hyperactivation of the downstream mTOR pathway, resulting in increased cell growth and proliferation.	Not conclusive	57
PTEN	10q23.31	Cowden disease.	Mutation of gene *PTEN*	Not conclusive	30
DHCR7	11q13.4	Smith-Lemli-Opitz syndrome	Mutations of gene *DHCR*, leading to a deficiency of cholesterol synthesis and an accumulation of 7-dehydrocholesterol	15–50% 3%	58-60 61, 62
CACNA1C	12p13.33	Timothy syndrome.	Missense mutations in the calcium channel gene *CACNA1H*	Not conclusive	63
UBE3A	15q11.2	Angelman syndrome	Maternal deletion, paternal UPD, deletions and epimutations at IC, mutations of *UBE3A*, Lack of expression of maternally expressed gene *UBE3A*	Not conclusive	32, 33
TSC2	16p13.3	Tuberous Sclerosis type II	Mutation in gene *TSC2* and subsequent hyperactivation of the downstream mTOR pathway, resulting in increased cell growth and proliferation.	Not conclusive	57
NF1	17q11.2	Neurofibromatosis	Polymorphisms within the intron-27, including the (AAAT)(n) and two (CA)n	Not conclusive	35
DMD	Xp21.2	Duchenne muscular dystrophy	Mutations of *DMD* gene resulting in absence of dystrophin protein	Not conclusive	64
ARX	Xp21.3	LIS, XLID, EPI, ASD	Naturally occurring mutations. Nonsense mutations, polyalanine tract expansions and missense mutations	Not conclusive	65
FMR1	Xq27.3	Fragile X syndrome	CGG repeat expansion and DNA methylation of FMR1 gene, reduced FMR1 expression	60–67% in males, 23% in female	66
MECP2	Xq28	Rett syndrome	Mutations in *MECP2* and *CDKL5*	Overlap in symptoms Infancy	67, 68

Abbreviations: LIS, lissencephaly; XLID, X-linked intellectual disability; EPI, epilepsy; OCD, obsessive compulsive disorder; TS, Tourette syndrome; ADHD, attention deficit hyperactivity disorder.

Table 2. Autism plus syndromic ASD caused by rare, single-gene disorders

Gene	Chromosome	Phenotype (human/mouse)	Mechanism involved in ASD	Reference
NRXN1	2p16.3	ASD, ID, SCZ, Language delay	De novo 320-kb deletion that removes the promoter and initial coding exons of the *NRXN1* gene, resulting in deletion of neurexin 1a	39
			Missense structural variants in the neurexin 1b signal peptide region	40
			CNV	69, 70
			Translocations and intragenic rearrangements in or near *NRXN1*gene	71, 72
FOXP1	3p13	ID, ASD, SLI	*De novo* intragenic deletion encompassing exons 4-14 of *FOXP1*, *de novo* nonsense mutation (c.1573C>T) in the conserved fork head DNA-binding domain	73
GRIK2	6q16.3	ASD, Recessive ID	SNP1 and SNP2 of gene *GRIK2* were associated with autism	74
FOXP2	7q31.1	ASD, SLI	Directly bind intron 1 of the *CNTNAP2* gene and regulate its expression	74
	11p15.5	Beckwith-Wiedemann syndrome	Overexpression of paternally expressed *IGF2*, due to a gain of DNA methylation at paternal allele of *IC1* and suppression of maternally expressed suppressing factor *CDKN1C*	75
	15q11-q13	Prader-Willi syndrome	Paternal deletions, maternal UPD at15q11–13, deletions and epimutations of *IC*, translocations disrupting *SNRPN*	76, 77
		Maternal duplication of 15q11-13 region	Maternal duplications of 15q11-13 region	78
SHANK3	22q13.33	ASD	Mutation at an intronic donor splice site, one missense mutation in the coding region	79
NLGN4X	Xp22.32-p22.31	ASD, ID, TS, ADHD	Frameshift mutation (1186insT)	37
NLGN3	Xq13.1	ASD	R451C mutation within the esterase domain of neuroligin 3	36, 37

Abbreviations: ID, intellectual disability; SCZ, schizophrenia; TS, Tourette syndrome; SLI, speech and language impairment; ADHD, attention deficit hyperactivity disorder

Table 3. Severe and specific phenotype with rare variants of genes

6. Copy number variation (CNV): A paradigm shift in autism

The strong genetic contribution shown in family studies and the association of cytogenetic changes, but apparent lack of common risk factors in autism, led to a hypothesis that rare sub-microscopic unbalanced changes in the form of CNVs likely contribute to the autism phenotype. With the development of microarrays capable of scanning the genome at sub-microscopic resolution, there is accumulating evidence that multiple CNVs contribute to the genetic vulnerability to autism [80]. *de novo* CNV has been identified in up to 7–10% of sporadic autism [81, 82], but are less frequent in multiplex families, in which CNV accounts only for about 2% of families screened [80, 83]. This could possibly suggest different genetic liabilities in simplex and multiplex autism. Recurrent CNVs at 15q11-13 (1-3% of autism patients), 16p11 (1% of autism patients), and 22q11-13 have been confirmed in multiple studies [80, 83-86]. This hypothesis also has been proven largely successful in identifying autism-susceptibility candidate genes, including gains and losses at *SHANK2* [87], *SHANK3* [88], *NRXN1* [13], *NLGN3* and *NLGN4* [37], and *PTCHD1* [89, 90]. Neurexins and neuroligins are synaptic cell-adhesion molecules (CAMs) that connect pre- and postsynaptic neurons at synapses, mediate trans-synaptic signaling, and shape neural network properties by specifying synaptic functions. The Shank family of proteins provides scaffolding for signaling molecules in the postsynaptic density of glutamatergic synapses. Genes encoding CAMs play crucial roles in modulating or fine-tuning synaptic formation and synaptic specification. Localization and interacting proteins at the synapse is shown in Figure 1.

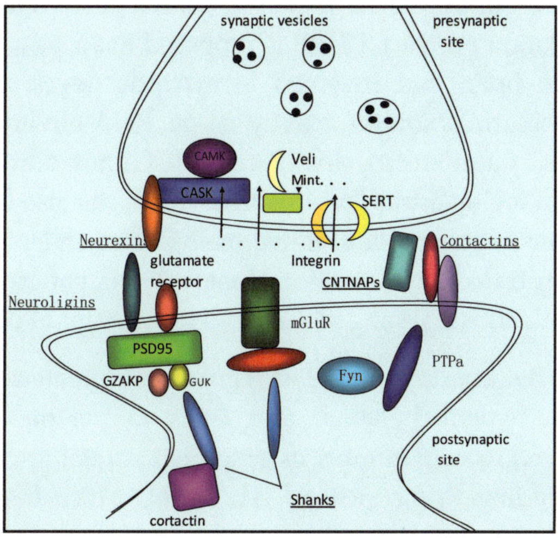

Figure 1. Localization of cell-adhesion molecules and their interacting proteins at the synapse. Proteins associated with ASD are underlined.

It is apparent that many different loci, each with a presumably unique yet subtle contribution to neurodevelopment, underlie the phenotype of autism. These observations have resulted in a paradigm shift away from the previously held "common disease-common variant" hypothesis to a "common disease-rare variant" model for the genetic architecture of autism. The central tenet of this model suggests a role for multiple, rare, highly penetrant, genetic risk factors for ASD, many of which are in the form of CNV. To make sense of the contribution of CNVs to autism, a "threshold" model has been proposed [80]. The model posits that different CNVs exhibit different penetrance depending on the dosage sensitivity and function (relative to autism) of the gene(s) they affect. Some CNVs have a large impact on autism susceptibility and these are typically *de novo* in origin, cause more severe autistic symptoms, are more prevalent among sporadic forms of autism, and are less influenced by other factors like gender and parent of origin. Other CNVs have moderate or mild effects that probably require other genetic (or non-genetic) factors to take the phenotype across the autistic threshold.

7. Epigenetics plays an important role in autism

In addition to structural genetic factors that play causative roles for autism, environmental factors also play an important role in autism by influencing fetal or early postnatal brain development, directly or *via* epigenetic modifications. Epigenetic modifications include cytosine methylation, post-translational modification of histones, small interfering RNA and genomic imprinting. Involvement of epigenetic factors in autism is demonstrated by the central role of epigenetic regulatory mechanisms in the pathogenesis of Rett syndrome and fragile X syndrome (FXS), both are the monogenic disorders resulted from single gene defects and commonly associated with autism [38-40]. FXS is a result of a triplet expansion of CGG repeats at the 5′ untranslated region of *FMR1* gene, which encodes the FMRP (fragile X mental retardation protein). FMRP is proposed to act as a translation regulator of specific mRNAs in the brain and involved in synaptic development and maturation, through its nucleo-cytoplasmic shuttle activity as an RNA-binding protein. It has been shown that FMRP uses its arginine-glycine-glycine (RGG) box domain to bind a subset of mRNA targets that form a G-quadruplex structure. FMRP has also been shown to undergo the post-translational modifications of arginine methylation and phosphorylation [91, 92]. Our recent study demonstrated that alteration of methylation patterns at loci of *Neurex1* and *ENO2* are associated with autism [Wang and Zhong, manuscript in preparation].

Genomic imprinting is the classic example of regulation of gene expression *via* epigenetic modifications, such as hypemethylation, that leads to parent of origin-specific gene expression. In addition, a growing number of genes that are not imprinted are regulated by DNA methylation, including Reelin (*RELN*) [41, 93-96], which has been considered as a candidate for autism. Several of the linkage peaks overlap or are in close proximity to regions that are subject to genomic imprinting on chromosomes 15q11-13, 7q21-31.31, 7q32.3-36.3 and possibly 4q21-31, 11p11.2-13 and 13q12.3, with the loci on chromosomes15q and 7q demonstrating the most compelling evidence for a combination of genetic and epigenetic factors that confer risks for autism [97-101]. Genes in the imprinted cluster on chromosome 15q11–13 include *MKRN3, ZNF127AS, MAGE12, NDN, ATP10A, GABRA5, GABRB3,* and *GABRG3* [102, 103]. Genes in the imprinted cluster on chromosome 7q21.3 include *SGCE, PEG10, PPP1R9A, DLX5, CALCR, ASB4, PON1, PON2,* and *PON3* [104, 105].

Research has recently focused on the connections between the immune system and the early development of brain, including its possible role in the development of autism [106]. Immune aberrations consistent with a deregulated immune response may target neuronal development and differentiation [107, 108]. Our study has suggested that a close contact with natural rubber latex (NRL) could trigger an immunoreaction to Hevea brasiliensis (Hev-b) proteins in NRL and resulted in autism [109]. This led us to a hypothesis that immune reactions triggered by environmental factors could damage synapse formation and neuronal connections, which would result in missing normal structure or function of synaptic proteins that are encoded by genes *NLGNs, NRXN1, CNTNAPs, SHANKs, or in deregulation of gene expression of FMR1, PTEN, FOXPs,* and *GRIK2.*

8. Converging molecular pathways of autism

Autism is a heterogeneous disorder with a fundamental question of whether autism represents an etiologically heterogeneous disorder in which a myriad of genetic or environmental risk factors perturb common underlying molecular pathways in the brain [110]. Two recent studies have suggested there could be convergence at the level of molecular mechanisms in autism. The first study on molecular convergence in autism identified protein interactors of known autism or autism-associated genes [111]. This interactome revealed several novel interactions, including between two autism candidate genes, *SHANK3* and *TSC1*. The biological pathways identified in this study include synapse, cytoskeleton and GTPase signaling, demonstrating a remarkable overlap with those identified by the gene expression. The second, an analysis of gene expression in postmortem autism brain, provides strong evidence for a shared set of molecular alterations in a majority of cases of autism. This included disruption of the normal gene expression pattern that differentiates frontal and temporal lobes and two groups of genes deregulated in autistic brains: one related to neuronal function, and the other related to immune/inflammatory responses [111]. Genes associated with neuronal function were enriched in metabolic signal pathways, providing evidence that these changes were causal, rather than the consequence of the disease [112]. In contrast, the immune/inflammatory changes did not show a strong genetic signal, indicating a non-genetic etiology for this process and implicating environmental or epigenetic factors instead. These results provide strong evidence for converging molecular abnormalities in autism, and implicating transcriptional and splicing deregulation as underlying mechanisms of neuronal dysfunction in this disorder.

9. In summary

Autism is a heterogeneous set of brain developmental disorders with complex genetics, involving interactions between genetic, epigenetic and environmental factors. The heterogenerous genetics involves many genes/loci and different genetic variations in autism, such as deletion, translocation, SNP and CNV. Recent studies have also suggested there could be convergence at the level of molecular mechanisms in autism. Although the genetic basis is well documented, considering phenotypic and genotypic heterogeneity, correspondences between genotype and phenotype have yet to be well established.

Author details

Yu Wang[1], Nanbert Zhong [1,2,3,*]

[1]*Shanghai Children's Hospital Affiliated to Shanghai Jiaotong University, Shanghai, China*

[2]*Peking University Center of Medical Genetics, Beijing, China*

[3]*New York State Institute for Basic Research in Developmental Disabilities, Staten Island, New York, USA*

Acknowledgement

This work was supported in part by the "973" program (2012CB517905) granted by the Chinese Ministry of Science and Technology, the Shanghai Municipal Department of Science and Technology (2009JC1412600), and the New York State Office of People with Developmental Disabilities (OPWDD).

10. References

[1] Geschwind DH (2009) Advances in autism. Annu Rev Med. 60: 367–380.

[2] Kogan MD, Blumberg SJ, Schieve LA (2007) Prevalence of parent-reported diagnosis of autism spectrum disorderamong children in the US. Pediatrics. 124: 1395–1403.

[3] Kim YS, Leventhal L, Koh YJ (2011) Prevalence of autism spectrum disorders in a total population sample. Am. J. Psychiatry. 168: 904–912.

[4] Ganz ML (2006) The Costs of Autism In Moldin, SO and Rubenstein, JLR (eds), Understanding Autism: from Basic Neuroscience to Treatment. CRC Press, Boca Raton, FL, pp. 476–498.

[5] Lord C, Pickles A, McLennan J (1997) Diagnosing autism: analyses of data from the Autism Diagnostic Interview. Autism Dev Disord. 27: 501-517.

[6] Lord C, Risi S, Lambrecht L (2000) The autism diagnostic observation schedule-generic: a standard measure of social and communication deficits associated with the spectrum of autism. Autism Dev Disord. 30: 205-223.

[7] Schopler E, Reichler R, Renner BR (1991) The childhood autism rating scale. Los Angeles: Western Psychological Services; 1988, Psychol Monogr. 117: 313-357.

[8] Robins D, Fein D, Barton M, Green J (2001) The Modified Checklist for Autism in Toddlers: an initial study investigating the early detection of autism and pervasive developmental disorders. Autism Dev Disord. 31: 131-151.

[9] Pinto MJ, Levy S (2004) Early diagnosis of autism spectrum disorders. Curr Treat Options Neurol. 6: 391-400.

[10] Gillberg C and Coleman M (2000) The biology of autistic syndromes, 3rd ed. Mac Keith, London. 22p.

[11] Fombonne E (2001) Is there an epidemic of autism? Pediatrics. 107: 411–412.

---

* Corresponding Author

[12] Szatmari P, Jones MB, Zwaigenbaum L (1998) Genetics of autism: overview and new directions. J Autism and Dev Disord. 28: 351–368.
[13] Abrahams BS, Geschwind DH (2008) Advances in autism genetics: on the threshold of a new neurobiology. Nat Rev Genet. 9: 341–355.
[14] Zwaigenbaum L, Bryson S, Roberts W (2005) Behavioral markers of autism in the first year of life. Intern J. Dev Neurosci. 23: 143–152.
[15] Bailey A, Le Couteur A, Gottesman I (1995) Autism as a strongly genetic disorder: Evidence from a British twin study. Psychological Medicine. 25: 63–77.
[16] Rosenberg RE, Law JK, Yenokyan G (2009) Characteristics and concordance of autism spectrum disorders among 277 twin pairs. Arch Pediatr Adolesc Med. 163: 907–914.
[17] Hallmayer J, Cleveland S, Torres A (2011) Genetic heritability and shared environmental factors among twin pairs with autism. Arch Gen Psychiatry. 68: 1095-1102.
[18] Bolton P, Macdonald H, Pickles A (1994) A case-control family history study of autism. Child Psychol Psychiatry. 35: 877–900.
[19] Glessner JT, Wang K, Cai G (2009) Autism genome-wide copy number variation reveals ubiquitin and neuronal genes. Nature. 459: 569–573.
[20] Wang K, Zhang H, Ma D (2009) Common genetic variants on 5p14.1 associate with autism spectrum disorders. Nature. 459: 528–533.
[21] Bucan M, Abrahams BS, Wang K (2009) Genome-wide analyses of exonic copy number variants in a family-based study point to novel autism susceptibility genes. PLoS Genet. 5: e1000536.
[22] Maddalena A, Richards CS, McGinniss MJ (2001) Technical standards and guidelines for Fragile X: The first of a series of disease-specific supplements to the Standards and Guidelines for Clinical Genetics Laboratories of the American College of Medical Genetics. Quality assurance subcommittee of the laboratory practice committee. Genet Med. 3: 200-205.
[23] Pfeiffer BE, Huber KM (2009) The state of synapses in fragile X syndrome. Neuroscientist. 15: 549-567.
[24] Tan H, Li H, Jin P (2009) RNA-mediated pathogenesis in fragile X-associated disorders. Neurosci Lett. 466: 103-108.
[25] Goffin D, Allen M, Zhang L (2011) Rett syndrome mutation MeCP2 T158A disrupts DNA binding, protein stability and ERP responses. Nat Neurosci. 15: 274-283.
[26] Strauss KA, Puffenberger EG, Huentelman MJ (2006) Recessive symptomatic focal epilepsy and mutant contactin-associated protein-like 2. N Engl J Med. 354: 1370–1377.
[27] Bakkaloglu B, O'Roak BJ, Louvi A (2008) Molecular cytogenetic analysis and resequencing of contactin associated protein-like 2 in autism spectrum disorders. Hum Genet. 82: 165–173.
[28] O'Roak BJ, Deriziotis P, Lee C (2011) Exome sequencing in sporadic autism spectrum disorders identifies severe de novo mutations. Nat Genet. 46: 585–589.
[29] Nord AS, Roeb W, Dickel DE (2011) Reduced transcript expression of genes affected by inherited and de novo CNVs in autism. Eur J Hum Genet. 19: 727–731.

[30] Conti S, Condò M, Posar A (2011) Phosphatase and Tensin Homolog (PTEN) Gene Mutations and Autism: Literature review and a case report of a patient with Cowden Syndrome, Autistic Disorder and Epilepsy. J. Child Neurol. 29: 123-126.
[31] Splawski I, Yoo DS, Stotz SC (2006) CACNA1H mutations in autism spectrum disorders. J. Biol Chem. 281: 22085-22091.
[32] Guffanti G, Strik Lievers L, Bonati MT (2011) Role of UBE3A and ATP10A genes in autism susceptibility region 15q11-q13 in an Italian population: a positive replication for UBE3A Psychiatry Res. 185: 33-38.
[33] Nurmi EL, Bradford Y, Chen Y (2001) Linkage disequilibrium at the Angelman syndrome gene UBE3A in autism families. Genomics. 77: 105-113.
[34] FJ Serajee, R Nabi, H Zhong (2003) Association of INPP1, PIK3CG, and TSC2 gene variants with autistic disorder: Implications for phosphatidylinositol. J Med Genet. 40: 119-123.
[35] Marui T, Hashimoto O, Nanba E (2004) Association between theNeurofibro matosis-1 (NF1) locus and autism in the Japanese population. Am J Med Genet B Neuropsychiatr Genet. 131B: 43-47.
[36] Jamain S, Quach H, Betancur C (2003) Mutations of the X-linked genes encoding neuroligins NLGN3 and NLGN4 are associated with autism. Nat Genet. 34: 27–29.
[37] Comoletti D, De Jaco A, Jennings LL (2004) The Arg451 Cys- neuroligin-3 mutation associated with autism reveals a defect in protein processing. J Neurosci. 24: 4889–4893.
[38] Friedman JM, Baross A, Delaney AD (2006) Oligonucleotide microarray analysis of genomic imbalance in children with mental retardation. Am J Hum Genet. 79: 500–513.
[39] Zahir FR, Baross A, Delaney AD (2008) A patient with vertebral, cognitive and behavioural abnormalities and a de novo deletion of N RXN1a. Med Genet. 45: 239–243.
[40] Feng J, Schroer R, Yan J (2006) High frequency of neurexin 1 signal peptide structural variants in patients with autism. Neurosci Lett. 409: 10–13.
[41] Hamdan FF, Daoud H, Rochefort D (2010) De novo mutations in FOXP1 in cases with intellectual disability, autism, and language impairment. Am J Hum Genet. 87: 671-678.
[42] Li H, Yamagata T, Mori M (2005) Absence of causative mutations and presence of autism-related allele in FOXP2 in Japanese autistic patients. Brain Dev. 27: 207-210.
[43] Mukamel Z, Konopka G, Wexler E (2011) Regulation of MET by FOXP2, genes implicated in higher cognitive dysfunction and autism risk. J Neurosci. 31: 11437-11442.
[44] Jamain S, Betancur C, Quach H (2002) Linkage and association of the glutamate receptor 6 gene with autism. Mol Psychiatry. 7: 302-310.
[45] Durand CM, Perroy J, Loll F (2012) SHANK3 mutations identified in autism lead to modification of dendritic spine morphology via an actin-dependent mechanism. Mol Psychiatry. 17: 71-84.
[46] Kolevzon A, Cai G, Soorya L (2011) Analysis of a purported SHANK3 mutation in a boy with autism: clinical impact of rare variant research in neurodevelopmental disabilities. Brain Res. 1380: 98-105.
[47] Chen CP, Lin SP, Chern SR (2010) A de novo 7.9 Mb deletion in 22q13.2→qter in a boy with autistic features, epilepsy, developmental delay, atopic dermatitis and abnormal immunological findings. Eur J Med Genet. 53: 329-332.

[48] Chiocchetti A, Klauck SM (2011) Genetic analyses for identifying molecular mechanisms in autism spectrum disorders. Encephale. 37: 68-74.

[49] Bonnet-Brilhault F. (2011) Genotype/phenotype correlation in autism: genetic models and phenotypic characterization. Encephale. 37: 68-74.

[50] Eapen V (2011) Genetic basis of autism: is there a way forward? Curr Opin Psychiatry. 24: 226-236.

[51] Vernes SC, Newbury DF, Abrahams BS (2008) A functional genetic link between distinct developmental language disorders. N Engl J Med. 359: 2337–2345.

[52] Newbury DF, Paracchini S, Scerri TS (2011) Investigation of dyslexia and SLI risk variants in reading- and language-impaired subjects. Behav Genet. 41: 90–104.

[53] Poot M, Beyer V, Schwaab I (2010) Disruption of CNTNAP2 and additional structural genome changes in a boy with speech delay and autism spectrum disorder. Neurogenetics. 11: 81–89.

[54] Sehested LT, Møller RS, Bache I (2010) Deletion of 7q34-q36.2 in two siblings with mental retardation, language delay, primary amenorrhea, dysmorphic features. Am J Med Genet. 152A: 3115–3119.

[55] Teramitsu I, Kudo LC, London SE (2004) Parallel FoxP1 and FoxP2 expression in songbird and human brain predicts functional interaction. Neurosci. 24: 3152–3163.

[56] Panaitof SC, Abrahams BS, Dong H (2010) Language-related Cntnap2 gene is differentially expressed in sexually dimorphic song nuclei essential for vocal learning in songbirds. Comp. Neurol. 518: 1995–2018.

[57] Shoubridge C, Tan MH, Fullston T (2010) Mutations in the nuclear localization sequence of the Aristaless related homeobox; sequestration of mutant ARX with IPO13 disrupts normal subcellular distribution of the transcription factor and retards cell division. Pathogenetics. 3: 1.

[58] Hartshorne TS, Grialou TL, Parker KR (2005) Autistic-like behavior in CHARGE syndrome. Am J Med Genet A. 133A: 257-261.

[59] Johansson M, Rastam M, Billstedt E (2006) Autism spectrum disorders and underlying brain pathology in CHARGE association. Dev Med Child Neurol. 48: 40-50.

[60] Smith IM, Nichols SL, Issekutz K (2005) Behavioral profiles and symptoms of autism in CHARGE syndrome: preliminary Canadian epidemiological data. Am J Med Genet A. 133A: 248-256.

[61] Skuse DH, James RS, Bishop DV (1997) Evidence from Turner's syndrome of an imprinted X-linked locus affecting cognitive function. Nature. 387: 705-708.

[62] Bianconi SE, Conley SK, Keil MF (2011) Adrenal function in Smith-Lemli-Opitz syndrome. Am J Med Genet A. 155A: 2732-2738.

[63] Depil K, Beyl S, Stary-Weinzinger A(2011) Timothy mutation disrupts the link between activation and inactivation in Ca(V)1.2 protein. J Biol Chem. 286: 31557-31564.

[64] Klymiuk N, Thirion C, Burkhardt K (2011) 238 tailored pig model of Duchenne muscular dystrophy. Reprod Fertil Dev. 24: 231.

[65] Valerio N, Romina M, Paolo C (2009) Recent advances in neurobiology of Tuberous Sclerosis Complex. Brain Dev. 31: 104-113.

[66] Bianconi SE, Conley SK, Keil MF (2011) Adrenal function in Smith-Lemli-Opitz syndrome. Am J Med Genet A. J. 155A: 2732-2738.

[67] Coutinho AM, Oliveira G, Katz C (2007) MECP2 coding sequence and 3′UTR variation in 172 unrelated autistic patients. Am J Med Genet B Neuropsychiatr Genet.144B: 475-483.

[68] Shibayama A, Cook EH, Feng J (2004) MECP2 structural and 3′-UTR variants in schizophrenia, autism and other psychiatricdiseases: a possible association with autism. Am J Med Genet B Neuropsychiatr Genet. 128B: 50-53.

[69] Glessner JT, Wang K, Cai G (2009) Autism genome-wide copy number variation reveals ubiquitin and neuronal genes.Nature. 459: 569–573.

[70] Szatmari P, Paterson AD, Zwaigenbaum L (2007) Mapping autism risk loci using genetic linkage and chromosomal rearrangements.Nat Genet. 39: 319–328.

[71] Kim HG, Kishikawa S, Higgins AW (2008) Disruption of neurexin 1 associated with autism spectrum disorder. Am J Hum Genet. 82: 199–207.

[72] Wisniowiecka KB, Nesteruk M, Peters SU (2010) Intragenic rearrangementsin NRXN1 in three families with autismspectrum disorder, developmental delay, and speech delay. Am J Med Genet B Neuropsychiatr Genet. 153B: 983–993.

[73] Hamdan FF, Daoud H, Rochefort D (2010) De novo mutations in FOXP1 in cases with intellectual disability, autism, and language impairment. Am J Hum Genet. 87: 671-678.

[74] Casey JP, Magalhaes T, Conroy JM (2011) Regan RA novel approach of homozygous haplotype sharing identifies candidate genes in autism spectrum disorder. Hum Genet. 131: 565-579.

[75] Kent L, Bowdin S, Kirby GA (2008) Beckwith Weidemann syndrome: a behavioral phenotype-genotype study.Am J Med Genet B Neuropsychiatr Genet. 147B: 1295-1297.

[76] Descheemaeker MJ, Govers V, Vermeulen PJ (2006) Pervasive developmental disorders in Prader-Willi syndrome: the Leuven experience in 59 subjects and controls. Am J Med Genet A. 140: 1136-1142.

[77] Veltman MW, Thompson RJ, Roberts SE (2004) Prader-Willi Syndrome-a study comparing deletion and uniparental disomy cases with reference to autism spectrum disorders. Eur Child Adolesc Psychiatry. 13: 42-50.

[78] Hogart A, Wu D, Lasalle JM (2010) The comorbidity of autism with the genomic disorders of chromosome 15q11.2-q13. Neurobiol Dis. 38: 181-191.

[79] Gauthier J, Champagne N, Lafrenière RG (2010). De novo mutations in the gene Encoding the synaptic scaffolding protein SHANK3 in patients ascertained for schizophrenia. Proc Natl Acad Sci. 107: 7863-7868.

[80] Cook EH, Scherer SW (2008) Copynumber variations associated with neuropsychiatric conditions. Nature. 16: 919–923.

[81] Sebat J, Lakshmi B, Malhotra D (2007) Strong association of de novo copy number mutations with autism. Science. 316: 445-449.

[82] Marshall CR, Noor A, Vincent JB (2008) Structural variation of chromosomes in autism spectrum disorder. Am J Hum Genet. 82: 477-488.

[83] Morrow EM, Yoo SY, Flavell SW (2008) Identifying autism loci and genes by tracing recent shared ancestry. Science. 321: 218-223.

[84] Szatmari P, Paterson AD, Zwaigenbaum L (2007) Mapping autism risk loci using genetic linkage and chromosomal rearrangements. Nat Genet. 39: 319-328.

[85] Weiss LA, Shen Y, Korn JM (2008) Association between microdeletion and microduplication at 16p11.2 and autism. N Engl J Med. 358: 667-675.

[86] Kumar RA, KaraMohamed S, Sudi J (2008) Recurrent 16p11.2 microdeletions in autism. Hum Mol Genet. 17: 628-638.

[87] Berkel S, Marshall CR, Weiss B (2010) Mutations in the SHANK2 synaptic scaffolding gene in autism spectrum disorder and mental retardation.Nature Genetics. 42: 489–491.

[88] Durand CM, Betancur C, Boeckers TM (2007) Mutations in the gene encoding the synaptic scaffolding protein SHANK3 are associated with autism spectrum disorders. Nature Genetics. 39: 25–27.

[89] Pinto D, Pagnamenta AT, Klei L (2010) Functional impact of global rare copy number variation in autism spectrum disorder. Nature. 466: 368-372.

[90] Noor A, Whibley A, Marshall CR (2010) Disruption at the PTCHD1 locus on Xp22.11 in autism spectrum disorder and intellectual disability. Sci Transl Med. 2: 49ra68.

[91] Auerbach BD, Osterweil EK, Bear MF(2011) Mutations causing syndromic autism define an axis of synaptic pathophysiology. Nature. 480: 63-68.

[92] Evans TL, Blice-Baum AC, Mihailescu MR (2012) Analysis of the Fragile X mental retardation protein isoforms 1, 2 and 3 interactions with the G-quadruplex forming semaphorin 3F mRNA. Mol Biosyst. 8: 642-649.

[93] Noh JS, Sharma RP, Veldic M (2005) DNA methyltransferase1 regulates reelin mRNA expression in mouse primary cortical cultures. Proc Natl Acad Sci USA. 102: 1749–1754.

[94] Grayson DR, Chen Y, Costa E (2006) The human reelin gene: Transcription factors (t), repressors (2) and the methylation switch(t/2) in schizophrenia. Pharmacol. Ther. 111: 272–286.

[95] Sato N, Fukushima N, Chang R (2006) Differential and epigenetic gene expression profiling identifies frequent disruption of the RELN pathway in pancreatic cancers.Gastroenterology. 30: 548–565.

[96] Serajee FJ, Zhong H, Mahbubul AH (2006) Association of Reelin gene polymorphisms with autism. Genomics. 87: 75–83.

[97] Numachi Y, Yoshida S, Yamashita M (2004) Psychostimulant alters expression of DNA methyltransferase mRNA in the rat brain. Ann. NY Acad Sci. 1025: 102–109.

[98] Huang CH, Chen CH. (2006) Absence of association of a polymorphic GGC repeat at the 50 untranslated region of the reelin gene with schizophrenia. Psychiatry Res. 142: 89–92.

[99] Skaar DA, Shao Y, Haines JL (2005) Analysis of the RELN gene as a genetic risk factor for autism. Mol. Psychiatry. 10: 563–571.

[100] Li J, Nguyen L, Gleason C (2004) Lack of evidence for an association between WNT2 and RELN polymorphisms and autism. Am J Med Genet B Neuropsychiatr. Genet. 126: 51–57.

[101] Bonora E, Beyer KS, Lamb JA (2003) Analysis of reelin as a candidate gene for autism. Mol. Psychiatry. 8: 885–892.

[102] Lee S, Walker CL, Karten B (2005) Essential role for the Prader-Willi syndrome protein necdin in axonal outgrowth. Hum Mol Genet. 14: 627–637.

[103] Kashiwagi A, Meguro M, Hoshiya H (2003) Predominant maternal expression of the mouse Atp10c in hippocampus and olfactory bulb. Hum Genet. 48: 194–198.

[104] Draganov DI, Teiber JF, Speelman A (2005) Human paraoxonases (PON1, PON2 and PON3) are lactonases with overlapping and distinct substrate specificities. Lipid Res. 46: 1239–1247.

[105] Terry-Lorenzo RT, RoadcapDW, Otsuka T (2005) Neurabin/protein phosphatase-1 complex regulates dendritic spine morphogenesis and maturation. Mol Biol Cell. 16: 2349–2362.

[106] Croen LA, Grether JK, Yoshida CK (2005) Maternal autoimmune diseases, asthma, and allergies, and childhood autism spectrum disorders. Arch Pediatr Adolesc Med. 159: 151–157.

[107] Braunschweig D, Ashwood P, Krakowiak P (2008) Autism: maternally derived antibodies specific for fetal brain proteins. NeuroToxicology. 29: 226–231.

[108] Singer HS, Morris CM, Gause CD (2008) Antibodies against fetal brain in sera of others with autistic children. Neuroimmunol. 194: 165–172.

[109] Shen C, Zhao XL, Zhong N. (2010) A proteomic investigation of B lymphocytes in an autisc faily: A pilot study of exposure to natural rubber latx (NRL) may lead to autism. J Mol Neurosci. 43: 443-452.

[110] Glessner JT, Wang K, Cai G (2009) Autism genome-wide copy number variation reveals ubiquitin and neuronal genes. Nature. 459: 569–573.

[111] Sakai Y, Shaw CA, Dawson BC (2011) Protein interactome reveals converging molecular pathways among autism disorders. Sci Transl Med. 3: 86ra49.

[112] Voineagu I, Wang X, Johnston P (2011) Transcriptomic analysis of autistic brain reveals convergent molecular pathology. Nature. 474: 380–384.

Chapter 12

Bioinformatics Approaches to the Functional Profiling of Genetic Variants

Biao Li, Predrag Radivojac and Sean Mooney

Additional information is available at the end of the chapter

http://dx.doi.org/10.5772/45900

1. Introduction

In the search for genetic mutations susceptible to human diseases, researchers take either genome-wide approaches or candidate gene approaches [1]. Traditional techniques in both approaches, such as chromosomal scan on the pedigree data and case-control design for a small number of genes of interest, however, have limitations in either achieving high resolution to identify specific genes, or obtaining whole genome coverage. Discoveries from pedigree linkage usually pointed to one or a few chromosomal regions related to the phenotype of interest, and these regions generally harbor many (perhaps hundreds) of genes, which rendered pinpointing actual genetic causes a daunting task. On the other hand, association studies typically focused on a couple of genes, some of which may participate in the same pathway, and the number of interrogated variants was always experimentally manageable. However, technical advances have brought high-throughput approaches within the reach of more and more scientists, increasing the volume of variants that researchers can interrogate by genotyping array and next-generation sequencing techniques at an exponential pace. A recent dbSNP build (build 135), a large public-domain database of single-nucleotide polymorphisms (SNPs), hosts more than 41.7 million validated human mutations, and with ongoing large-scale efforts such as the 1000 Genomes Project [2], that number is poised to grow significantly larger.

Of all genomic variants, those occurring in the protein-coding genes and resulting in amino acid substitutions hold special interest, as we have more knowledge about coding genes and their products than other genomic elements. Amino acid substitutions, or nonsynonymous SNPs (nsSNPs), not only change primary protein sequence but also have the potential for altering protein structure and disrupting or creating functional sites. These consequences can be tested experimentally, although doing so is costly and time-consuming.

Currently, about 1.2 million nsSNPs have been mapped to NCBI RefSeq proteins (2012/06), but we only have knowledge for a small fraction of them. The Human Gene Mutation

Database (HGMD; [3]) logs roughly 69,000 nsSNPs that are associated with diseases or traits; UniProt documents 37,000 nsSNPs as being neutral. For every six nsSNPs deposited in the public databases, five will have no disease or phenotype association. This gap will even grow larger as the emerging personal genome projects (www.personalgenomes.org) and whole-exome sequencing [4, 5] discover more rare variants.

Accompanying the compilation of a myriad of variants, a natural question arises about interpreting them in the context of human health. More specifically, how do we assess the disease risk for individual variants based on available biomedical information? Population studies, such as genome-wide association studies, have in recent years provided estimates of an odds ratio by comparing the frequencies of hundreds of thousands of genomic variants between disease/trait patients and healthy controls. One centralized resource, namely the Catalog of Published Genome-Wide Association Studies from the National Human Genome Research Institute [6], has collected published association studies involving at least 100,000 variants from 2008. The latest version (2012/06) records 8,063 significant mutation-trait associations from 1,287 studies. Most of these associations present a modest effect size with a median odds ratio (OR) of 1.36 (interquartile range [IQR]: 1.19–2.02). One clear observation from these studies is that the majority of variants occur in non-coding regions where the two most frequent locations are intergenic regions (43 percent) and introns (40 percent). In sharp contrast, only 368 nsSNPs associated with 177 diseases/traits were reported, with a slightly stronger effect size: a median OR of 1.52 (IQR: 1.21–3.33). This examination makes clear that the number of cohort studies will not keep pace with the increase in nsSNP data generation, suggesting that computational approaches may provide an important aid to our understanding of mutation-disease relationships.

Among all genome-level characteristics, scientists have collected the most knowledge about protein-coding genes, and they have published many investigations into the impacts of missense variants. Through mapping disease-associated nsSNPs and amino acid changes without disease annotations to the multispecies sequence alignment, researchers have observed that mutations related to monogenic diseases occurred significantly more frequently at slow-evolving positions, while neutral nsSNPs were enriched at fast-evolving positions [7, 8]. This observation therefore suggests that evolutionary rate could act as an indicator for discriminating diseases from neutral mutations. Also, the availability of crystal structure for numerous proteins provides us an opportunity to examine nsSNP consequences in the steric context. For example, p53, a well-studied tumor suppressor protein, is involved in many critical cell processes, such as DNA repair and cell-cycle regulation; p53 is inactive in half of all cancers [9]. Six mutation hot spots, such as R175H, R273H, and R282W, have been mapped to the p53 DNA-binding core domain that is critical to its activation, and most of them destabilize protein structure, leading to the degradation of p53 [10]. Intriguingly, certain mutations introduced to the mutant p53 could counteract this reduced stability and potentially rescue its functionality [11]. For example, nsSNP N268D in mutant p53 results in a hydrogen bond which bridges two strands and ultimately leads to an increase in thermodynamic stability. Finally, nsSNPs could influence a broad array of functional sites, including protein- and ligand-binding sites, catalytic residues, and numerous post-translational modification (PTM) sites. N-linked glycosylation, one type of PTM, is essential for the folding of some proteins. Proteins subjected to N-linked glycosylation contain an `NX[ST]` motif recognized by enzymes.

For example, amino acid substitution T183A, identified in the prion protein (PRNP), can cause spongiform encephalopathy by disrupting the consensus sequence `NX[ST]` through the loss of the threonine [12].

Many computational tools aiming to establish that nsSNPs cause disease are based on evolutionary characteristics, structural consequences, or functional impact, alone or in combination. One early and established method, SIFT (sort intolerant from tolerant substitutions; [13]), estimates the predisposition to disease for mutation solely by exploiting conservation information from sequence homology. Another well-known tool, PolyPhen-2 [14], uses predicted physicochemical features based on protein sequence in a naive Bayes classifier, in addition to sequence alignment.

In this chapter, we discuss the structural and functional impact of nsSNPs on the underlying proteins. We will provide concrete examples of both aspects, showing mechanisms through which amino acid substitutions affect proteins and contribute to disease phenotypes. We describe algorithms for predicting stability changes and for assigning probabilities to putative phosphorylation sites. We then apply these concepts/tools to the problem of distinguishing deleterious mutations from neutral ones. Finally, we will present another nsSNP prediction approach, MutPred, and apply it to a subset of dbSNP. Through these efforts, we aim to characterize a variety of computational approaches to the problem of inferring disease consequences for genetic variants, and demonstrate that these approaches are fruitful.

2. Structural impact of mutations

A classic disease that results from protein structural change via amino acid substitution is sickle cell anemia [15]. Replacement of a hydrophilic glutamic acid residue with a strong hydrophobic valine on the sixth amino acid of hemoglobin subunit beta causes the protein to aggregate and form rigid molecules, which in turn reshape the red blood cells as sickle-like [16]. The sickle cells die prematurely and thus result in anemia. Other possible structural abnormalities that nsSNPs can induce include changes of secondary structure, gain or loss of protein stability, and other physicochemical property alterations. In this section, we will illustrate two mutations on a cancer-related gene, BRCA1, and then describe an algorithm for predicting protein stability; finally, we will discuss its application to discriminating neutral and deleterious mutations.

BRCA1 is a well-known suppressor of breast and ovarian cancer tumors. Two C-terminal sequence repeats (BRCT) are essential for BRCA1's function, since mutations of stop codon and missense substitutions on these regions were observed in breast cancer patients [17, 18]. The crystal structure of the BRCT segments [19] shows that these two domains pack to each other in a tandem manner where one helix on the N-terminal domain and two helices on the C-terminal domain form an inner-domain interaction surface (Figure 1).

Two amino acid substitutions occur on this interface at A1708E, located near the end of the $\alpha1$ helix, and at M1775R, located near the beginning of the $\alpha2$ helix. At position 1708, the mutant glutamic acid is much larger than the original alanine (having a molecular weight of 147 versus 89) and introduces negative charge. Because M1708 lies near the center of the interaction surface, the compact core cannot accommodate this mutation sterically. Thus,

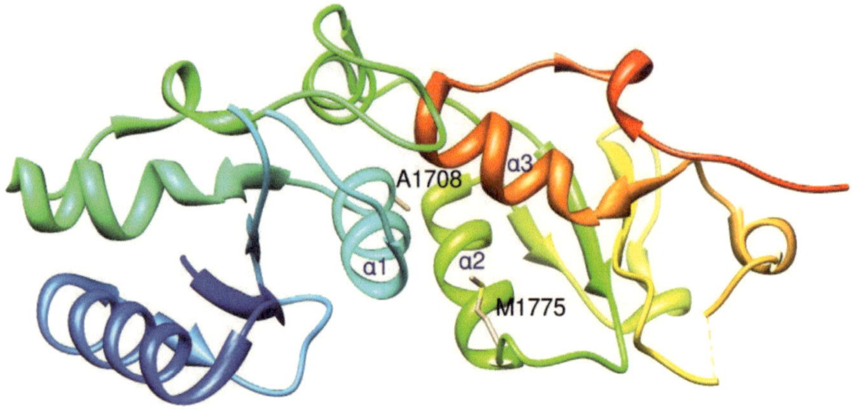

Figure 1. The crystal structure of human BRCT domains (PDB ID: 1JNX). The N-terminus is shown in blue; the C-terminus, in red. Residues A1708 and M1775 are depicted as ball and stick models. Three helices, $\alpha 1$ from the N-terminus and both $\alpha 2$ and $\alpha 3$ from the C-terminus, pack into a hydrophobic core that is important to the folding of BRCT domains.

A1708E would destabilize the BRCT interaction. On the other hand, although R1775 could be placed on the edge of the BRCT interface spatially, it positions a positive charge against the nearby R1835. Thus, both mutations would destabilize the BRCT core through either sterical incompatibility or disruption of electrostatic interactions [19]. This explanation found support from a mutation sensitivity assay that measures the stability of the inner domain interaction subject to proteolytic degradation. The wild-type protein resists the digestion by trypsin, elastase, and chymotrypsin, whereas the mutant with M1775R was partially degraded and A1708E was almost completely degraded [19]. The BRCT structure and in vitro experiments suggest that the genetic variants A1708E and M1775R cause the BRCA1 defect by destabilizing its inner-domain interaction.

From this example, we can see that crystal structure can be a powerful tool in interpreting possible consequences of nsSNPs by physicochemical principles. However, we cannot reasonably expect every protein and its mutants to have high-resolution three-dimensional (3D) structures or homology models available, either because of difficulties in structural determination, such as for membrane proteins, or because some proteins are intrinsically disordered [20].

To overcome this severe limitation, many computational tools aiming to predict structural properties use sequence information as input, either by direct use of sequence or through derived features such as amino acid composition and sequence motifs. Here, we describe a stability prediction method proposed by [21], namely MUpro, which was based on a sophisticated machine learning technique–Support Vector Machine (SVM)–and which achieved good performance.

In traditional molecular dynamics simulation, potential functions from a force field were usually calculated to obtain $\Delta\Delta G$, which was mainly influenced by interactions between nonlocal amino acids [22]. Although it is generally difficult, if not completely impossible, to infer protein structural architecture accurately based solely on amino acid sequence, pioneering work from [23, 24] showed that protein sequence was effective in the prediction of secondary structure and solvent accessibility. MUpro fit a set of features derived from protein sequence to an experimental stability data by nonlinear transformation through SVM. The ProTherm database [25] collects from the literature a range of experimentally measured thermodynamic parameters, such as Gibbs free energy changes for wild-type and mutant proteins, with experimental conditions, including pH and temperature. From ProTherm MUpro used protein sequences and mutations for training and test purposes, along with numeric energy changes.

MUpro adopted a standard binary classification scheme in feature generation by selecting a window centered on a mutant position and then encoding each amino acid in the window as a vector of 20 elements. In this kind of vector, each element corresponds to one of 20 standard amino acids and takes a value of 1 if the corresponding amino acid is identical to the one observed or else 0. MUpro considered a window of seven amino acids for each mutation, thereby representing the feature set by a 140-element vector. The first 20-element vector records information about wild-type and mutant amino acids at the mutant position, and the final six vectors document the six flanking amino acids.

In a two-dimensional space, linear classifiers are designed to separate two classes of data points by a straight line. As illustrated in Figure 2 (left plot), any lines passing through the space between two parallel lines can separate the blue points (one class) from the orange (the other class) perfectly, and thus would be a good choice for linear classification. However, SVM algorithms [26] would select the dashed line, which distances two lines equally, as the class boundary. In other words SVMs optimize a margin separator that maximizes its distance to data points. Figure 2 shows the margin m between two classes, which is the optimization object in SVMs algorithm. Mathematically, larger m is expected to provide the classifier greater generalization, which measures how well the classifier performs on new, unseen data points.

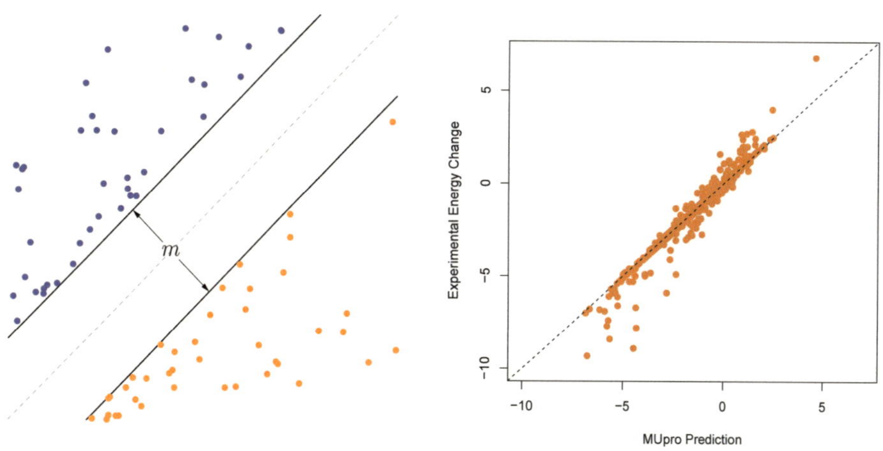

Figure 2. The left plot illustrates a linear classification on separable data with two classes (blue and orange). The class boundary (dashed line) is the middle line between two parallel lines. The right plot shows MUpro predictions against experimental values for 1,008 nsSNPs; points on the diagonal represent exact predictions.

When data sets overlap, SVMs still try to optimize a new objective function that considers both m and penalties from misclassification. Regardless of the separability of the data, m depends only on points located on the parallel lines (completely separable) or points located between them (partially separable). These points are called support vectors.

Besides data classification, SVMs can perform regression for data points with continuous response values, where the objective function measures the difference between prediction and actual values. But unlike typical linear regression, SVM regressions do not penalize differences falling within a predefined range.

The abilities of SVMs, however, go beyond linear classification and regression. By projecting the original data points into higher dimensional spaces, SVMs actually create additional, and usually more complex, features from the input points. By using the same linear settings as described above in these newly high-dimensional spaces, SVMs can effectively capture highly nonlinear relationships among data which otherwise would be missed.

MUpro applied a popular SVM implementation, SVM^{light} [27], to carry out energy change sign classification and regression. In 1,008 training mutations, MUpro performed rather well against true energy changes, with a root-mean-square deviation (RMSD) of 0.39 (Figure 2, right plot). Moreover, it made more accurate predictions with less dramatic actual stability changes between wild-type and mutant amino acids. Generally, MUpro tended to underestimate larger energy changes.

In one early comprehensive examination of the effects of nsSNPs on protein function, [28] catalogued nsSNP effects according to structural and sequence changes caused by the introduction of mutant amino acids. That study extracted 262 disease-causing missense variants from the HGMD and 42 neutral variants from hypertension-associated genes. Proteins harboring these variants either had 3D structures deposited in the Protein Data Bank (PDB) or they could find homologous ones with a sequence similarity of at least 40 percent. They then modeled both wild-type and mutant protein structures based on available 3D structures. By examining a broad range of physicochemical parameters from built models, including loss of hydrogen bonds, loss of a salt bridge, over-packing, and disruption of binding, Wang *et al.* could compare distributions of effects observed in disease-causing and neutral variants (Table 1). Their results clearly demonstrated that loss of stability accounts for many more disease-causing variants than neutral variants (83 versus 26 percent) and that 70 percent of neutral variants cause no measurable effects on the protein structure.

Effect	Disease	Neutral
Stability	83	26
Ligand binding	5	2
Other	2	2
No effect	10	70

Table 1. Percentage of effects from missense variants on protein function (adapted from Figure 2 in [28])

This survey suggests that nsSNPs giving rise to stability changes will more likely be disease-related than not, and this property might be useful in distinguishing disease-causing from neutral nsSNPs. Moreover, computational tools like MUpro capable of predicting stability greatly facilitate this task by applying to virtually any protein with sequences available.

3. Functional impact of mutations

Besides structural consequences, variants can disrupt molecular functional sites, such as catalytic residues and DNA/protein binding sites, which are usually position-specific or share consensus motifs. Those disruptions, however, do not necessarily involve disruption of structure. A prominent class of sites that variants would affect consists of diverse PTM sites, of which some of the most frequent types are phosphorylation, glycosylation, acetylation, methylation, and ubiquitination. PTMs play an important role in cellular signal transduction and regulation, and activating and inactivating certain key proteins rely on precise modulation of PTMs in cell activities. For instance, without environmental stress, p53 is suppressed through ubiquitination catalyzed by E3 ubiquitin ligases, while in the presence of stress, such as DNA damage, p53 is activated by a variety of PTM enzymes, including acetylation and phosphorylation on its flexible DNA-binding domain [29]. PTM sites and flanking residues generally form consensus sequences with a high degree of variety, and therefore variants within these enzyme-specific motifs could abolish known functionalities or create new ones. This section starts by detailing two concrete examples of functional changes due to variants, followed by a description of DisPhos (Disorder-enhanced Phosphorylation sites predictor), an established phosphorylation predictor, and then explain how the concepts of gain and loss of phosphorylation can be used to analyze a cancer data.

FGFR2 (fibroblast growth factor receptor 2), one of four members of FGFR family of receptor tyrosine kinases, plays an important role in transmembrane signal transduction. Recent research identified one missense mutation, A628T, as being involved in LADD syndrome through severely impairing the kinase activity of FGFR2 [30]. Residue A628 is in the center of the catalytic pocket in the tyrosine kinase domain of FGFR2. A mutant structure, A628T-FGFR2 [31], reveals that the substitution of the smaller amino acid alanine at position 628 with the larger, polar threonine pushes one of the key residues, R630, out of the catalytic pocket; that movement disrupts the hydrogen bond between D626 and R630 existed in the wild-type structure (Figure 3, left). Although the position of D626 remains almost unchanged, R630 is too far away from the catalytic pocket and fails to stabilize the interaction with substrates, which consequently greatly compromises the catalytic ability of FGFR2. Compared with wild-type FGFR2, the A628T-FGFR2 mutant has roughly the same structure but highly reduced kinase activity.

It has been observed that amino acid substitutions occurred on non-PTM-sites could spread their influence to neighboring PTM sites on the same protein. One of such examples is PTPS, human PTP (protein tyrosine phosphatase) synthase, which catalyzes triphosphate elimination. PTPS participates in the biosynthetic pathway for tetrahydrobiopterin (BH4). Lack of PTPS catalytic activity causes a deficiency of BH4, which in turn leads to hyperphenylalaninemia (HPA), an autosomal recessive disorder. Missense mutation R16C was associated with HPA and resulted in reduced activity of PTPS [32]. Moreover, phosphorylation of S19 on PTPS is required for maximal enzyme activity [33]. So how does R16C affect phosphorylation on S19? There are multiple potential explanations. One is that the structure of PTPS shows the exposure of both R16 and S19 on the surface of the protein (Figure

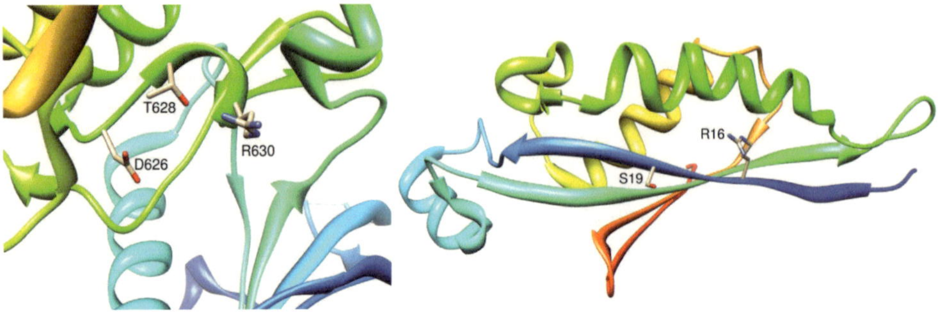

Figure 3. The crystal structure of the catalytic pocket of the A628T-FGFR2 mutant (left, PDB ID: 3B2T) and ribbon view of human PTPS structure (right, PDB ID: 3I2B). In both cases, the N-terminus is colored in blue and the C-terminus in red. Residues of interest are depicted as ball and stick models.

3, right; [34]) that forms the consensus sequence $R_{16}XXS_{19}$ for cGMP protein kinase II. The substitution C16 disrupts this kinase-recognizable motif and thus hinders phosphorylation, which ultimately leads to the inactivation of PTPS. Another explanation is that a removal of R16 prevents a salt bridge between it and a phosphate group when attached, which in turn results the loss of stability of the modified protein.

As with the stability prediction tool MUpro, described in the previous section, experimental difficulties have promoted the development of computational approaches to estimating many common PTM sites based on protein sequence. For the prediction of phosphorylation, DisPhos differs from other available methods like NetPhos [35] and ScanSite [36], since its model explicitly includes a range of characteristic features from the predicted disorder region around the phosphorylation site [37].

In some cases, researchers have found phosphorylation sites located on intrinsically disordered regions or have observed disorder-to-order or order-to-disorder conformational changes upon phosphorylation [38]. DisPhos exploited such observations by integrating predicted disorder information with the motif profile to improve its predictive performance.

Because phosphorylation occurs on residues S, T, and Y (S/T/Y), DisPhos assembled three pairs of positive-negative data sets, with each pair corresponding to one residue-specific predictor. First, it extracted proteins with phosphorylation annotations from UniProt (Universal Protein Resource); it then combined this data with data from Phospho.ELM [39]. DisPhos placed a 25-residue segment centered on each annotated S/T/Y into a positive set, while placing the same length segment around every non-annotated S/T/Y on the same protein into a negative set. To reduce the sequence bias caused by homologs or duplications, DisPhos only kept entries with a pairwise sequence similarity of less than 30 percent, which means that it allowed up to seven matches from alignment without gap. Due to the small size of experimentally verified phosphorylation sites, the filtered data sets were highly unbalanced (Table 2).

DisPhos used a broad range of features to discriminate positive from negative sites (Table 3).

To cope with the highly dimensional, yet sparse feature space, DisPhos performed feature selection by applying a permutation test to binary features and applying principal component

Residue	Positive Sites (P)	Negative Sites (N)	N/P Ratio
S	613	10,798	17.6
T	140	9,051	64.7
Y	136	5,103	37.5

Table 2. Data sets used in DisPhos (adapted from Table 1 in [37])

Type	Features	Dimension
Amino acid composition	Binary coding	480
Amino acid frequency	Binary coding	20
Disorder	VLXT, VL2, VLV, VLC, VLS	5
Secondary structure	Helix, loop and sheet	7
Sequence property	Complexity and flexibility	2
Residue property	Net charge, aromatic content, Hydrophobic moment, Hydrophobicity, exposed/buried	5

Table 3. Descriptive and predicted features used in DisPhos training.

analysis (PCA) to continuous features and then fitted logistic regression models to the transformed data sets.

Generally, binary classifiers work best in settings of balanced or close to balanced data sets in terms of accuracy, sensitivity, and specificity. For a classification in which the class boundary is determined by a solution that maximizes accuracy–the default configuration for many popular classifiers–training on highly unbalanced data sets inevitably results in extreme values for sensitivity or specificity, ultimately leading to poor generalization. DisPhos adopted an ensemble strategy to correct this issue in the S/T/Y data sets.

The combination of data filtering, feature selection, and sophisticated training and test configurations enabled DisPhos to achieve accuracy ranges between 70 and 80 percent, an improvement over the accuracy of other similar predictors. Moreover, the features derived from disorder predictions improved the accuracy by two percent on average, and these improvements showed the usefulness of disorder features in the prediction of phosphorylation sites.

DisPhos represents outcomes as probabilities, which quantitatively measure the likelihood that the underlying residues are phosphorylation sites. This characteristic facilitated the definition of gain and loss of phosphorylation for a specific site [40], and since these concepts can be interpreted readily, they may help provide insight into the underlying molecular mechanisms of mutations associated with diseases. Actually, the definitions of gain and loss are not limited to phosphorylation sites and can apply just as well to many other functional and structural properties.

Using bioinformatics tools that predict functional and structural attributes on both wild-type and mutant protein sequences provides us with two probabilistic estimates for a property p: $P(p = 1 \text{ at } s_i^w)$ and $P(p = 1 \text{ at } s_i^m)$ at site s_i, with s_i^w denoting a wild type site and s_i^m denoting a mutant site. Then, conceptually, we have

$$P(\text{loss of property } p \text{ at site } s_i) = P(p = 1 \text{ at } s_i^w \text{ AND } p = 0 \text{ at } s_i^m). \quad (1)$$

Given that s^w and s^m are actually different molecules, we consider that $P(p = 1 \, \text{at} \, s_i^w)$ and $P(p = 0 \, \text{at} \, s_i^m)$ are not dependent because of any underlying process. Therefore, we can expand the right hand of equation (1) as a product:

$$\begin{aligned} P(p = 1 \, \text{at} \, s_i^w \, \text{AND} \, p = 0 \, \text{at} \, s_i^m) &= P(p = 1 \, \text{at} \, s_i^w) \cdot P(p = 0 \, \text{at} \, s_i^m) \\ &= P(p = 1 \, \text{at} \, s_i^w) \cdot [1 - P(p = 1 \, \text{at} \, s_i^m)] \end{aligned} \tag{2}$$

By substituting equation (1) with equation (2), we get

$$P(\text{loss of property } p \text{ at site } s_i) = P(p = 1 \, \text{at} \, s_i^w) \cdot [1 - P(p = 1 \, \text{at} \, s_i^m)] \tag{3}$$

Likewise, we can define gain of a property as

$$P(\text{gain of property } p \text{ at site } s_i) = [1 - P(p = 1 \, \text{at} \, s_i^w)] \cdot P(p = 1 \, \text{at} \, s_i^m) \tag{4}$$

Figure 4 shows the contour of gain of a property. Note that we can still compute gain/loss even if the predictions for the property are the same for wild-type and mutant sequences. The value of gain/loss varies from 0 to 0.25 when both predictions take a value of 0 through 0.5.

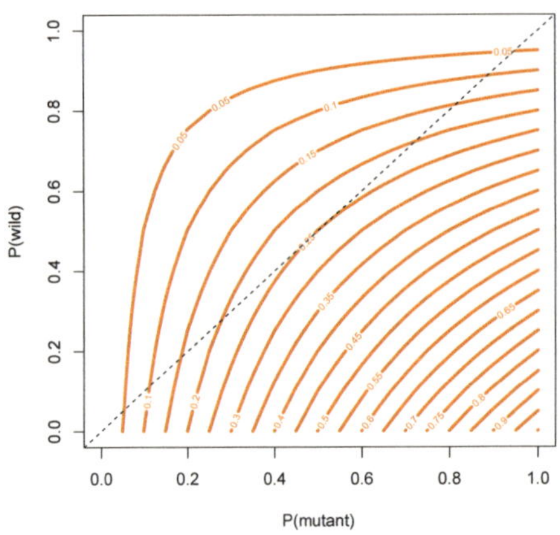

Figure 4. The contour of gain of property with respect to probability on mutant sequence–x-axis, $P(\text{mutant})$–and wild-type sequence–y-axis, $P(\text{wild})$). The dashed line denotes sites with equal probabilities for the two types of sequences.

[40] showed one application of gain and loss of phosphorylation. An experiment in their study collected 1,099 breast and colorectal cancer nsSNPs occurring on 847 proteins from a large-scale cancer-tumor-sequencing project [41]. Radivojac *et al.* then paired control and mutation data by randomly mutating on the same set of 847 wild-type proteins at the codon level. Their study then calculated gain and loss of phosphorylation for each mutation in both data sets, and found that disease-associated nsSNPs were significantly more likely to be involved in adding new phosphorylation sites (Table 4).

Phosphorylaiton change	Disease nsSNPs	Control nsSNPs	*P*-value
Gain	1.91	0.86	0.014
Loss	1.70	1.50	0.59

Table 4. Percentage of mutations predicted to have undergone gain or loss of phosphorylation. *P*-values were computed by *t*-test.

This survey showed how the concepts of gain and loss of phosphorylation could distinguish cancer-associated from neutral somatic mutations; it also suggested that they could serve as useful features for discriminating between general disease-related nsSNPs and neutral ones.

4. Mutation prediction: MutPred

In light of the above observations on the wide variety of consequences of a single mutation, we developed a large range of features for each variant and employed a popular machine learning technique, random forest, to distinguish disease-associated mutations from neutral ones. We called the model MutPred [42].

In a supervised learning scenario, we collected two sets of disease-associated mutations. One set came from the HGMD [3], in which 95 percent of mutations were annotated to monogenic diseases. We extracted the other set from a cancer-sequencing project [41]. Also, we created two corresponding control data sets (Table 5). For the HGMD data, we took a set of variants from UniProt that were annotated as polymorphisms to serve as controls (SPP). We identified all neutral mutations that occurred on the same proteins observed in the cancer data set and used them as the cancer controls. On average, HGMD proteins harbored 7.3 times as many variants as SPP proteins, while we observed a much less dramatic difference between cancer data set and its controls.

Data set	Mutations	Proteins	Type
HGMD	39,218	1,879	Disease
SPP	26,439	9,305	Neutral
Cancer	653	519	Disease
Cancer control	1,016	312	Neutral

Table 5. Summary of disease and neutral data sets.

We generated a total of 130 numeric attributes based on protein sequences for each mutation and utilized them as the input into a random forest classifier. These attributes can be divided into three major types (Table 6). Other evolutionary attributes include position-specific scoring matrix (PSSM) generated by PSI-BLAST, Pfam domain profile, and transition frequency from SNAP [43].

As the PTPS example shows, the influence of nsSNPs could spread to neighboring PTM sites. Accordingly, we expanded the definitions for gain/loss of structural and functional properties to pick up the largest gain/loss changes within an 11-residue window centered on the mutant position.

Random forest is an ensemble learning technique based on a population of binary decision trees, each of which is grown on a proportion of randomly chosen features and bootstrapped samples [54]. For classification, the outcome is the majority voting of individual trees.

Type	Property	Software
Functional properties	DNA-binding residues	DBS-PRED [44]
	Catalytic residues	†
	MoRFs	[45]
	Phosphorylation sites	DisPhos [37]
	Methylation sites	[46]
	Glycosylation sites	†
	Ubiquitination sites	[47]
Structure and dynamics	Secondary structure	PHD/Prof [48]
	Solvent accessibility	PHD/Prof [48]
	Stability	MUpro [21]
	Intrinsic disorder	DISPROT [49]
	B-factor	[50]
	Transmembrane helix	HMMTOP [51]
	Coiled-coil structure	marcoil [52]
Evolutionary information	Sequence Conservation	SIFT [13]
		Conservation index‡[53]

Table 6. Major attributes used in MutPred. † unpublished in-house program. ‡ used in latest version of MutPred.

Compared to a normal single decision tree, each subtree within a random forest uses only partial features and samples, which results in small correlations among subtrees and effectively reduces the overall variance of the model. Moreover, random forests inherit some attractive properties from decision trees, such as robustness to outliers and ease of interpretation.

In our model, we specified 1,000 trees to build the classifier between disease and neutral mutations. The HGMD achieved better accuracy than the somatic cancer data, suggesting that monogenic disease-related mutations are more suited to MutPred than somatic cancer mutations (Table 7). This is likely due to the large number of passenger variants (not causative) in tissue cancer sequencing data sets. Also, in terms of area under the curve (AUC) MutPred observed 0.86 in HGMD and 0.69 in cancer data sets (Figure 5, left).

Data set	Sensitivity	Specificity	Accuracy
HGMD	76.8	79.0	77.7
Cancer	60.9	68.4	65.5

Table 7. Percentage of classification performance measurement for HGMD and cancer data sets.

MutPred can provide not only comparable predictions for a mutation's predisposition to cause diseases [55], but it also allows the estimation of the significance level for individual gain/loss of properties (Figure 5, right). It is reasonable to assume that the distribution of property p in the neutral data set provides an unbiased approximation of the true null distribution, given the fact that UniProt provided the largest available set of curated neutral variants. Therefore, we could generate hypotheses about the molecular mechanism underlying variants at three different confidence levels: (1) actionable hypotheses: $0.78 \geq$ MutPred score > 0.5 AND property score < 0.05; (2) confident hypotheses: MutPred score > 0.78 AND $0.01 \leq$ property

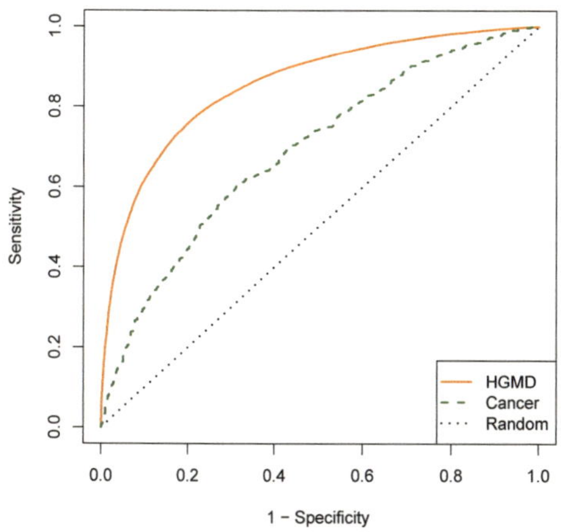

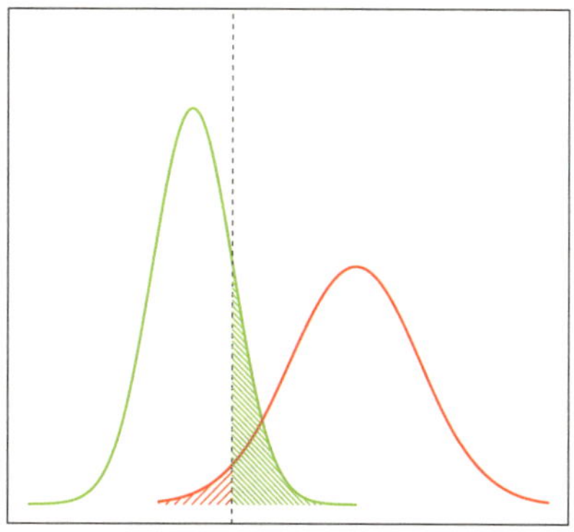

Figure 5. The Receiver Operating Characteristic (ROC) curves for HGMD and cancer data sets (left), and example distributions of gain/loss property *p* in neutral and disease sets (green and red, respectively; right). An empirical distribution of the putatively neutral substitutions can be used to define a threshold *r* on the false positive rate that, in turn, can be used to accept/reject the null hypothesis on new substitutions. The area shaded in green represents the *P*-value threshold (corresponding to the score *r*) that is used by MutPred to hypothesize molecular cause of disease. A particular area under the right tail of the neutral distribution is referred to as the property score.

score < 0.05; (3) very confident hypotheses: MutPred score > 0.78 AND property score < 0.01, where 0.78 corresponds to specificity 0.95 in HGMD data set.

We applied MutPred to 203,899 nsSNPs deposited in the dbSNP (build 135) and examined the score distribution and frequent hypotheses behind predicted deleterious mutations. In general, 35 percent of mutations were predicted with scores higher than 0.5; thus, we classified them as disease-associated (Figure 6). Of these deleterious mutations, 19.6 percent got at least one functional or structural hypothesis of possible molecular mechanism. The top three hypotheses all pointed to structural changes: gain of disorder (9.7 percent), loss of stability (8.5 percent), and loss of disorder (6.2 percent). This result agrees with [28]–at least in the sense that these changes are the most frequently seen. On the other hand, common functional alterations involved in disease included loss of MoRF binding (6.0 percent), gain of methylation (5.9 percent), and gain of catalytic residue (5.6 percent).

5. Conclusion

Understanding mutation data generated in biomedical research stimulates the development of computational methods. Previous studies have revealed structural and functional impacts on underlying proteins from variants, and research has proven that these impacts can differentiate between disease-associated and neutral mutations. Most current prediction tools have taken advantage of these characteristics, along with evolutionary information readily available from sequence alignment. Such tools have demonstrated impressive classification

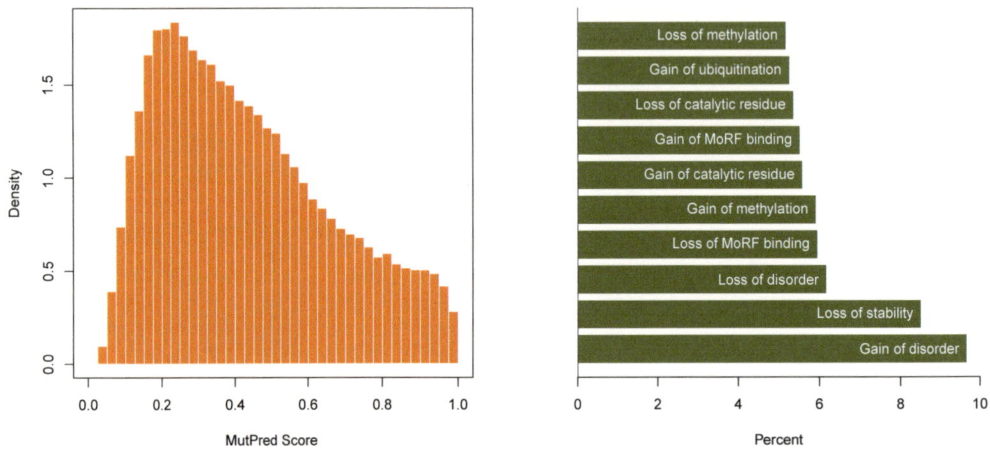

Figure 6. The distribution of MutPred scores for nsSNPs from dbSNP (left), and the top ten hypotheses for disease-associated mutations (right). The density on the left is a normalized frequency to ensure a total area in the bar plot equals one.

accuracy in monogenic disease-associated mutations but have performed less well for cancer somatic mutations. One explanation from an evolutionary perspective for this descrepency is that cancers usually arise late in life, so they are subjected to less purifying selection. This makes conservation information in cancers less useful than in monogenic diseases [56]. This field faces two immediate challenges: (1) How can we improve these tools to improve performance with somatic mutations? If the consensus opinion holds that tools depending on evolutionary knowledge are less effective than when applied to monogenic-disease-related mutations, it seems that research should explore other avenues. Inclusion of the mutation context in the model–e.g., pathways containing disease proteins–might offer a starting point for new directions. (2) How can we more accurately elucidate the molecular mechanisms for predicted deleterious mutations? MutPred has demonstrated this concept through definitions of gain/loss of individual properties. Similar features should be considered once they prove capable of reliably discriminating between disease-associated and neutral mutations. By continuously improving our computational tools, we can obtain better and more accurate understandings of biology and human health.

Author details

Biao Li
The Buck Institute for Research on Aging, Novato, CA 94945, USA

Predrag Radivojac
Indiana University, Bloomington, IN 47405, USA

Sean Mooney
The Buck Institute for Research on Aging, Novato, CA 94945, USA

6. References

[1] David Altshuler, Mark J. Daly, and Eric S. Lander. Genetic mapping in human disease. *Science*, 322(5903):881–888, 2008.

[2] 1000 Genomes Project Consortium. A map of human genome variation from population-scale sequencing. *Nature*, 467(7319):1061–73, 2010.

[3] Peter D Stenson, Matthew Mort, Edward V Ball, Katy Howells, Andrew D Phillips, Nick St Thomas, and David N Cooper. The human gene mutation database: 2008 update. *Genome Med*, 1(1):13, 2009.

[4] Jamie K Teer and James C Mullikin. Exome sequencing: the sweet spot before whole genomes. *Hum Mol Genet*, 19(R2):R145–51, 2010.

[5] Jens G. Lohr, Petar Stojanov, Michael S. Lawrence, Daniel Auclair, Bjoern Chapuy, Carrie Sougnez, Peter Cruz-Gordillo, Birgit Knoechel, Yan W. Asmann, Susan L. Slager, Anne J. Novak, Ahmet Dogan, Stephen M. Ansell, Brian K. Link, Lihua Zou, Joshua Gould, Gordon Saksena, Nicolas Stransky, Claudia Rangel-Escareño, Juan Carlos Fernandez-Lopez, Alfredo Hidalgo-Miranda, Jorge Melendez-Zajgla, Enrique Hernández-Lemus, Angela Schwarz-Cruz y Celis, Ivan Imaz-Rosshandler, Akinyemi I. Ojesina, Joonil Jung, Chandra S. Pedamallu, Eric S. Lander, Thomas M. Habermann, James R. Cerhan, Margaret A. Shipp, Gad Getz, and Todd R. Golub. Discovery and prioritization of somatic mutations in diffuse large b-cell lymphoma (dlbcl) by whole-exome sequencing. *Proceedings of the National Academy of Sciences*, 109(10):3879–3884, 2012.

[6] Lucia A. Hindorff, Praveen Sethupathy, Heather A. Junkins, Erin M. Ramos, Jayashri P. Mehta, Francis S. Collins, and Teri A. Manolio. Potential etiologic and functional implications of genome-wide association loci for human diseases and traits. *Proceedings of the National Academy of Sciences*, 106(23):9362–9367, 2009.

[7] C D Bottema, R P Ketterling, S Ii, H S Yoon, J A Phillips, 3rd, and S S Sommer. Missense mutations and evolutionary conservation of amino acids: evidence that many of the amino acids in factor ix function as "spacer" elements. *Am J Hum Genet*, 49(4):820–38, Oct 1991.

[8] M. P. Miller and S. Kumar. Understanding human disease mutations through the use of interspecific genetic variation. *Hum Mol Genet*, 10(21):2319–28, 2001.

[9] C Prives. How loops, beta sheets, and alpha helices help us to understand p53. *Cell*, 78(4):543–6, 1994.

[10] Y Cho, S Gorina, PD Jeffrey, and NP Pavletich. Crystal structure of a p53 tumor suppressor-dna complex: understanding tumorigenic mutations. *Science*, 265(5170):346–355, 1994.

[11] Andreas C. Joerger, Mark D. Allen, and Alan R. Fersht. Crystal structure of a superstable mutant of human p53 core domain. *Journal of Biological Chemistry*, 279(2):1291–1296, 2004.

[12] E Grasbon-Frodl, Holger Lorenz, U Mann, R M Nitsch, Otto Windl, and H A Kretzschmar. Loss of glycosylation associated with the t183a mutation in human prion disease. *Acta Neuropathol*, 108(6):476–84, Dec 2004.

[13] P C Ng and S Henikoff. Predicting deleterious amino acid substitutions. *Genome Res*, 11(5):863–874, 2001.

[14] Ivan A Adzhubei, Steffen Schmidt, Leonid Peshkin, Vasily E Ramensky, Anna Gerasimova, Peer Bork, Alexey S Kondrashov, and Shamil R Sunyaev. A method and server for predicting damaging missense mutations. *Nat Methods*, 7(4):248–9, 2010.

[15] L Pauling and H A Itano. Sickle cell anemia a molecular disease. *Science*, 110(2865):543–8, 1949.

[16] B C Wishner, K B Ward, E E Lattman, and W E Love. Crystal structure of sickle-cell deoxyhemoglobin at 5 a resolution. *J Mol Biol*, 98(1):179–94, 1975.

[17] Y Miki, J Swensen, D Shattuck-Eidens, P A Futreal, K Harshman, S Tavtigian, Q Liu, C Cochran, L M Bennett, and W Ding. A strong candidate for the breast and ovarian cancer susceptibility gene brca1. *Science*, 266(5182):66–71, 1994.

[18] L S Friedman, E A Ostermeyer, C I Szabo, P Dowd, E D Lynch, S E Rowell, and M C King. Confirmation of brca1 by analysis of germline mutations linked to breast and ovarian cancer in ten families. *Nat Genet*, 8(4):399–404, 1994.

[19] R S Williams, R Green, and J N Glover. Crystal structure of the brct repeat region from the breast cancer-associated protein brca1. *Nat Struct Biol*, 8(10):838–42, 2001.

[20] A K Dunker, J D Lawson, C J Brown, R M Williams, P Romero, J S Oh, C J Oldfield, A M Campen, C M Ratliff, K W Hipps, J Ausio, M S Nissen, R Reeves, C Kang, C R Kissinger, R W Bailey, M D Griswold, W Chiu, E C Garner, and Z Obradovic. Intrinsically disordered protein. *J Mol Graph Model*, 19(1):26–59, 2001.

[21] Jianlin Cheng, Arlo Randall, and Pierre Baldi. Prediction of protein stability changes for single-site mutations using support vector machines. *Proteins*, 62(4):1125–1132, 2006.

[22] D Gilis and M Rooman. Predicting protein stability changes upon mutation using database-derived potentials: solvent accessibility determines the importance of local versus non-local interactions along the sequence. *J Mol Biol*, 272(2):276–90, 1997.

[23] P Y Chou and G D Fasman. Prediction of protein conformation. *Biochemistry*, 13(2):222–45, Jan 1974.

[24] N Qian and T J Sejnowski. Predicting the secondary structure of globular proteins using neural network models. *J Mol Biol*, 202(4):865–84, Aug 1988.

[25] M D Shaji Kumar, K Abdulla Bava, M Michael Gromiha, Ponraj Prabakaran, Koji Kitajima, Hatsuho Uedaira, and Akinori Sarai. Protherm and pronit: thermodynamic databases for proteins and protein-nucleic acid interactions. *Nucleic Acids Res*, 34(Database issue):D204–6, 2006.

[26] Trevor Hastie, Robert Tibshirani, and J. H Friedman. *The elements of statistical learning: data mining, inference, and prediction*. Springer series in statistics. Springer, New York, NY, 2nd edition, 2009.

[27] Thorsten Joachims. *Learning to classify text using support vector machines*, volume SECS 668. Kluwer Academic Publishers, Boston, 2002.

[28] Z Wang and J Moult. Snps, protein structure, and disease. *Hum Mutat*, 17(4):263–270, 2001.

[29] Christopher L Brooks and Wei Gu. p53 ubiquitination: Mdm2 and beyond. *Mol Cell*, 21(3):307–15, 2006.

[30] Imad Shams, Edyta Rohmann, Veraragavan P Eswarakumar, Erin D Lew, Satoru Yuzawa, Bernd Wollnik, Joseph Schlessinger, and Irit Lax. Lacrimo-auriculo-dento-digital syndrome is caused by reduced activity of the fibroblast growth factor 10 (fgf10)-fgf receptor 2 signaling pathway. *Mol Cell Biol*, 27(19):6903–12, 2007.

[31] Erin D Lew, Jae Hyun Bae, Edyta Rohmann, Bernd Wollnik, and Joseph Schlessinger. Structural basis for reduced fgfr2 activity in ladd syndrome: Implications for fgfr autoinhibition and activation. *Proc Natl Acad Sci U S A*, 104(50):19802–7, 2007.

[32] B Thöny, W Leimbacher, N Blau, A Harvie, and C W Heizmann. Hyperphenylalaninemia due to defects in tetrahydrobiopterin metabolism: molecular characterization of mutations in 6-pyruvoyl-tetrahydropterin synthase. *Am J Hum Genet*, 54(5):782–92, 1994.

[33] T Scherer-Oppliger, W Leimbacher, N Blau, and B Thöny. Serine 19 of human 6-pyruvoyltetrahydropterin synthase is phosphorylated by cgmp protein kinase ii. *J Biol Chem*, 274(44):31341–8, 1999.

[34] T Oppliger, B Thöny, H Nar, D Bürgisser, R Huber, C W Heizmann, and N Blau. Structural and functional consequences of mutations in 6-pyruvoyltetrahydropterin synthase causing hyperphenylalaninemia in humans. phosphorylation is a requirement for in vivo activity. *J Biol Chem*, 270(49):29498–506, 1995.

[35] N Blom, S Gammeltoft, and S Brunak. Sequence and structure-based prediction of eukaryotic protein phosphorylation sites. *J Mol Biol*, 294(5):1351–62, 1999.

[36] M B Yaffe, G G Leparc, J Lai, T Obata, S Volinia, and L C Cantley. A motif-based profile scanning approach for genome-wide prediction of signaling pathways. *Nat Biotechnol*, 19(4):348–53, 2001.

[37] Lilia M Iakoucheva, Predrag Radivojac, Celeste J Brown, Timothy R O'Connor, Jason G Sikes, Zoran Obradovic, and A Keith Dunker. The importance of intrinsic disorder for protein phosphorylation. *Nucleic Acids Res*, 32(3):1037–1049, 2004.

[38] D P Teufel, M Bycroft, and A R Fersht. Regulation by phosphorylation of the relative affinities of the n-terminal transactivation domains of p53 for p300 domains and mdm2. *Oncogene*, 28(20):2112–8, 2009.

[39] Holger Dinkel, Claudia Chica, Allegra Via, Cathryn M Gould, Lars J Jensen, Toby J Gibson, and Francesca Diella. Phospho.elm: a database of phosphorylation sites–update 2011. *Nucleic Acids Res*, 39(Database issue):D261–7, 2011.

[40] Predrag Radivojac, Peter H Baenziger, Maricel G Kann, Matthew E Mort, Matthew W Hahn, and Sean D Mooney. Gain and loss of phosphorylation sites in human cancer. *Bioinformatics*, 24(16):i241–7, 2008.

[41] Tobias Sjöblom, Siân Jones, Laura D Wood, D Williams Parsons, Jimmy Lin, Thomas D Barber, Diana Mandelker, Rebecca J Leary, Janine Ptak, Natalie Silliman, Steve Szabo, Phillip Buckhaults, Christopher Farrell, Paul Meeh, Sanford D Markowitz, Joseph Willis, Dawn Dawson, James K V Willson, Adi F Gazdar, James Hartigan, Leo Wu, Changsheng Liu, Giovanni Parmigiani, Ben Ho Park, Kurtis E Bachman, Nickolas Papadopoulos, Bert Vogelstein, Kenneth W Kinzler, and Victor E Velculescu. The consensus coding sequences of human breast and colorectal cancers. *Science*, 314(5797):268–74, 2006.

[42] Biao Li, Vidhya G Krishnan, Matthew E Mort, Fuxiao Xin, Kishore K Kamati, David N Cooper, Sean D Mooney, and Predrag Radivojac. Automated inference of molecular mechanisms of disease from amino acid substitutions. *Bioinformatics*, 25(21):2744–50, 2009.

[43] Yana Bromberg and Burkhard Rost. Snap: predict effect of non-synonymous polymorphisms on function. *Nucleic Acids Res*, 35(11):3823–35, 2007.

[44] Shandar Ahmad, M Michael Gromiha, and Akinori Sarai. Analysis and prediction of dna-binding proteins and their binding residues based on composition, sequence and structural information. *Bioinformatics*, 20(4):477–86, 2004.

[45] Predrag Radivojac, Slobodan Vucetic, Timothy R O'Connor, Vladimir N Uversky, Zoran Obradovic, and A Keith Dunker. Calmodulin signaling: analysis and prediction of a disorder-dependent molecular recognition. *Proteins*, 63(2):398–410, 2006.

[46] Kenneth M. Daily, Predrag Radivojac, and A. Keith Dunker. Intrinsic disorder and protein modifications: building an svm predictor for methylation. In *IEEE Symposium on Computational Intelligence in Bioinformatics and Computational Biology, CIBCB 2005*, pages 475–481, 2005.

[47] Predrag Radivojac, Vladimir Vacic, Chad Haynes, Ross R Cocklin, Amrita Mohan, Joshua W Heyen, Mark G Goebl, and Lilia M Iakoucheva. Identification, analysis, and prediction of protein ubiquitination sites. *Proteins*, 78(2):365–80, 2010.

[48] B Rost. Phd: predicting one-dimensional protein structure by profile-based neural networks. *Methods Enzymol*, 266:525–39, 1996.

[49] Kang Peng, Predrag Radivojac, Slobodan Vucetic, A Keith Dunker, and Zoran Obradovic. Length-dependent prediction of protein intrinsic disorder. *BMC Bioinformatics*, 7:208, 2006.

[50] Predrag Radivojac, Zoran Obradovic, David K Smith, Guang Zhu, Slobodan Vucetic, Celeste J Brown, J David Lawson, and A Keith Dunker. Protein flexibility and intrinsic disorder. *Protein Sci*, 13(1):71–80, 2004.

[51] A Krogh, B Larsson, G von Heijne, and E L Sonnhammer. Predicting transmembrane protein topology with a hidden markov model: application to complete genomes. *J Mol Biol*, 305(3):567–80, 2001.

[52] Mauro Delorenzi and Terry Speed. An hmm model for coiled-coil domains and a comparison with pssm-based predictions. *Bioinformatics*, 18(4):617–25, 2002.

[53] J Pei and N V Grishin. Al2co: calculation of positional conservation in a protein sequence alignment. *Bioinformatics*, 17(8):700–12, 2001.

[54] Leo Breiman. Random forests. *Machine Learning*, 45(1):5–32, 2001.

[55] Janita Thusberg, Ayodeji Olatubosun, and Mauno Vihinen. Performance of mutation pathogenicity prediction methods on missense variants. *Hum Mutat*, 32(4):358–68, 2011.

[56] Sudhir Kumar, Joel T Dudley, Alan Filipski, and Li Liu. Phylomedicine: an evolutionary telescope to explore and diagnose the universe of disease mutations. *Trends Genet*, 27(9):377–86, 2011.

Chapter 13

Anderson's Disease/Chylomicron Retention Disease and Mutations in the *SAR1B* Gene

A. Sassolas, M. Di Filippo, L.P. Aggerbeck, N. Peretti and M.E. Samson-Bouma

Additional information is available at the end of the chapter

http://dx.doi.org/10.5772/45976

1. Introduction

Anderson's Disease (AD)/Chylomicron Retention Disease (CMRD) (OMIM #607689) is a rare autosomal recessively inherited lipid malabsorption syndrome characterized by hypocholesterolemia associated with failure to thrive, diarrhea, steatorrhea and abdominal distension that presents most frequently in young infants. Charlotte Anderson first published a description of the disorder in 1961 [1] based upon observations of a young girl of seven months of age who manifested a characteristic macroscopic and microscopic appearance of the intestinal mucosa which was filled with fat. Forty two years later, in 2003, Jones and colleagues [2], in 8 families, identified mutations in the *SAR1B* gene, which encodes for the intracellular trafficking protein SAR1b, and proposed that this was the molecular defect in the disorder. The disease is very rare. From the first clinical description of the disease up to the identification of the causal gene, only 39 patients from 24 families were described in the literature [3-21]. From 2003 to the present, 23 new patients from 14 additional families have been identified. In all, 16 different mutations in the *SAR1B* gene now have been described in 34 patients from 21 families [2, 22-27]. Here, we provide an overview of this disease, including the description of 4 new patients from 3 new families (one new mutation), and we describe the predicted molecular impact on the SAR1b protein of novel or previously-described mutations in the *SAR1B* gene.

2. Clinical features

The first symptoms of AD/CMRD, which most frequently occurr within a few months after birth, consist of failure to thrive, diarrhea with steatorrhea and abdominal distension. Of the 62 patients described in the literature, only 4 were diagnosed as adults; two sisters presented with diarrhea that was found to have begun in infancy [21, 23], the third adult had severe neurological signs in infancy [6] and the past medical history of the last adult revealed some clumsiness in walking and running and very loose bowel movements in infancy [7]. These patients may have spontaneously avoided the fat in their diets to minimize symptoms. Non specific malabsorptive diarrhea is present in almost all cases with steatorrhea, even when a low fat diet is observed [28]. The diagnosis is sometimes delayed (often for several years) because the symptoms are non-specific and are attributed to chronic diarrhea (cystic fibrosis or coeliac disease). Thus, 39/45 patients exhibited the first symptoms before one year of age, whereas only 21/52 received the proper diagnosis without undue delay. As consequence of diarrhea, failure to thrive (-1 to -4DS for height and/or weight) is also frequent (45/51 patients) and persists if a low fat diet is not instituted. Other digestive symptoms, such as vomiting or a grossly distended abdomen are commonly observed. Usually, if a low fat diet supplemented with lipid soluble vitamins is instituted, the growth starts again; however, some patients with a delayed diagnosis do not attain a normal height and weight [29]. Tolerance to fat in the diet has been reported in a few cases [14, 16, 22, 24, 27]; however, in most instances, diarrhea begins again when fat is reintroduced in the diet [29].

Hepatic and neurological abnormalities, although sometimes reported in young patients, generally are tardive manifestations, particularly when the diagnosis and the implementation of dietary vitamin supplements are delayed. Several cases of transient hepatomegaly have been described [6, 9, 11, 16, 17, 22] and one or both amino-transaminases (ASAT and ALAT) are frequently reported to be increased (13/15 patients of Charcosset [22]) but confirmed hepatic steatosis are infrequent (three cases described) [11, 25]. However, no instance of cirrhosis has been reported. In young adults or older patients, neurological abnormalities consist mainly of areflexia [11, 12, 14, 22]. In some cases, more severe neurological degeneration consisting of ataxia, sensory neuropathy and/or tremor has been reported [6, 7, 11, 19]. Mild defects in color vision and retinal function also have been observed [11, 14, 28] but no retinis pigmentosa has been reported. Acanthocytosis is very rare and usually transient [6, 12, 17, 27].

Mild muscular abnormalities have been described in several patients and consist mainly of muscular pain and cramps; one patient was described with myopathy [6]. Creatine kinase (CK) levels are often found to be elevated (1,5-2,5 times normal) [23, 27]. Jones et al (2003) have shown that high levels of SAR1B mRNA expression occurs in tissues other than intestine [2] and, therefore, extra-intestinal clinical manifestations might occurr in AD/CMRD. Silvain et al have described a cardiomyopathy in an adult and documented the accumulation of lipids in some muscle fibers [23]. Consequently, clinical evaluation and follow-up of these patients should include CK levels and cardiac examination.

Poor mineralization and delayed bone maturation may be present and vitamin D levels may be normal or decreased [5, 12, 18, 21, 23, 28]. Several patients also have exhibited associated infectious diseases [14, 16].

AD/CMRD patients exhibit a particular recessive hypocholesterolemia which differs from other familial hypocholesterolemias. The hypocholesterolemia manifests itself by a decrease of plasma LDL (LDLc) and HDL (HDLc) cholesterol (both by approximately 50%) associated with a normal level of triglycerides (Table 1). The severe decrease of HDLc (the mean level in patients is 0,49mM) associated with a normal triglyceride level is pathognomonic of AD, if all the secondary causes of malabsorption such as celiac disease, exocrine pancreatic insufficiency (cystic fibrosis or Shwachman-Diamond syndrome), and the Mc Kusick syndrome (small height and malabsorption with exactly the same lipid profile as AD) have been ruled out. Further, other causes of familial hypocholesterolemias must be carefully ruled out; for example, some patients with AD/CMRD have low levels of triglycerides and high levels of HDLc that are similar to those found in atypical abetalipoproteinemia [30, 31] or homozygous hypobetalipoproteinemia (data not shown). Plasma levels of vitamin E, measured before supplementation in patients diagnosed during the last decade, are usually low or very low (but detectable, from 0,5 to 6,8 μM, 3 of 19 patients had undetectable levels). In patients described previously, the undetectable levels were probably due to technical limitations (reported values range from 0, 23 to 11,3 μM, and 13 of 28 patients had undetectable levels). Mild decreases of vitamin A have also been found [5, 6, 11, 12, 18, 21, 24, 27] but there are normal levels of other fat soluble vitamins in most of the AD/CMRD patients.

Patients data	All published cases	Published cases with mutations
N	62	34
age at onset	56% < 3 mths, 87% < 1 year	53% < 3 mths, 84% < 1 year
age at diagnosis	60% > 1 year, 23% > 10 years	50% > 1 year, 23% > 10 years
major clinical data	90% diarrhea, 88% failure to thrive	90% diarrhea, 57% failure to thrive
TC mM	n=54 M=1,75 (0,86-3,38)	n=34 M=1,81 (1,11-2,82)
TG mM	n=48 M=0,87 (0,36-2,06)	n=33 M=0,92 (0,36-1,98)
HDLc mM	n=26 M=0,49 (0,32-0,83)	n=23 M=0,50 (0,32-0,83)
LDLc mM	n=26 M=0,87 (0,26-1,61)	n=23 M=0,88 (0,31-1,61)
apoB g/l	n=37 M=0,44 (0,20-0,82)	n=21 M=0,49 (0,20-0,82)
apoA1 g/l	n=31 M=0,52 (0,26-0,90)	n=18 M=0,52 (0,38-0,90)
Vitamin E μM	n=43 M=2,74 (0 – 11,3)	n=23 M=2,81 (0 – 7,6)

(TC: total cholesterol, TG: triglycerides, HDLc: HDL cholesterol, LDLc: LDL cholesterol)

Table 1. Mean data for all the published cases

In most cases, an essential fatty acid (FA) deficiency has been not investigated, nevertheless, a decrease of linoleic acid (C18:2 n-6) and normal levels of n-3 FA have been found in two files of patients [10, 28]. For all the patients, the lipid profiles of the heterozygous parents were normal.

Four new cases of AD/CMRD in 3 families have recently been discovered (Table 2, 3). All the individuals presented with diarrhea and failure to thrive (4/4 patients). Interestingly, one of the patients presented with tremor at diagnosis (Table 2). The plasma lipids and vitamin E exhibit a wide range of levels and, in particular, the triglycerides and total and LDL cholesterol values which is an other characteristic of AD.

The inability of the enterocytes to secrete chylomicrons and apoB 48 after a fat load is a common clinical feature of AD/CMRD, ABL (abetalipoproteinemia) and, generally, homozygous FHBL (familial hypobetalipoproteinemia). When observed with video-endoscopy, the intestine of AD/CMRD patients shows a white mucosa (*"gelée blanche"*). This typical white stippling, like hoar frosting, covers the mucosal surface of the small intestine (Fig 1A, B) even in the fasted state in contrast to healthy individuals. When intestinal biopsies from patients who have fasted are observed by light microscopy, they appear to have a normal number of *villi* of appropriate length. However, the enterocytes are overloaded with birefringent droplets in the cytoplasm (Fig 1 C, D) [1, 5, 6, 8, 9, 11, 12, 14, 16-18, 20, 25, 27]. These droplets are present, mainly, in the upper one-third of the *villus* of the enterocyte and they stain positively with oil red O indicating that they are fat droplets (mainly triglyceride) (Fig 1D, E). In some cases, the droplets are seen to be present preferentially on one side of the *villus* as opposed to both sides, whereas, in other cases (or sometimes in the same case), they may be present on both sides [32]. When the biopsies are examined by electron microscopy, two types of lipid-containing structures, in fact, are observed in the cytoplasm which alter the normal architecture of the cells.Very large lipid droplets (1025 nm average diameter), not in a membrane-bound compartment, are present along with smaller lipoprotein–sized particles (305 nm average diameter) which are present in membrane-bound structures (Fig 2 A, B) [32]. This is in contrast to enterocytes in biopsies

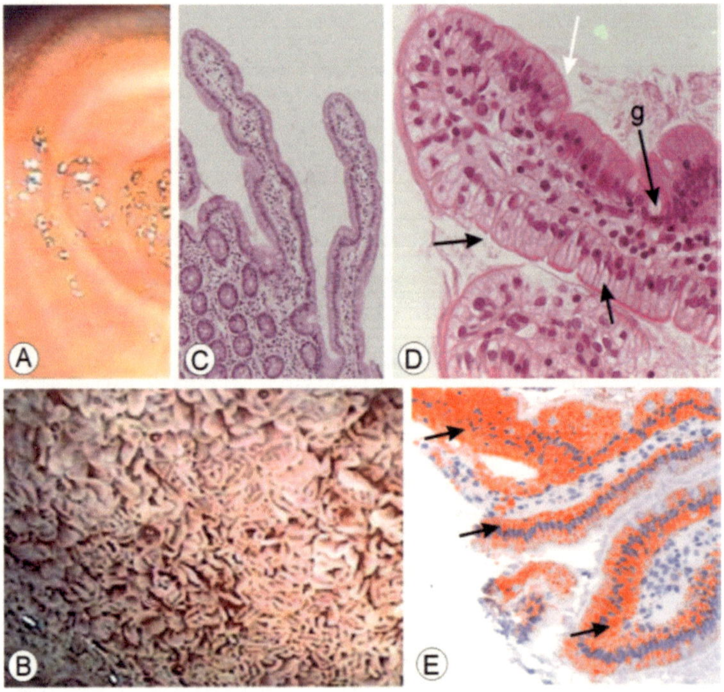

Intestinal endoscopy after a 12-hour fast. In contrast to what is observed in a normal subject (A), video-endoscopy of the duodenum (D) of patient AD2 (B), shows the typical « white hoary frosting » on the small intestinal mucosa. In contrast with a normal subject(C), light microscopy of the duodenal biopsy from AD2 (D) shows the typical vacuolated enterocytes (black arrows) that stain positively with oil red O (E, black arrows). Note the typical heterogeneous aspect of the villi either fat loaded (black arrows) or without lipid droplets (white arrows).
Goblet cells are normal (D, arrow g). (C ×100; D ×400; E ×200).

Figure 1. Intestinal endocopy after a 12-hour fast (A, B, C, D, E) (from A. Georges [27])

from patients with ABL which exhibit only (or predominantly) the very large lipid droplets whereas the smaller lipoprotein-sized particles, in membrane bound structures, are absent. In the enterocytes of both AD/CMRD and ABL patients, the Golgi apparatus is often distended but it is, generally, empty and free of lipoprotein-like particles. Further, in AD/CMRD, lipoprotein-like particles are observed, although in only a few cases, in the intercellular spaces between the enterocytes in contrast to ABL where they are never observed in intercellular spaces.

In addition to the lipid profiles of the patient and the parents, the diagnosis is supported by the absence of secretion of chylomicrons after a fat load, the presence of white duodenal mucosa upon endoscopy, the presence of cytosolic lipid droplets and lipoprotein-sized particles in the enterocytes of the intestinal biopsy and, finally, the discovery of a mutation in *SAR1B* gene. It should be noted, however, that the AD/CMRD phenotype has been observed in patients for which there is no mutation in the coding sequence of the *SAR1B* gene ([33] and unpublished data).

3. Functions of the SAR1B protein

SAR1 is a well-known GTPase (guanine tri-phosphatase) which belongs to the ARF (ADP-ribosylation factor) family of small GTPases [34, 35]. SAR1 initiates the assembly of COPII (coat protein complex II) in the endoplasmic reticulum (ER) by binding to SEC12. Then, SAR1-GDP is converted into SAR1-GTP which undergoes a large conformational change in the two switch regions. The residue Threonine 56, in switch 1, forms bonds to the y phosphate and Mg2+ and the residue Glycine 78, in switch 2, binds to the y phosphate. The movements expose the amino terminal, amphipatic $\alpha1$ helix (« the membrane anchor ») which then inserts into the ER membrane [36]. Mg2+ has an important regulatory role in this conformational change, mostly related to switch 1 [37]. The membrane-bound SAR1 recruits SEC23-SEC24 and triggers the formation of the pre-budding complex which then recruits SEC13-SEC31 to form the COPII vesicle [36, 38]. SEC24 interacts with specific cargo proteins and concentrates them into the COPII vesicle [39]. SAR1 GTP hydrolysis is stimulated by SEC23 and SEC31 and permits vesicle fission, allowing transport to the Golgi, and eventual disassembly of the coat for recycling of the components [40-42]. SED4p, a protein with 45% homology to SEC12p, accelerates the dissociation of SEC23-24 from the membrane if no cargo is transported with COPII vesicles and it has been proposed that this restricted disassembly might play a role in concentrating cargoes into COPII vesicles [43].

The typical size of the COPII vesicles ranges from 60 to 70 nm in diameter, which would appear to prohibit these vesicles from carrying chylomicrons (250 nm average diameter) from the ER to the Golgi apparatus [44]. Another vesicle (350-500 nm in diameter), the pre-chylomicron transport vesicle (PCTV), has been shown to be able to transport chylomicrons [45]. The PCTV is composed of several proteins: VAMP7 (vesicle-associated membrane protein 7) which is the v-SNARE (vesicle-associated soluble N-ethylmaleimide-sensitive factor attachment protein receptor), apoprotein B48 (a cargo), FABP1 (also called liver fatty acid- binding protein, LFABP) (budding initiator), the fatty acid transporter CD36 (a fatty

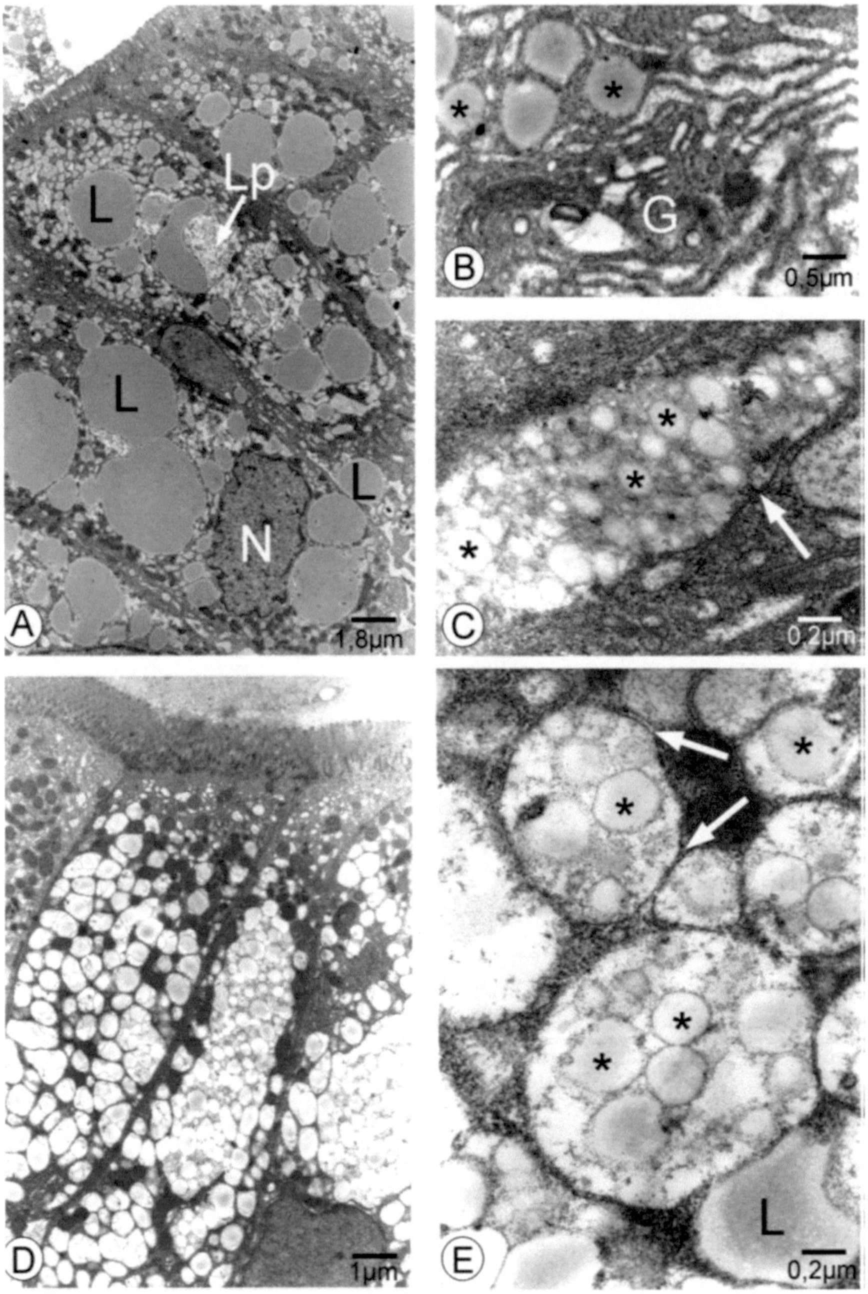

Electron microscopy of duodenal biopsies of patients with AD. As shown for AD3 (A, B, C) and AD2 (D, E), two types of particles are apparent in the enterocytes in these patients (A, D): large lipid droplets, free in the cytoplasm (L), and smaller, lipoprotein-sized like particles (Lp), surrounded by a membrane. A higher magnification shows in (B) some individual lipoprotein-sized particles surrounded by a membrane (*)near a Golgi apparatus (G) which appears distended but devoid of particles and in (C, E) numerous lipoprotein-sized particles accumulated in membrane bound compartment (membrane, white arrow). The intercellular spaces are empty. The cell nucleus is labelled N.

Figure 2. Electron microscopy of duodenal biopsies of patients with AD (from A. Georges ref 27)

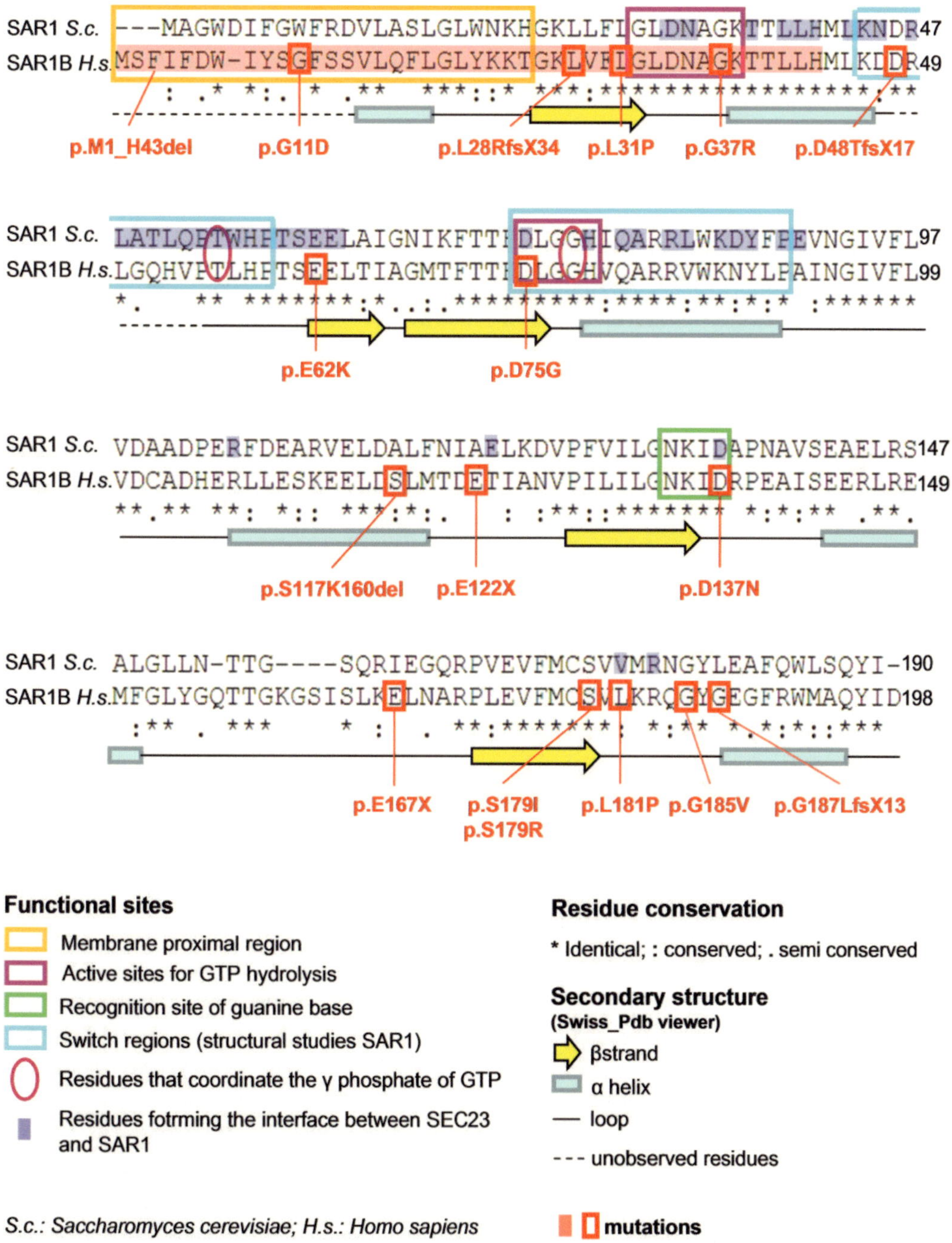

Figure 3. Sequence alignment of SAR1B protein with functional regions

acid translocase) and the COPII proteins [46]. PCTV budding does not require GTP (and, consequently, SAR1) but rather ATP [44]. Further, VAMP7 is necessary for the fusion of the PCTV with the Golgi [44, 47]. The role of Sar1 in the budding of PCTV has been clarified, recently, in an elegant study by Siddiqi and Mansbach (2012) [47]. They showed that the binding of FABP1 to intestinal ER generates PCTV. A cytosolic multi-protein complex (composed of SAR1b, SEC13, SVIP (Small VPC/p97- Interactive Protein) binds all the FABP1 which is subsequently liberated by the phosphorylation of SAR1b by PKCζ (Protein Kinase C Zeta).

These findings raise a number of questions as to the mechanism by which *SAR1B* gene mutations could affect PCTV transport to produce AD/CMRD. In particular, it is not clear how mutations that are located in regions involved in the binding and hydrolysis of GDP/GTP (and for which the effect on COPII mediated transport is evident) would affect PCTV transport (see below: Predicted impact of the mutations). Since SAR1b plays a role in both vesicle budding and vesicle fusion to the Golgi apparatus, further studies will be necessary to completely understand the apparently multiple roles that SAR1b plays in PCTV transport. Recently, L Jin and coll showed that the ubiquitylation by CUL3-KLHL2 allow the formation of COPII vesicle of a size sufficient to transport collagen (300-400 nm) [48]. It is of interest to know whether this mechanism also could permit the transport of chylomicrons. These recent data provide novel insights into the possible mechanisms for the transport of chylomicrons (either by PCTVs or COPII vesicles) and are very interesting because impaired COPII function results not only in AD/CMRD but also in collagen deposition defects [49] and lenticulo-structural dysplasia (SEC23A mutation). However, given the ubiquitous expression and essential roles of COPII components such as SAR1 and SEC23 as well as other proteins involved in trafficking between ER and Golgi, it is still not entirely clear as to how mutations in these proteins produce diseases with such marked tissue specific effects and low incidence.

4. Structure of the SAR1b protein

Although the SAR1 protein is included in the GTPase superfamily (and, in particular, the RAS superfamily) members of which are present in most living cells, from bacteria to vertebrates, it is only slightly related to other RAS or ARF proteins and is distant from the RAB/YPT1/SEC4 subclass [50, 51]. SAR1 is conserved from an evolutionary standpoint and appears to present in all eukaryotes. However, whereas yeast and insects have a single SAR1 protein, higher organisms express two forms, SAR1b and SAR1a (both with 198 amino acids), which differ by 20 amino-acid residues [52].The function of SAR1a has not been elucidated yet and, to date, no variant in the *SAR1A* gene has been described. The sequence alignment of SAR1b as compared to SAR1p (Figure 3) illustrates the different regions that are highly conserved across species and shows the different functional motifs in SAR1b that participate in vesicle budding, in GDP/GTP binding and hydrolysis and in interactions with other COP proteins.

Five X-ray crystallographic-derived structures for SAR1b bound to GDP or GTP, alone or complexed with other COPII components, have been deposited in the Protein Data Bank. Three of these structures are derived from *S. cerevisiae* (yeast) recombinant protein and two from *Cricetulus griseus* (hamster) recombinant protein. These structures provide insights into the structural changes that SAR1b may undergo upon GDP/GTP binding as well as demonstrating which parts of the protein constitute interfaces with other COPII components. No X-ray derived structures of SAR1b complexed with components of the PCTV are available to our knowledge. There is also one X-ray derived structure for SAR1a using human recombinant protein.

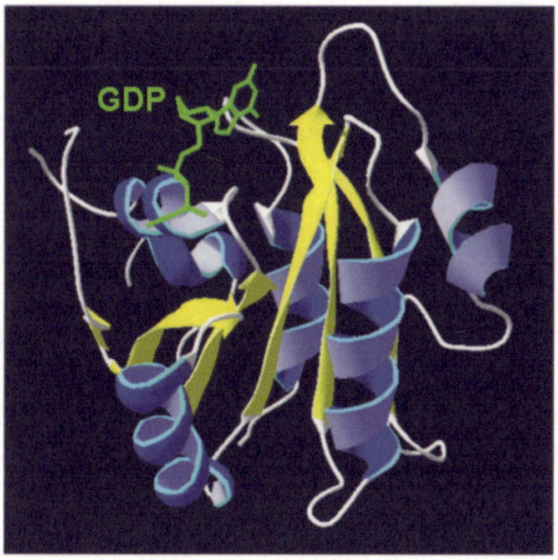

Using the 1F6B model Cricetulus griseus SAR1b [53]
(which lacks the first twelve AA)
and Swiss pdb Viewer:
two residues were modified (I80V, V163I)
in order to produce a structural module
having a sequence identical to that of human SAR1b.
In yellow: **β strands**
In blue: **α helixes**
In white: **loops**
In green: **GDP**

Figure 4. Three dimensional structure of SAR1B protein

The X-ray structures show that SAR1b has six central β strands (5 parallel, β2 antiparallel) that are sandwiched between three α helixes on each side (Figure 4). In SAR1-GDP (the inactive form), the α1helix is retracted into a pocket formed by the β2- β3 hairpin. The β strands 1-2-3 are approximately parallel to the membrane allowing their juxtaposition with the membrane (the N and C terminus and β2- β3 hairpin would participate in this membrane interaction) [36]. The Mg2+ ion is coordinated by an oxygen atom of the phosphate of the GDP and the hydroxyl oxygen of Threonine residue 39 (in SAR1-GDP) [37]. Many H bonds stabilize the structure and could be altered by mutations (see discussion below), for example Ser 179 with Asp 137 and Leu 181 [2].

The X-ray data also provide insights into the roles played by the different parts of the structure in SAR1b functions (see the protein alignment Figure 3). The amino- (N) terminal part of SAR1b contains the STAR (SAR1 NH2 Terminal Activation Recruitment) motif, a hydrophobic sequence of amino acids (AA) (1-9), a structure different from other ARF superfamily GTPases, which recruits SEC12, and the α1 amphipathic helix (AA 15-19, residues VLNFL). The role of the α1 amphipathic helix is fundamental as demonstrated by the loss of all export activity of SAR1B following the substitution of the 4 hydrophobic AA by 4 Alanine [53]. Between the STAR motif and the α1 helix, a short domain (AA 9-14, YSGFS) participates in deforming the ER membrane [38]. Three other regions contact the membrane, one each in the N- (AA 1-25) and carboxyl- (C) (AA 195-198) terminii and a central motif in the β2- β3 strand (AA 65-70) [36, 38]. There is one motif that recognizes the guanine base (AA 134-137, NKXD) and two active sites for GTP hydrolysis (AA 32-38, motif GXXXXGK and AA 75-78, motif DXXG) [54]. Close to the GTP hydrolysis site, Threonine 39 is a highly conserved residue and the substitution T39N inhibits SAR1 function by interfering with activation by SEC12 [53].

The two switch regions (AA 48-59 and AA 78-94) contain two very important residues, the Threonine at position 56 and the Glycine at position 78, respectively [53]. A second unique structural region of SAR1, not observed in the ARF GTPases, is a long surface-exposed loop (AA 156-171) which connects the α4 helix and the β6 strand and which regulates the function of SAR1b. The substitution Thr158Ala abolishes the activity of SAR1 [53]. A specific C-terminal motif (AA 171-181, PXEVFMC/VSV/L), present in the β6 strand, targets SAR1b to the ER [55].

The three-dimensional structure was obtained by crystallography [36, 53] and then by a computational approach. By crystallography (without the nine first and the 48-55 residues), SAR1-GDP appeared as a dimer [37, 53]. Nothing is available about an in vivo GTPase activity with this dimer structure. Moreover, Long and coll (2010) showed that SAR1b may function as a monomer [56], so we will only consider the monomer form.

5. Predicted impact of the mutations in the *SAR1B* gene on the structure and function of the protein

Currently, including the 4 new cases belonging to 3 new families reported here (one new missense mutation), mutations in the *SAR1B* gene have been established for 43 individuals with AD/CMRD (belonging to 24 families). There are only 17 unique mutations. The majority of individuals are homozygous for their mutation (38/43) and 5 individuals from 4 families are compound heterozygous. There are a total of 7 nonsense and 10 missense mutations (Table 2). Since structural information concerning SAR1b in PCTV vesicles is not available, the discussion of the possible effects of *SAR1B* gene mutations upon protein function will be limited to the COPII vesicle transport system.

Recently we identified the same mutation (del exon2) as the Algerian family (n°2) in 3 patients from 2 Tunisian families (to be published).

SAR1B	DNA variant	protein mutation	ethnic origin	Family number	sex	status	age dg	references
exon 2 (1-58 bp)	c.32 G>A	p.G11D	thaï	1	M	comp Hz	11m	24
	c.-4482_58 +1406 del 5946 ins 15bp (*named* del exon 2)	p.M1_H43del	algerian	2	F	Ho	6y	22
		p.M1_H43del	algerian	2	M	Ho	8y	22
exon 3 (59-178bp)	c.83_84 delTG	p.L28R fsX34	french canad	3	F	comp Hz	?	2, 11
	c.83_84 delTG	p.L28R fsX34	morrocan	4	F	Ho	7m	25
	c.83_84 delTG	p.L28R fsX34	morrocan	5	F	Ho	8m	27
	c.92 T>C	p.L31P	morrocan	6	M	Ho	3m	*this article*
	c.92 T>C	p.L31P	morrocan	6	M	Ho	15y	*this article*
	c.109 G>A	p.G37R	algerian	7	F	Ho	3,5y	2, 13
	c.109 G>A	p.G37R	algerian	7	M	Ho	3m	2, 13
	c.109 G>A	p.G37R	morrocan	8	M	Ho	3y	2, 12
	c.142 delG	p.D48T fsX17	turkish	9	M	Ho	10m	27
	c.142 delG	p.D48T fsX17	turkish	9	F	Ho	1m	27
exon 4 (179-244bp)	c.184 G>A	p.E62K	tunisian	10	F	Ho	7y	26
	c.224 A>G	p.D75G	thaï	1	M	comp.Hz *(see family 1 exon 2)*		
exon 6 (349-480bp)	c.349-1 G>C	p.S117K160del	italian	11	M	Ho	12y	2, 19
	c.349-1 G>C	p.S117K160del	italian	11	M	Ho	19y	2, 19
	c.364 G>T	p.E122X	turkish	12	M	Ho	3m	22
	c.364 G>T	p.E122X	turkish	12	F	Ho	6y	22
	c.364 G>T	p.E122X	turkish	12	F	Ho	8y	22
	c.364 G>T	p.E122X	turkish	12	M	Ho	11y	22
	c.409 G>A	p.D137N	french canad	13	M	Ho	?	2, 11
	c.409 G>A	p.D137N	french canad	13	F	Ho	?	2, 11
	c.409 G>A	p.D137N	french canad	3	F	comp.Hz *(see family 3 exon 3)*		
	c.409 G>A	p.D137N	french canad	14	M	Ho	3m	22
	c.409 G>A	p.D137N	french canad	14	M	Ho	2m	22
	c.409 G>A	p.D137N	french canad	15	M	Ho	3m	22
	c.409 G>A	p.D137N	french canad	16	F	comp Hz	2w	22
	c.409 G>A	p.D137N	french canad	16	M	comp Hz	3,5m	22
	c.409 G>A	p.D137N	french canad	17	F	Ho	50y	*this article*
	c.409 G>A	p.D137N	caucasian	18	M	Ho	8m	*this article*
exon 7 (481-597bp)	c.499 G>T	p.E167X	caucasian	19	F	Ho	34y	21, 23
	c.499 G>T	p.E167X	caucasian	19	F	Ho	38y	23
	c.536 G>T	p.S179I	pakistan	20	F	comp Hz	6m	2
	c.537 T>A	p.S179R	french canad	16	F	comp.Hz *(see family 16 exon 6)*		
	c.537 T>A	p.S179R	french canad	18	M	comp.Hz *(see family 16 exon 6)*		
	c.537 T>A	p.S179R	french canad	21	F	Ho	10y	22
	c.537 T>A	p.S179R	french canad	21	M	Ho	2m	22
	c.537 T>A	p.S179R	french canad	22	F	Ho	5m	22
	c.542 T>C	p.L181P	pakistan	20	F	comp.Hz *(see family 20 exon 7)*		
	c.554 G>T	p.G185V	portuguese	23	F	Ho	2y	22
	c.555-557 dupTTAC	p.G187LfsX13	turkish	24	F	Ho	1y	2, 16
	c.555-557 dupTTAC	p.G187LfsX13	turkish	24	M	Ho	1y	2, 16

(Ho: homozygous, comp Hz: compound heterozygous, age dg: age at diagnosis, m months, y years, w weeks)

Table 2. All published mutations in *SAR1B* gene

5.1. Nonsense mutations

Among the seven non-sense mutations, one deletes exon 2 (p.1-4482_58+1406 del 5946 ins 15bp, named "del exon 2") and one eliminates exon 6 (p.S117K160del), two are stop codons (p.E122X, p.E167X) which lead to truncated proteins, and two deletions and an insertion produce frameshifts followed by stop codons (p.L28RfsX34, p.D48TfsX17, p.G187LfsX13) leading to truncated proteins and modified C-terminal sequences. The major deletion (5943bp) of exon 2 (family 2 and new Tunisian patients) potentially leads to 4 different proteins [22] each of which lacks part of the N-terminus. The largest fragment lacks the first 43 residues, including the STAR motif, the $\alpha 1$ helix, the active site for GTP hydrolysis and Threonine 39. The deletion of exon 6 eliminates the recognition site for the guanine base (AA 134-137) thus abolishing the function of SAR1b. The five other nonsense mutations (resulting in stop codons) produce truncated proteins lacking the C-terminus. The shortest fragment is predicted to have about 33 AA and the longest contains 187/198 AA but, interestingly, all are predicted to abolish the function of the protein in the same manner. This suggests that the C terminal part of the protein plays a major role in the function of SAR1.

5.2. Missense mutations

The Swiss-pdb Viewer 3.1 program ([57], available on http://www.expasy.org/spdbv/) was used to calculate atomic resolution structural models for SAR1b having missense mutations (Table 3). First, using the 1F6B model [53] and PDB for *Cricetulus griseus* SAR1b (which lacks the first twelve AA and the 48-55 residues), two residues were modified (I80V, V163I) in order to produce a structural module having a sequence identical to that of human SAR1b. The effects of the missense mutations of AD/CMRD on this "humanized" structure were then modelled.

All the missense mutations are located on the exterior of the three dimensional structure, in strategic places near the recognition, binding and hydrolysis sites for the guanine base (in the N- and C-terminii) and/or affect a highly conserved residue in SAR1/Arf proteins. From the N- to the C- terminus the predicted effects may be summarized as the following (Figure 3). The p.G11D mutation is located in the membrane interacting site (anchorage of the N-terminal part of the molecule) and probably prevents binding to SEC12 and fixation to the ER membrane. The substitution G11P, associated with Y9F and S14F, has been described as being deleterious for vesicle release [38], however no model is available for this mutation (since the coordinates of the first 12 residues of the protein could not be established by the X-ray study leading to the 1F6B structure). The new mutation p.L31P affects the AA just before the active site of GTP and could decrease the GTP hydrolysis. The substitution of a linear (leucine) by a cyclic (proline) residue could lead to steric hindrance (Figure 5). The p.G37R and the p.D75G mutations are located in two different GDP hydrolysis sites. Replacement of glycine 37 by arginine creates steric hindrances with C178 and N134 and the replacement of the aspartic acid 75 by glycine abolishes the H bond with L38. All four of these mutations reduce or eliminate the affinity of SAR1b for GDP/GTP and are expected to

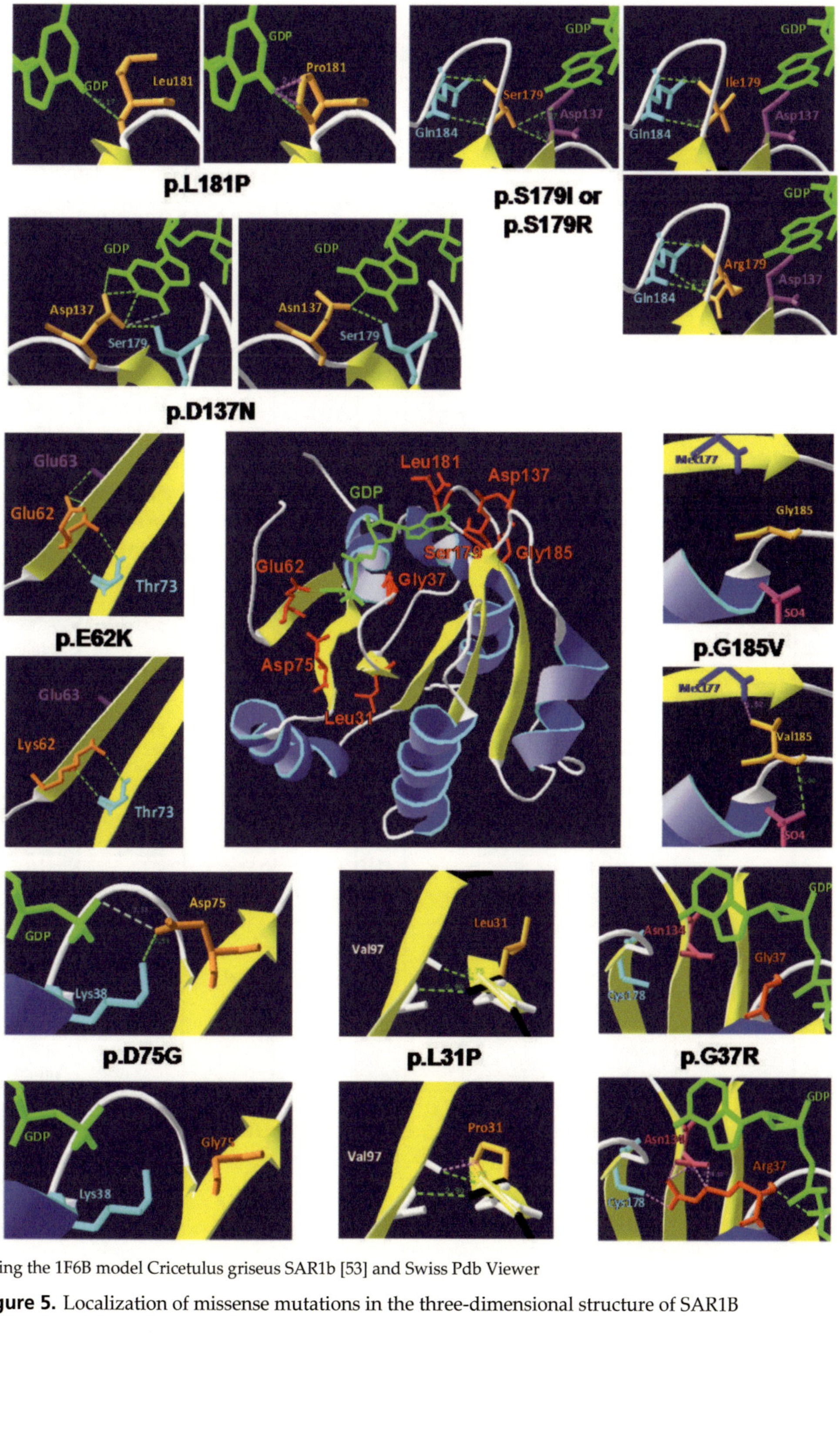

Using the 1F6B model Cricetulus griseus SAR1b [53] and Swiss Pdb Viewer

Figure 5. Localization of missense mutations in the three-dimensional structure of SAR1B

	Energy kJ/mol [a]	Grantham distance [b]	Consequence of mutation on prot. (concerned residue) [a]	Residue conservation [c]				PolyPhen prediction (Score) [d]	SIFT prediction (Score)[e]
				Sar1b prot.	Sar1 prot.	Sar1/ Arf family prot.	Small GTP binding prot.		
wild type	-9 749								
G11D	no modelisation	94	no modelisation	?	0	0	0	possibly damaging (0,927)	affect protein (0,03)
L31P	-6560	98	steric hindrance (Val97)	+	c	c	c	probably damaging (1,0)	affect protein (0,02)
G37R	75988	125	steric hindrances (Asn134, Cys178)	+	+	+	+	probably damaging (1,0)	affect protein (0,00)
E62K	-7777	56	loss of one H- (Glu63)	+	c	+	0	possibly damaging (0,955)	affect protein (0,00)
D75G	-9406	94	loss of one H- (Lys38)	+	+	+	+	probably damaging (0,99)	affect protein (0,00)
D137N	-10 086	23	loss of one H-bond (GDP)	+	+	+	+	probably damaging (1,0)	affect protein (0,00)
S179I	-8867	142	loss of : one weak H-bond (GDP) and one H-bond (Asp137)	+	+	s	0	probably damaging (1,0)	affect protein (0,00)
S179R	-7550	110	loss of : one weak H-bond (GDP) and one H-bond (Asp137)		+	s	0	probably damaging (1,0)	affect protein (0,00)
L181P	-9023	98	steric hindrances with GDP	c	0	0	0	beningn (0,281)	affect protein (0,00)
G185V	127 288	109	Steric hindrance (Met177)	+	+	+	0	probably damaging (1,0)	affect protein (0,00)

a Swiss Pdb Viewer 3.7 based upon the template 1F6b lacking the first 12 residues of SAR1b *C.g.* (resolution: 1,70Å, R value: 0,220, homolgy 98,9%) modified (p.I80V and p.V163I: homology 100%)
b Grantham distance (Alamut)
c http://www.ebi.ac.uk/clustalw/
residue conservation: +, identical; c, conserved substitution; s, semi conserved substitution
d PolyPhen-2 v2.2.2r395 http://genetics.bwh.harvard.edu/pph/
e Sorting Intolerant From Tolerant: http://blocks.fhcrc.org/sift/SIFT.html

Table 3. Molecular impact of missense mutations

affect the stability of the protein. The substitution p.E62K affecting a well-conserved AA belongs to some residues forming the interface with SEC23 [36], abolishes the H-bond with Glu63 and is predicted to be deleterious by "in silico" analysis (Polyphen, available on http://genetics.bwh.harvard.edu/pph2/ [58] and SIFT available on http://sift.jcvi.org/ [59-63]). A H-bond with the guanine in the guanine recognition site is abolished by the p.D137N mutation (Figure 5). Similarly the p.S179I and p.S179R mutations abolish the H-bonds with Asp 137 and with the guanine base. The substitution of a leucine for a proline (L181P) leads to steric hindrance with the guanine base and p.G185V modifies a highly conserved residue in the Arf/Sar1 family and is predicted to be deleterious by *"in silico"* analysis (Polyphen, SIFT). The last four mutations modify the α helix and β strands in the C-terminus and could affect the stability as well as the conformation of the protein.

6. Possible founder effects:

Founder effects are likely in the North African and French Canadian families (Table 2); it is likely that the same founder effect is responsible for the mutations of the North African patients (del exon 2, c.109 G>A). However, it is more uncertain for the c.409G>A and c.83_84delTG mutations, since the pedigrees of these families are not available. Perhaps there are hot spots, or different founder effects at the same place in the gene.

7. The biological and clinical impact of SAR1b mutations:

Table 4 provides the lipid profiles of the patients for which mutations in *SAR1B* have been established. As is typical for individuals affected with AD/CMRD, the mean values of total and HDL-cholesterol, apoAI and apoB are decreased, LDL-cholesterol is mildly decreased and triglycerides are in the normal range, however there is a large range of values for each of these parameters. As previously discussed, some patients present with low triglycerides or apoB levels and could be confused with atypical abetalipoproteinemia (familes 7, 12), and those with normal HDL cholesterol (family 10) could be confused with heterozygous FHBL. In homozygous patients, missense mutations are more frequent (12 families) than nonsense (8) and are as severe as nonsense mutations, except for the patient in family 10 (p.E62K) who has a normal HDL cholesterol level. The clinical data are not different among patients with different mutations. Several patients have been diagnosed later (adult or teenager) probably because of a mild intestinal syndrome and false diagnoses. Nevertheless, among the late diagnoses (10 patients after 10 years of age), only 3 have a missense mutation.

It has been suggested previously [22] that there is no apparent correlation between the genotype and the phenotype in AD/CMRD patients. For example, patients (from different families) with the same homozygous *SAR1B* mutation (for example the D137N mutation) exhibit different lipid profiles and vitamin E levels as do patients from the same families with the same mutations (the E122X and the S179R mutations). It is possible that modifier genes could be a cause of the different phenotypes. For example, a decrease in the transcriptional factor SREBP (Sterol Regulatory Element Binding Protein) has been shown to block the incorporation of SCAP (SREBP chaperone) in COPII vesicles and an acute depletion of cellular cholesterol concentration has been shown to decrease COPII transport [64, 65]. Other genes that modulate cholesterol homeostasis could interfere such as *MTTP* (microsomal triglycerides transfert protein), *APOB, ABCG5/G8* (ATP Binding Cassette G5/G8).

mutation	ethnic origin	family	sex	status	TC	TG	HDLC	LDLC	apoB	apoA1	vitE	references
p.G11D	thaï	1	M	comp Hz	1,81	1,29			0,54	0,43	1,5	24
p.M1_H43del	algerian	2	F	Ho	2,01	1,44	0,32	1,04	0,5	0,42	3,3	22
p.M1_H43del	algerian	2	M	Ho	2,32	0,78	0,4	1,57	0,55	0,45	2,6	22
p.L28R fsX34	french canad	3	F	comp Hz	2,2	0,73					1,4	2, 11
p.L28R fsX34	morrocan	4	F	Ho	1,45	0,77	0,36	0,73	0,39	0,4	1,2	25
p.L28R fsX34	morrocan	5	F	Ho	2,31	1,36	0,7	1	0,82	0,5	2,4	27
p.L31P	morrocan	6	M	Ho	1,96	0,89	0,77	0,79	0,37	0,91	1,34	*this article*
p.L31P	morrocan	6	M	Ho	2,09	0,93	0,59	1,31			3,75	*this article*
p.G37R	algerian	7	F	Ho	1,26	0,67			0,2	0,39	7,6	2, 13
p.G37R	algerian	7	M	Ho	1,79	1,44			0,33	0,38		2, 13
p.G37R	morrocan	8	M	Ho	1,55	0,59			0,36	0,64	2,9	2, 12
p.D48T fsX17	turkish	9	M	Ho	2,61	1,24	0,57	1,48	0,56	0,7	4,4	27
p.D48T fsX17	turkish	9	F	Ho	2,72	1,36	0,83	1,28	0,43	0,9	6,8	27
p.E62K	tunisian	10	F	Ho	2,59		1,3	1,14	0,4			26
p.D75G	thaï	1	M	comp Hz								24
p.S117K160del	italian	11	M	Ho	2,07	0,94	0,52	0,78			1	2, 19
p.S117K160del	italian	11	M	Ho	2,43	1,28	0,7	1,22			5	2, 19
p.E122X	turkish	12	M	Ho	1,99	0,43	0,57	1,23	0,36		4,71	22
p.E122X	turkish	12	F	Ho	1,26	0,5	0,53	0,51	0,38	0,43	0,88	22
p.E122X	turkish	12	F	Ho	1,37	0,72	0,39	0,66	0,33	0,51	1,44	22
p.E122X	turkish	12	M	Ho	1,36	0,45	0,45	0,71	0,35	0,59	1,42	22
p.D137N	french canad	13	M	Ho	1,85	0,94					0	2, 11
p.D137N	french canad	13	F	Ho	2,08	0,59					1,6	2, 11
p.D137N	french canad	2	F	comp Hz								2, 11
p.D137N	french canad	14	M	Ho	1,3	0,45	0,49	0,61				22
p.D137N	french canad	14	M	Ho	0,86	0,37	0,38	0,31				22
p.D137N	french canad	15	M	Ho	1,24	0,82	0,41	0,46				22
p.D137N	french canad	16	F	comp Hz	1,39	0,91	0,36	0,62				22
p.D137N	french canad	16	M	comp Hz	1,11	0,54	0,45	0,42				22
p.D137N	french canad	17	F	Ho	2,52	1,35	0,53	1,38				*this article*
p.D137N	caucasian	18	M	Ho	1,41	0,85	0,35	0,68	0,24	0,57	2,5	*this article*
p.E167X	caucasian	19	F	Ho	1,86	0,43			0,44	0,57	<1	21, 23
p.E167X	caucasian	19	F	Ho	2,15	0,36			0,55	0,62	<1	23
p.S179I	pakistan	20	F	comp Hz	1,4	0,79	0,44	0,6	0,59			2
p.S179R	french canad	16	F	comp Hz								22
p.S179R	french canad	16	M	comp Hz								22
p.S179R	french canad	21	F	Ho	2,82	1,36	0,59	1,61				22
p.S179R	french canad	21	M	Ho	1,5	0,78	0,56	0,59				22
p.S179R	french canad	22	F	Ho	1,78	1,28	0,56					22
p.L181P	pakistan	20	F	comp Hz								2
p.G185V	portuguese	23	F	Ho	2,36	1,98	0,49	0,98	0,61	0,46	2,5	22
p.G187L fsX13	turkish	24	F	Ho	2	1,6			0,7	0,5	6,6	2, 16
p.G187L fsX13	turkish	24	M	Ho	1,5	1,5			0,5	0,5	3,6	2, 16

(TC total cholesterol, TG triglycerides, LDLc LDL cholesterol, HDLc HDL cholesterol : mM; apoB, apoA1: g/l; vitE vitamin E: μM)

Table 4. Biological data in described cases with mutations

Recently a polymorphism of *PCSK9* (proprotein convertase subtilisin/kexin type 9), p.L15_16insL, has been reported in an AD patient [27]. This polymorphism is frequent (25% heterozygous in normal individuals and 34% in cases of HBL) and weakly hypocholesterolemic (-14%) [66]. Further, mutations or polymorphisms in other COPII and PCTV genes could contribute to the different phenotypes by modifying the network of all their corresponding proteins. However, none of these mutations have been described in cases of AD/CMRD. The search for polymorphisms in multiple proteins is very time-consuming but could be facility by the new sequencing methods. Rare polymorphisms in the coding regions of the *SAR1B* and *SAR1A* genes have been described but none of these has been observed in the *SAR1A* gene in any of our patients and only one polymorphism (heterozygous) has been found in the *SAR1B* gene (L45L) in our patients. This polymorphism is found with the same frequency in the patients as in normal individuals (0,18 versus 0,19, respectively). The impact of this polymorphism has not been studied.

8. Management of AD/CMRD (for details, see the guidelines of Peretti, 2010 [29])

Treatment consists primarily of a low fat diet, with the appropriate amounts of n-6 and n-3 fatty acids, supplemented with fat soluble vitamins. The failure to thrive of the children is the most important clinical feature and catch-up growth is not observed systematically [29]. The neurological and ophtamological complications may be less severe than in other familial hypocholesterolemias and may depend upon the levels of the fat soluble vitamins and when vitamin supplementation is instituted. Myolysis and cardiac abnormalities have been observed in some AD/CMRD patients [23] and consequently, measurement of the serum CK level should be included in the evaluation and follow-up of the patients. A moderate degree of fat liver is common, but until now no case of cirrhosis has been published.

9. Conclusions and future prospects

Significant advances in the diagnosis of AD/CMRD and in the understanding of lipoprotein secretion have occurred over the last decade. However, many questions remain to be answered. SAR1b is a ubiquitous protein, essential for the trafficking of proteins between the ER and the Golgi. Why do the mutations in *SAR1B,* that have been reported to date, apparently affect only the intestine and the transport of chylomicrons in the enterocyte? Although an increase of *SAR1A* mRNA was measured in enterocytes containing mutated *SAR1B* [27], the AD/CMRD phenotype was still manifested by a lack of chylomicron secretion. Under what conditions, if any, could SAR1a replace SAR1b? Is SAR1a the veritable GTPase for COPII vesicles? Do some mutations or polymorphisms in other regulator genes explain the lack of correlation between genotype and phenotype in AD/CMRD? There are some CMRD patients without mutations of *SAR1B, SAR1A, VAMP7, MTTP* genes (unpublished data). What gene mutations could explain the AD/CMRD phenotype in these patients? Novel technologies (such as whole exome and whole genome sequencing) may provide a better understanding of this disease and open novel diagnostic approaches.

Author details

A. Sassolas[1,2], M. Di Filippo[1,2], L.P. Aggerbeck[3], N. Peretti[2,4] and M.E. Samson-Bouma[5]
[1]*Department of Biochemistry, GHE, Hospices Civils de Lyon, France*
[2]*INSERM U1060 CarMeN, University of Lyon, Lyon, France*
[3]*INSERM UMR-S747, University Paris Descartes, Paris France*
[4]*Department of Pediatric Gastroenterology, GHE, Hospices Civils de Lyon, Lyon, France*
[5]*INSERM U698, University Denis Diderot, Centre Hospitalier Universitaire Xavier Bichat, Paris, France*

Acknowledgement

We thank the physicians Dr C. Vilain, Dr Damaj and others who have referred new patients for molecular investigation. We thank S. Dumont for technical assistance. This study was partially supported by a grant from French Health Ministry, Rare Diseases Plan.

10. References

[1] Anderson C, Townley R, Freemann J, Johansen P (1961) Unusual causes of steatorrhoea in infancy and childhood. Med J Aust 48:617-622.

[2] Jones B, Jones EL, Bonney SA, Patel HN, Mensenkamp AR, Eichenbaum-Voline S, et al. (2003) Mutations in a Sar1 GTPase of COPII vesicles are associated with lipid absorption disorders. Nat Genet. 34:29-31.

[3] Silverberg M, Kessler J, Neumann PZ, Wiglesworth FW (1968) An intestinal lipid transport defect. A possible variant of hypo-beta-lipoproteinemia. Gastroenterology. 54:1271.

[4] Polonovski C, Navarro J, Fontaine JL, de Gouyon F, Saudubray JM, Cathelineau L (1970) [Anderson's disease]. Ann Pediatr (Paris). 17:342-354.

[5] Costil J (1976) Maladie d'Anderson. Journées parisiennes de pédiatrie. 229-239.

[6] Scott BB, Miller JP, Losowsky MS (1979) Hypobetalipoproteinaemia--a variant of the Bassen-Kornzweig syndrome. Gut. 20:163-168.

[7] Gauthier S, Sniderman A (1983) Action tremor as a manifestation of chylomicron retention disease. Ann Neurol. 14:591.

[8] Bouma ME, Beucler I, Aggerbeck LP, Infante R, Schmitz J (1986) Hypobetalipoproteinemia with accumulation of an apoprotein B-like protein in intestinal cells. Immunoenzymatic and biochemical characterization of seven cases of Anderson's disease. J Clin Invest. 78:398-410.

[9] Polanco I, Mellado MJ, Lama R, Larrauri J, Zapata A, Redondo E, et al. (1986) [Anderson's disease. Apropos of a new case]. An Esp Pediatr. 24:185-188.

[10] Levy E, Marcel Y, Deckelbaum RJ, Milne R, Lepage G, Seidman E, et al. (1987) Intestinal apoB synthesis, lipids, and lipoproteins in chylomicron retention disease. J Lipid Res. 28:1263-1274.

[11] Roy CC, Levy E, Green PH, Sniderman A, Letarte J, Buts JP, et al. (1987) Malabsorption, hypocholesterolemia, and fat-filled enterocytes with increased intestinal apoprotein B. Chylomicron retention disease. Gastroenterology. 92:390-399.

[12] Lacaille F, Bratos M, Bouma ME, Jos J, Schmitz J, Rey J (1989) [Anderson's disease. Clinical and morphologic study of 7 cases]. Arch Fr Pediatr. 46:491-498.

[13] Pessah M, Benlian P, Beucler I, Loux N, Schmitz J, Junien C, et al. (1991) Anderson's disease: genetic exclusion of the apolipoprotein-B gene in two families. J Clin Invest. 87:367-370.

[14] Strich D, Goldstein R, Phillips A, Shemer R, Goldberg Y, Razin A, et al. (1993) Anderson's disease: no linkage to the apo B locus. J Pediatr Gastroenterol Nutr. 16:257-264.

[15] Patel S, Pessah M, Beucler I, Navarro J, Infante R (1994) Chylomicron retention disease: exclusion of apolipoprotein B gene defects and detection of mRNA editing in an affected family. Atherosclerosis. 108:201-207.

[16] Nemeth A, Myrdal U, Veress B, Rudling M, Berglund L, Angelin B (1995) Studies on lipoprotein metabolism in a family with jejunal chylomicron retention. Eur J Clin Invest. 25:271-280.

[17] Benavent MO, Chirivella Casanova M, Pereda Pérez A, Ribes Konickx C, Ferrer Calvete J (1997) Enfermedad de Anderson (esteatorrea por retencion de quilomicrones): Criterios diagnosticos. An Esp Pediatr. 47:195-198.

[18] Dannoura AH, Berriot-Varoqueaux N, Amati P, Abadie V, Verthier N, Schmitz J, et al. (1999) Anderson's disease: exclusion of apolipoprotein and intracellular lipid transport genes. Arterioscler Thromb Vasc Biol. 19:2494-2508.

[19] Aguglia U, Annesi G, Pasquinelli G, Spadafora P, Gambardella A, Annesi F, et al. (2000) Vitamin E deficiency due to chylomicron retention disease in Marinesco-Sjogren syndrome. Ann Neurol. 47:260-264.

[20] Boldrini R, Biselli R, Bosman C (2001) Chylomicron retention disease--the role of ultrastructural examination in differential diagnosis. Pathol Res Pract. 197:753-757.

[21] Mignard S, Calon E, Hespel JP, Le Treut A (2004) [A severely disturbed lipid profile]. Ann Biol Clin (Paris). 62:330-333.

[22] Charcosset M, Sassolas A, Peretti N, Roy CC, Deslandres C, Sinnett D, et al. (2008) Anderson or chylomicron retention disease: molecular impact of five mutations in the SAR1B gene on the structure and the functionality of Sar1b protein. Mol Genet Metab. 93:74-84.

[23] Silvain M, Bligny D, Aparicio T, Laforet P, Grodet A, Peretti N, et al. (2008) Anderson's disease (chylomicron retention disease): a new mutation in the SARA2 gene associated with muscular and cardiac abnormalities. Clin Genet. 74:546-552.

[24] Treepongkaruna S, Chongviriyaphan N, Suthutvoravut U, Charoenpipop D, Choubtum L, Wattanasirichaigoon D (2009) Novel missense mutations of SAR1B gene in an infant with chylomicron retention disease. J Pediatr Gastroenterol Nutr. 48:370-373.

[25] Cefalu AB, Calvo PL, Noto D, Baldi M, Valenti V, Lerro P, et al. (2010) Variable phenotypic expression of chylomicron retention disease in a kindred carrying a mutation of the Sara2 gene. Metabolism. 59:463-467.

[26] Fancello T, Najah M, Magnolo AL, Jelassi A, Di Leo E, Slimene N, et al. Novel mutations in SAR1B and MTP genes in chylomicron retention disease and abetalipoproteinemia (2011) 74th European Atherosclerosis Society Congress. Gothenburg. 2011.

[27] Georges A, Bonneau J, Bonnefont-Rousselot D, Champigneulle J, Rabes JP, Abifadel M, et al. (2011) Molecular analysis and intestinal expression of SAR1 genes and proteins in Anderson's disease (Chylomicron retention disease). Orphanet J Rare Dis. 6:1.

[28] Peretti N, Roy CC, Sassolas A, Deslandres C, Drouin E, Rasquin A, et al. (2009) Chylomicron retention disease: a long term study of two cohorts. Mol Genet Metab. 97:136-142.

[29] Peretti N, Sassolas A, Roy CC, Deslandres C, Charcosset M, Castagnetti J, et al. (2010) Guidelines for the diagnosis and management of chylomicron retention disease based on a review of the literature and the experience of two centers. Orphanet J Rare Disl. Available: http://www.ojrd.com/content/5/1/24. Accessed 2012 Mar 23.

[30] Sakamoto O, Abukawa D, Takeyama J, Arai N, Nagano M, Hattori H, et al. (2006) An atypical case of abetalipoproteinaemia with severe fatty liver in the absence of steatorrhoea or acanthocytosis. Eur J Pediatr. 165:68-70.

[31] Di Filippo M, Crehalet H, Samson-Bouma ME, Bonnet V, Aggerbeck LP, Rabes JP, et al. (2012) Molecular and functional analysis of two new MTTP gene mutations in an atypical case of abetalipoproteinemia. J Lipid Res. 53:548-555.

[32] Dannoura AH, Berriot-Varoqueaux N, Amati P, Abadie V, Verthier N, Schmitz J, et al. (1999) Anderson's disease : exclusion of apolipoprotein and intracellular lipid transport genes. Arterioscler Thromb Vasc Biol. 19:2494-2508.

[33] Okada T, Miyashita M, Fukuhara J, Sugitani M, Ueno T, Samson-Bouma ME, et al. (2011) Anderson's disease/chylomicron retention disease in a Japanese patient with uniparental disomy 7 and a normal SAR1B gene protein coding sequence. Orphanet J Rare Disl. Available: http://www.ojrd.com/content/6/1/78. Accessed 2012 Mar 23.

[34] Nakano A, Muramatsu M (1989) A novel GTP-binding protein, Sar1p, is involved in transport from the endoplasmic reticulum to the Golgi apparatus. J Cell Biol. 109:2677-2691.

[35] Barlowe C, Schekman R (1993) SEC12 encodes a guanine-nucleotide-exchange factor essential for transport vesicle budding from the ER. Nature. 365:347-349.

[36] Bi X, Corpina RA, Goldberg J (2002) Structure of the Sec23/24-Sar1 pre-budding complex of the COPII vesicle coat. Nature. 419:271-277.

[37] Rao Y, Bian C, Yuan C, Li Y, Chen L, Ye X, et al. (2006) An open conformation of switch I revealed by Sar1-GDP crystal structure at low Mg2+. Biochem Biophys Res Commun. 348:908-915.

[38] Bielli A, Haney CJ, Gabreski G, Watkins SC, Bannykh SI, Aridor M (2005) Regulation of Sar1 NH2 terminus by GTP binding and hydrolysis promotes membrane deformation to control COPII vesicle fission. J Cell Biol. 171:919-924.

[39] Mossessova E, Bickford LC, Goldberg J (2003) SNARE selectivity of the COPII coat. Cell. 114:483-495.

[40] Futai E, Hamamoto S, Orci L, Schekman R (2004) GTP/GDP exchange by Sec12p enables COPII vesicle bud formation on synthetic liposomes. Embo J. 23:4146-4155.

[41] Jensen D, Schekman R (2011) COPII-mediated vesicle formation at a glance. J Cell Sci. 124:1-4.

[42] Zanetti G, Pahuja KB, Studer S, Shim S, Schekman R (2011) COPII and the regulation of protein sorting in mammals. Nat Cell Biol. 14:20-28.

[43] Kodera C, Yorimitsu T, Nakano A, Sato K (2011) Sed4p stimulates Sar1p GTP hydrolysis and promotes limited coat disassembly. Traffic. 12:591-599.

[44] Mansbach CM, Siddiqi SA (2010) The biogenesis of chylomicrons. Annu Rev Physiol. 72:315-333.

[45] Siddiqi SA, Gorelick FS, Mahan JT, Mansbach CM, 2nd (2003) COPII proteins are required for Golgi fusion but not for endoplasmic reticulum budding of the pre-chylomicron transport vesicle. J Cell Sci. 116:415-427.

[46] Siddiqi S, Saleem U, Abumrad NA, Davidson NO, Storch J, Siddiqi SA, et al. (2010) A novel multiprotein complex is required to generate the prechylomicron transport vesicle from intestinal ER. J Lipid Res. 51:1918-1928.

[47] Siddiqi S, Mansbach CM (2012) Phosphorylation of Sar1b releases the Liver Fatty Acid Binding Protein from a Multiprotein Complex in intestinal cytosol enabling it to bind the Pre-Chylomicron Transport Vesicle. J Biol Chem. Paper in Press.

[48] Jin L, Pahuja KB, Wickliffe KE, Gorur A, Baumgartel C, Schekman R, et al. (2012) Ubiquitin-dependent regulation of COPII coat size and function. Nature. 482:495-500.

[49] Kim SD, Pahuja KB, Ravazzola M, Yoon J, Boyadjiev SA, Hammamoto S, et al. (2012) The SEC23-SEC31 interface plays a critical role for the export of procollagen from the endoplasmique reticulum. J Biol Chem. Paper in Press.

[50] Bourne HR, Sanders DA, McCormick F (1990) The GTPase superfamily: a conserved switch for diverse cell functions. Nature. 348:125-132.

[51] Kuge O, Dascher C, Orci L, Rowe T, Amherdt M, Plutner H, et al. (1994) Sar1 promotes vesicle budding from the endoplasmic reticulum but not Golgi compartments. J Cell Biol. 125:51-65.

[52] Shoulders CC, Stephens DJ, Jones B (2004) The intracellular transport of chylomicrons requires the small GTPase, Sar1b. Curr Opin Lipidol. 15:191-197.

[53] Huang M, Weissman JT, Beraud-Dufour S, Luan P, Wang C, Chen W, et al. (2001) Crystal structure of Sar1-GDP at 1.7 A resolution and the role of the NH2 terminus in ER export. J Cell Biol. 155:937-948.

[54] Dever TE, Glynias MJ, Merrick WC (1987) GTP-binding domain: three consensus sequence elements with distinct spacing. Proc Natl Acad Sci U S A. 84:1814-1818.

[55] d'Enfert C, Gensse M, Gaillardin C (1992) Fission yeast and a plant have functional homologues of the Sar1 and Sec12 proteins involved in ER to Golgi traffic in budding yeast. EMBO J. 11:4205-4211.

[56] Long KR, Yamamoto Y, Baker AL, Watkins SC, Coyne CB, Conway JF, et al. (2010) Sar1 assembly regulates membrane constriction and ER export. J Cell Biol. 190:115-128.

[57] Guex N, Peitsch MC (1997) SWISS-MODEL and the Swiss-PdbViewer: an environment for comparative protein modeling. Electrophoresis. 18:2714-2723.

[58] Adzhubei IA, Schmidt S, Peshkin L, Ramensky VE, Gerasimova A, Bork P, et al. (2010) A method and server for predicting damaging missense mutations. Nat Methods. 7:248-249.

[59] Ng PC, Henikoff S (2001) Predicting deleterious amino acid substitutions. Genome Res. 11:863-874.

[60] Ng PC, Henikoff S (2002) Accounting for human polymorphisms predicted to affect protein function. Genome Res. 12:436-446.

[61] Ng PC, Henikoff S (2003) SIFT: Predicting amino acid changes that affect protein function. Nucleic Acids Res. 31:3812-3814.

[62] Ng PC, Henikoff S (2006) Predicting the effects of amino acid substitutions on protein function. Annu Rev Genomics Hum Genet. 7:61-80.

[63] Kumar P, Henikoff S, Ng PC (2009) Predicting the effects of coding non-synonymous variants on protein function using the SIFT algorithm. Nat Protoc. 4:1073-1081.

[64] Espenshade PJ, Li WP, Yabe D (2002) Sterols block binding of COPII proteins to SCAP, thereby controlling SCAP sorting in ER. Proc Natl Acad Sci U S A. 99:11694-11699.

[65] Ridsdale A, Denis M, Gougeon PY, Ngsee JK, Presley JF, Zha X (2006) Cholesterol is required for efficient endoplasmic reticulum-to-Golgi transport of secretory membrane proteins. Mol Biol Cell. 17:1593-1605.

[66] Yue P, Averna M, Lin X, Schonfeld G (2006) The c.43_44insCTG variation in PCSK9 is associated with low plasma LDL-cholesterol in a Caucasian population. Hum Mutat. 27:460-466.

Chapter 14

Activating Mutations and Targeted Therapy in Cancer

Musaffe Tuna and Christopher I. Amos

Additional information is available at the end of the chapter

http://dx.doi.org/10.5772/48701

1. Introduction

Neoplasia, the accumulation of abnormal cells, occurs because tumor cells often lose control of proliferative signaling, escape growth suppression, can become invasive and metastasize and grow in abnormal environments, induce angiogenesis, withstand cell death, deregulate cellular energetic constraints, avoid immune destruction, promote inflammation and enhance genome instability and mutation (Hanahan and Weinberg 2011). Understanding the mechanisms underlying both the sensitivity and the resistance of tumor cells to anticancer agents first requires understanding the global view of the cancer genome (genetic, genomic, and epigenetic alterations) to identify driver events that decisively influence the viability and clinical behavior of a given tumor. This knowledge, together with an understanding of the mechanism of action of drugs, will lead to the identification of novel targets and the development of targeted therapeutics in the appropriate patient subpopulation.

By 1982, mutations and chromosomal translocations had been established as key genetic mechanisms that are capable of driving cancer. Then, the *MYC* proto-oncogene was found to be activated by translocation as well as amplification, and amplification thus became recognized as an additional cardinal mechanism of cancer gene deregulation (Collins and Groudine 1982; Taub, Kirsch et al. 1982; Vennstrom, Sheiness et al. 1982; Alitalo, Schwab et al. 1983). Epigenetic modifications of genomic DNA or histones by methylation or acetylation also became recognized as key mediators of the cancer phenotype (Esteller 2007).

One of the first pivotal discoveries of activating mutations was within *BRAF* (Figure 1), which encodes a serine/threonine kinase oncogene that transmits proliferative and survival signals downstream of RAS in the mitogen-activated protein (MAP) kinase cascade (Davies,

Bignell et al. 2002). This was after the discovery of *HRAS* mutations (Reddy, Reynolds et al. 1982; Tabin, Bradley et al. 1982) and similar mutations within *KRAS* (Capon, Seeburg et al. 1983; Shimizu, Birnbaum et al. 1983), *NRAS* (Bos, Toksoz et al. 1985), and other genes. Some of the driver mutations were found to be targets for therapy, whereas others play crucial roles in resistance to therapy. Here, we focus on activating mutations, small molecules that have been used to target mutated genes, and mutations that play crucial roles in resistance to certain therapeutic agents.

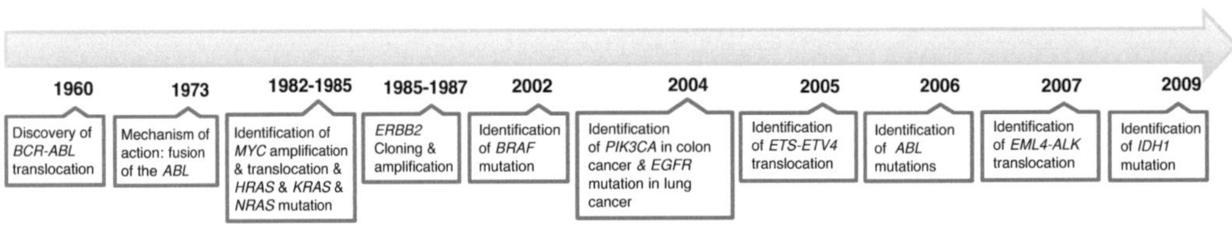

Figure 1. The historical timelines for discovery of driver translocation, mutation and amplification.

2. Types of mutations

Oncogenesis results from mutations or alterations of genes that regulate cell functions such as proliferation, growth, invasion, angiogenesis, metastasis, death, energy metabolism, genome stability, and replication. Simple mutations can be induced in DNA by exposure to a variety of mutagens, such as radiation and chemicals, or by spontaneous errors in DNA replication and repair. Genes with mutations that cause cancer can be grouped into two classes: oncogenes and tumor suppressor genes.

Oncogenes are the mutant form of proto-oncogenes, a class of normal cellular protein-coding genes that promote the growth and survival of cells. Oncogenes encode proteins such as:

a. Growth factors (e.g., *PDGF* and *IGF1*);
b. Growth factor receptors (e.g., *ERBB2*, *EGFR*, and *MET*);
c. Intracellular signal transduction factors (e.g., *RAS* and *RAF*);
d. Cell cycle factors (e.g., *CDK4*);
e. Transcription factors that control the expression of growth promoting genes (e.g., *FOS*, *JUN*, and *MYC*); and
f. Inhibitors of programmed cell death machinery (e.g., *BCL2*).

Tumor suppressor genes, which control cell growth, can be grouped into two classes: gatekeeper and caretaker tumor suppressor genes. Gatekeeper tumor suppressor genes (e.g., *RB1* and *TP53*) block tumor development by controlling cell division and survival, and caretaker tumor suppressor genes (e.g., *MSH2* and *MLH1*) protect the integrity of the genome.

Activation of proto-oncogenes (activating mutations) can occur either by large-scale alterations, such as gain/amplification, insertion, or chromosome translocation, or by small-scale mutations, such as point mutation. Inactivation of tumor suppressor genes (inactivating mutations) can occur either by small-scale mutation or by large-scale alterations, such as loss of region of tumor suppressor gene or whole chromosome.

Small-scale mutations can be grouped into the following classes on the basis of the effect of the mutation on the DNA sequence:

a. **Base substitution mutation** is the replacement (exchange) of a single nucleotide by another. Base substitutions can be either a **transition**—substitution of a pyrimidine by a pyrimidine (C↔T) or a purine by a purine (A↔G)—or a **transversion**—substitution of a pyrimidine by a purine or vice versa (A↔G, A↔C, G↔T, T↔C). Single nucleotide mutation can lead to qualitative rather than quantitative changes in the function of a protein. The biological activity can be retained, but the characteristics may differ, such as optimum pH and stability. Mutations that occur in coding DNA can be grouped into two classes:

i. **Synonymous (silent) mutations.** In this type of mutation, even if the sequence changes, the amino acid is not altered due to the degenerate genetic code, except if the mutations affect splicing by activating a cryptic splice site or by altering an exonic splice enhancer sequence. Because silent mutations usually confer no advantage or disadvantage to the organism in which they arise, they are also called neutral mutations.

ii. **Non-synonymous mutations.** In this type of mutation, the altered sequence changes the amino acid, which can be a polypeptide (gene product) or functional non-coding RNA. Non-synonymous mutations may have a harmful effect, no effect, or a beneficial effect in the organism. Non-synonymous mutations can be grouped into **nonsense** mutations, where the altered amino acid is replaced by a stop codon, which results in premature termination and is likely to cause loss of function or expression because of degradation of mRNA, and **missense** mutations, where the altered codon specifies a different amino acid, which may affect protein function or stability. **Splice site mutations** are likely to cause aberrant splicing, such as exon skipping or intron retention, and mutations in **promoter** sequences can result in altered gene expression. Finally, some mutations alter the normal stop codon, which terminates mRNA transcription so that a longer or shorter amino acid than normal is translated.

b. **Deletions.** In this type of mutation, one or more nucleotides are lost from a sequence.

i. Deletion of multiple codons (three bases) may affect protein function or stability.

ii. A frameshift mutation—not of a multiple of three bases (codon)—is likely to result in premature termination with loss of function.

iii. A large deletion—partial- or whole-gene deletion—is likely to result in premature termination with loss of function or expression.

c. **Insertions.** In this type of mutation, one or more nucleotides are added into a sequence.

i. Insertion of 3 nucleotides (a codon) or of multiple codons may affect protein function or stability.

ii. A frameshift mutation, which occurs when either <3 or >3 nucleotides are inserted, is likely to result in premature termination with loss of function.

iii. A large insertion, which is partial-gene duplication, is likely to result in premature termination with loss of function. Whole-gene duplication may have an effect because of increased gene dosage.

iv. A dynamic mutation, which is the expansion of a dinucleotide or a trinucleotide repeat, may alter gene expression or may alter protein stability or function.

Whereas mutations in coding DNA have a phenotypic effect, mutations in non-coding DNA are less likely to have a phenotypic effect, except when the mutation occurs in a regulatory sequence such as a promoter sequence and miRNAs. Mutations exert their phenotypic effect through either gain of function or loss of function. Loss-of-function mutations result in either reduced activity or complete loss of the gene product. Gain-of-function mutations can result in either an increased level of expression or the development of a new function of the gene product.

Important progress has been made in developing new technologies for identifying mutations. One of these is next-generation sequencing. This technology enables the identification of copy number changes, chromosomal alterations such as translocations and inversions, and point mutations.

3. Activating mutations and targeted therapies

Recent advances in molecular oncology and discoveries in genetic alterations have yielded new treatment strategies that target specific molecules and pathways in the cancer cell and thereby shed light on personalized therapy. In the past, treatment decisions were based on pathologic results. Now, diagnostic or therapeutic decisions are often also based on genetics/genomic alterations. Currently, the genomic view effectively guides cancer treatment decisions and predicts therapeutic response. Early clinical success was achieved with all-*trans* retinoic acid therapy in patients with acute promyelocytic leukemia (characterized by chromosomal translocations involving retinoic acid receptor α, the target of all-*trans* retinoic acid) (Huang, Ye et al. 1988; Castaigne, Chomienne et al. 1990), Herceptin (trastuzumab, a monoclonal antibody) and in patients with breast cancer in which *ERBB2* is amplified and/or overexpressed (Baselga, Tripathy et al. 1999; Slamon, Leyland-Jones et al. 2001; Vogel, Cobleigh et al. 2002). Also, imatinib mesylate and, subsequently, nilotinib (a selective ABL tyrosine kinase inhibitor [TKI]) have proved effective in patients with the *BCR-ABL* fusion gene, including most individuals (95%) with chronic myeloid leukemia (CML), which constitutively activates the ABL tyrosine kinase (Mauro, O'Dwyer et al. 2002). These successes motivated the discovery of new targets and selective inhibitors for those targets. Currently, targeted therapeutics are used to target receptor tyrosine kinases (*EGFR, ERBB2, FGFR1, FGFR2, FGFR3, PDGFRA, PDGFRB, ALK, c-MET, IGF1R, c-KIT, FLT3,* and *RET*), non-receptor tyrosine kinases (*ABL, JAK2,* and *SRC*), serine-threonine-lipid kinases (*BRAF, Aura A and B kinases, mTOR,* and *PIK3*), and DNA damage and repair genes (*BRCA1* and *BRCA2*), however not all therapeutics are selective inhibitors. Here, we focus on activating mutations that are targeted by selective inhibitors to inhibit only mutated genes; *EGFR, ALK, c-KIT, BCR-ABL, JAK2, BRAF, IDH1, IDH2, FLT3* and *PIK3CA* (Table 1).

EGFR	*BRAF*	*KRAS*	*PIK3CA*	*c-KIT*	*BCR-ABL*	*IDH1*	*JAK2*
G719A[12]	M117R[13]	G12C[5, 12]	E542K[4, 5, 6, 28, 29]	K642E[13, 22]	M244V[10]	R132C[2, 5, 8, 9, 19, 20, 21, 27]	V617F[8, 19, 20]
G719C[12]	I326T[4]	G12R[12]	E545K[4, 5, 6, 9, 12, 28, 29]	L576P[13]	L248V[10]	R132H[1, 2, 9, 21, 26, 27]	K539L[19]
G719S[12]	K439Q[12]	G12S[5, 12]	E545Q[4]	W557R[13]	G250E[10]	R132S[2, 9, 26]	N542-E543del[19]
T790M[12]	K439T[12]	G12A[5, 9, 12]	E545A[4]	V559A[13]	Q252H[10]	R132G[2, 9, 26]	F537-K539delinsK[19]
L858R[4, 12]	T440P[12]	G12D[5, 12]	E545G[4, 5, 29]	V560D[22]	Y253F[10]	R132L[2, 9, 26]	H538-K539delinsL[19]
L858Q[12]	V459L[12]	G12V[5, 12]	E545V[4]	D816H[13, 22]	Y253H[10]	R132V[2, 9]	F537-I546dupF547L[19]
L858L[21]	G469A[14]	G13C[5, 12]	Q546K[4, 6]	F504L[13]	E255K[10]	R132G[2]	E543del[19]
D761Y[12]	R462I[5]	G13R[12]	Q546E[4]	S502-Y503insFA[13]	E255V[10]	V71I[14, 24]	H538QK539L[19]
L747S[12]	I463S[5]	G13S[12]	Q546P[4]	K550N[13]	D276G[10]	G123R[24]	I540-E543delinsMK[19]
T854A[12]	G464E[5, 11, 17]	G13A[12]	Q546R[4, 6]	Y553N[13]	E279K[10]	G97D[9, 25]	F547V[19]
P782L[21]	G464V[5, 11, 17]	G13D[5, 12, 14]	Q546L[4]	556insL[13]	V299L[10]		H538DK539LI540S[19]
F788L[21]	G464R[5, 11, 17]	Q61K[10, 12, 13]	D549N[4]	K558N[13]	F311L[10]	***IDH2***	F537-F547dup[19]
R748K[21, 22]	G466A[6, 12, 13]	Q61L[5, 10, 12]	H1047L[4, 6, 29]	G565V[13]	T315I[10]		I540-N542delinsS[19]
L747–S752del	G466E[12, 13]	Q61R[12, 13]	H1047R[4, 5, 6, 9, 28, 29]	N566D[13]	T315A[10]	V294M[13]	V536-F547dup[19]
E746-A750del[4, 17, 28]	G466R[12, 13]	Q61H[5, 10, 12, 14]	Q1064R[6]	V569G[13]	F317L[10]	R172K[2, 9]	V536-I546dup[19]
S752-I759del[4]	G466V [12, 13]	A146T[5, 14]	A1066V[6]	R634W[13]	F317V[10]	R172M[2, 9]	
L707S[25]	F468C[5]	Y64D[14]	Y1021C[6]	V654A[13]	F317C[10]	R172G[2, 9]	
T710A[25]	G469A[3, 5, 10, 11, 12, 13,16]	L19F[14]	G12-R19del[6]	N655K[13]	M351T[10]	R172S[2]	***FLT3***
E711V[25]	G469E[3, 5, 10, 11, 12, 13,16]	K117N[14]	R38H[6]	D816H[13]	E355G[10]	R172W[2, 9]	
E749K[25]	G469R[3, 5, 10, 11, 12, 13,16]	E63K[14]	R88Q[4, 5, 6, 9]	D816V[2, 13]	F359V[10]	R140Q[2, 9, 19, 20]	Y592A[2]
E762G[25]	G469S[3, 5, 10, 11, 12, 13,16]	K147N[28]	G106A[6]	D820V[13]	F359C[10]	R140W[2]	
A767T[25]	G469V[3, 5, 10, 11, 12, 13,16]	G12F[10, 12]	E109del[6]	D820Y[13]	V379I[10]	R140L[2, 26]	Y599F[2]
K745R[28]	K475E[13]		V344G[6]	N822I[13]	L384M[10]		F691L[2]
G735S[24]	N581S[5]		E309NfsX10[6]	N822K[2, 13]	L387M[10]		
R108K[9]	E586K[17]		E453K[4, 6]	Y823D[13]	H396R[10]		
T263P[9]	D587A[5]		M1043V[6, 9]	A829P[13]	H396P[10]		D835N[2]
A289V[9]	D594G[5, 13, 16, 23]		M1043I[6]	I841V[13]	F486S[10]		D835Y[2]
G598V[9]	D594K[5, 13, 16, 23]		E81K[6]	S864F[13]	E459K		D835A[2]
L861Q[9]	D594V[5, 13, 16, 23]		H1048R[6]	V120F[29]			D835E[2]
R680G[9]	F595L[5, 11]		G1049R[6]	V560D[22]			D835H[2]
G136A[9]	G596R[5]		E418K[6]	Y503-F504insAY[22]			D835V[2]
G136C[9]	L597Q[11, 12, 13, 17]		C420R[6]	Y570-L576del[22]			D835F[2]
G323A[9]	L597R[11, 12, 13, 17]		H701P[6]	A599T[15]			I836F[2]
A787C[9]	L597S[11, 12, 13, 17]		LWGIHLM10del[9]	V833L[10, 30]			I836S[2]
C866A[9]	L597V[11, 12, 13, 17]		P18del[9]	P577S[10, 30]			M837P[2]
G865A[9]	T599I[5]		N345K[9]	V825A[10, 30]			Y842H[2]
C866T[9]	T599-ins(T-T)[13]		C420R[9]	L576P[30]			Y842D[2]
G971T[9]	V600D[3, 4, 5, 7, 9, 11, 12, 13, 17, 22, 23, 24]			E562K [30]			
G988A[9]	V600E[3, 4, 5, 7, 9, 11, 12, 13, 17, 22, 23, 24]			N564S[30]			
D1006Y[14]	V600G[3, 4, 5, 7, 9, 11, 12, 13, 17, 22, 23, 24]			D816V[2, 10, 17]			
M178I[28]	V600K[3, 4, 5, 7, 9, 11, 12, 13, 17, 18, 19, 23]			D816H[2, 10, 17, 26]			
I475V[28]	V600M[3, 4, 5, 8, 9, 11, 12, 13, 17, 22, 23, 24]			D816I[10]			
S492R[25]	V600R			D816G[10]			
F712S[25]	V600-K605 ins[13]			D816F[10]			
T725T[25]	K601E[5, 13, 22]			V825A[2]			
V742V[21, 25]	K601N[5, 13, 22]			D816Y[2, 17, 26]			
F795S[25]	R682Q[6]			R634R[30]			
G796S[25]	A728V[1]			D820G[19]			
G796V[21]				V825I[19]			
T751I[21]				E839K[19]			
R748K[21]				I957T[19]			
R836R[25]				P31L[19]			
T847I[4]				R956Q[19]			
Q820R[21]				T22A[19]			
E804G[21]				G961S[19]			
L828M[21]				K642E[13]			
F856Y[21]				V559D[22]			
F856L[21]				W557R[22]			

A839V[21]				V559G[22]			
G863D[12, 21]				V559D[13, 22]			
V851I[12, 21]				V540L[2]			
I821T[21]				M541L[2]			
I789I[21]							
H870N[21]							
V834A[21]							
T725M[17]							
L858R[17]							
R832C[17]							
A868D[17]							
T852M[17]							
T725A[17]							
L703P[17]							
S720F[17]							
N700S[17]							
R836S[17]							
G721S[17]							
L703P[17]							
K708G[17]							
P772-H773insV[12]							
R108K[9]							
L62R[9]							
V651M[9]							
R222C[9]							
T263P[9]							
A289T[9]							
A289V[9]							
A597P[9]							
G598V[9]							
C620Y[9]							
S703F[9]							

[1]Acute lymphocytic leukemia; [2]acute myleloid leukemia; [3]Barret's adenocarcinoma; [4]breast carcinoma; [5]colon carcinoma; [6]endometrial carcinoma; [7]ependymoma; [8]essential thrombocyte; [9]glioma; [10]leukemia; [11]hepatocellular carcinoma; [12]lung cancer; [13]melanoma; [14]multiple myeloma; [15]neuroblastoma; [16]non-hodgkins lymphoma; [17]ovarian carcinoma; [18]pancreas cancer; [19]polycythemia vera; [20]primary myelofibrosis; [21]prostate cancer; [22]sarcoma; [23]stomach cancer; [24]thyroid cancer; [25]colorectal cancer; [26]myelodysplastic syndromes; [27]paraganglioma; [28]H&N (head and neck) cancer; [29]esophageal cancer, [30]lymphoma.

Table 1. Mutations have been reported at *EGFR, BRAF, KRAS, PIK3C, c-KIT, ABL, IDH1, IDH2* and *JAK2* in variety of cancers (Garnett and Marais 2004; Lee, Vivanco et al. 2006; Loeffler-Ragg, Witsch-Baumgartner et al. 2006; Thomas, Baker et al. 2007; Balss, Meyer et al. 2008; The Cancer Genome Atlas Network 2008; Bleeker, Lamba et al. 2009; Hayes, Douglas et al. 2009; MacConaill, Campbell et al. 2009; Yan, Parsons et al. 2009; de Muga, Hernandez et al. 2010; Gravendeel, Kloosterhof et al. 2010; Green and Beer 2010; Reitman and Yan 2010; Yen, Bittinger et al. 2010; Chapman, Lawrence et al. 2011; Konopka, Janiec-Jankowska et al. 2011; Metzger, Chambeau et al. 2011; Murugan, Dong et al. 2011; Passamonti, Elena et al. 2011; Peraldo-Neia, Migliardi et al. 2011; Stransky, Egloff et al. 2011; Tanaka, Terai et al. 2011; The Cancer Genome Atlas Network 2011; Teng, Tan et al. 2011; Montagut, Dalmases et al. 2012; Weisberg, Sattler et al. 2010; *Catalog of Somatic Mutations in Cancer*: www.sanger.ac.uk/genetics/CGP/cosmic/)

3.1. Activating mutations at *BCR-ABL*

In a normal cell, ABL protein is located in the nucleus, but in cancer cells the BCR-ABL fusion protein is found in the cytoplasm and is constitutively active (Goldman and Melo 2008). Studies have shown that *BCR-ABL* is oncogenic in hematopoietic cells, promoting leukemic cell proliferation and inhibiting apoptosis (Lugo, Pendergast et al. 1990; Stoklosa, Poplawski et al. 2008). Notably, *BCR-ABL* activity has also been found to stimulate the generation of mutagenic reactive oxygen species and to inhibit DNA repair mechanisms (Koptyra, Falinski et al. 2006; Fernandes, Reddy et al. 2009).

The discovery of this oncogenic fusion protein led to the development of imatinib mesylate. Imatinib, an ABL kinase inhibitor, was the first therapeutically successful treatment for CML and gained U.S. Food and Drug Administration approval in 2001. However, a substantial proportion of patients with CML developed resistance to imatinib because of mutation in *BCR-ABL* fusion gene (>90 mutations that affect >55 amino acid residues in *BCR-ABL*) (Table 1) (Branford 2007). Interestingly, *BCR-ABL* mutations were found in 57% of patients with acquired resistance to imatinib compared with 30% of patients with primary resistance (Soverini, Colarossi et al. 2006). The point mutation(s) in the *BCR-ABL* kinase domain result in the resistance to imatinib by reducing the flexibility of the kinase domain and its binding to imatinib, and inhibiting the activity of the kinase (Burgess, Skaggs et al. 2005; O'Hare, Walters et al. 2005).

T315I is the most common imatinib-resistant mutation in *BCR-ABL;* among the other highly imatinib-resistant mutations are L248V, Y253F/H, E255K/V, H396P/R, and F486S (Houchhaus, La Rosee et al. 2011). These discoveries were followed by the development of second-generation TKIs to inhibit BCR-ABL: dasatinib, and nilotinib. The response rate to these second-generation BCR-ABL inhibitors in patients harboring imatinib-resistant mutations is variable, depending on the mutation: L248V (40%), G250E (33%), E255K (38%), and E255V (36%), but response rates are low in those harboring F317L (7%) or Q252H (17%) (Muller, Cortes et al. 2009). The following imatinib-resistant mutations are sensitive to nilotinib: M351T, G250E, M244V, H396R, F317L, E355G, E459K, F486S, L248V, D276G, E279K, and V299L. The following are sensitive to dasatinib: M351T, G250E, F359V, M244V, Y253H, H396R, E355G, E459K, F486S, L248V, D276G, E279K, Y253F, F359C, and F359I. The following mutations are resistant to dasatinib: V299L, T315A, and F317I/L. The following are resistant to nilotinib: Y253F/H, E255K/V, and F359C/V (Hochhaus, La Rosee et al. 2011). All three these inhibitors inhibit the catalytic activity of BCR-ABL by binding to the ATP-binding pocket of the ABL kinase domain.

3.2. Activating mutations at *BRAF*

One of the discoveries of mutations affecting cancer prognosis is *BRAF* mutations. *BRAF* has been discovered to be the most commonly mutated oncogene in melanoma (50–60%) (Davies, Bignell et al. 2002), papillary thyroid carcinoma (36–53%) (Yeang , McCormick et al. 2008), colon carcinoma (57%), serous ovarian carcinoma (~30%) (Yeang , McCormick et al. 2008), and hairy cell leukemia (100%) (Tiacci, Trifonov et al. 2011). To date, >60 distinct mutations in the *BRAF* gene have been identified (Table 1) (Garnett and Marais 2004; *Catalog of Somatic Mutations in Cancer*: www.sanger.ac.uk/genetics/CGP/cosmic/). The most prevalent mutation is a missense mutation in *BRAF,* which results in a substitution of glutamic acid to valine at codon 600 ($BRAF^{V600E}$) and occurs in 90% of all *BRAF* mutations (Garnett and Marais 2004). *BRAF* encodes BRAF, a member of the RAF family of cytoplasmic serine/threonine protein kinases. BRAF phosphorylates MEK protein and activates ERK signaling, downstream of RAS, which regulates multiple key cellular processes that are required for cell proliferation, differentiation, apoptosis, and survival. The *RAF* family (*A-RAF, B-RAF, C-RAF*) members are components of a signal transduction pathway downstream of the membrane-bound small G-protein RAS, which is activated by growth factors, hormones, and cytokines (Robinson and Cobb 1997).

MEK inhibitors suppress ERK signaling in all normal and tumor cells. In contrast, the RAF inhibitor vemurafenib inhibits the ERK pathway and cell proliferation only in tumor cells with mutant *BRAF*. Targeted therapy and selective inhibitors for certain altered genes are crucial to enable targeting of tumor cells but not normal cells.

Mutated *BRAF* activates and deregulates the kinase activity of BRAF. The recently developed BRAF inhibitor vemurafenib (PLX4032) inhibits RAF activation selectively only in cells carrying the *BRAF* V600E mutation. Clinically, vemurafenib has an 80% response rate in metastatic melanoma patients harboring the *BRAF* V600E mutation, but 18% of patients treated with vemurafenib develop at least one squamous-cell carcinoma of the skin or keratoacanthoma as an adverse event (Chapman, Hauschild et al. 2010). The remaining 20% of patients who harbor the *BRAF* V600E mutation, and also patients who do not harbor the *BRAF* V600E mutation, are resistant to vemurafenib. Other mechanisms that cause vemurafenib resistance are mutations in *NRAS* and *c-KIT* alterations. *c-KIT* alterations (mutations and/or amplifications) are found more frequently (28-39%) in melanomas from acral, mucosal, and chronically sun-damaged sites (Curtin, Busam et al. 2006), whereas uveal melanomas uniquely harbor activating mutations in the a-subunit of a G proteins of the Gq family, GNAQ and GNA11 (Van Raamsdonk, Bezrookove et al. 2009; Van Raamsdonk, Griewank et al. 2010). *NRAS* mutations are observed in 15–30% of cutaneous melanomas and are mutually exclusive of *BRAF* mutations; the most common change occurs at G12 or Q61 (Brose, Volpe et al. 2002). Currently, no selective inhibitor for those mutations exists. In contrast, *BRAF* mutations are also found in colon cancer (8%) (Hutchins, Southward et al. 2011), papillary thyroid cancer (44%) and anaplastic thyroid cancer (24%) (Xing, Westra et al. 2005), but limited study has reported to date. However, vemurafenib has limited therapeutic effects in *BRAF* (V600E) mutant colon cancers because inhibition of *BRAF* (V600E) causes a rapid feedback activation of EGFR, which induces continued proliferation in *BRAF* (V600E) inhibited cells. Therefore, blocking the *EGFR* by gefitinib, erlotinib or cetuximab has strong synergistic with inhibition of *BRAF* (V600E) by vemurafenib in colon tumor cell *in vivo* and *in vitro* (Prahallad, Sun et al. 2012). The question remains to answer whether the same BRAF selective inhibitor can be effective in other tumor types due to lack of evidence.

3.3. Activating mutations at *PIK3CA*

Shortly after *BRAF* mutations were found and selective inhibitors of the mutant *BRAF* were developed, activating point mutations were found in *PIK3CA* (Samuels, Wang et al. 2004) in a variety of cancers, including breast (20–30%) (Bachman, Argani et al. 2004; Campbell, Russell et al. 2004), colorectal (Parsons, Wang et al. 2005), endometrial (Samuels and Ericson

2006), ovarian, and hepatocellular cancers and medulloblastoma (Broderick, Di et al. 2004), among others (Kang, Bader et al. 2005; Lee, Soung et al. 2005). *PIK3CA* encodes the p110α catalytic subunit of phosphatidylinositol 3-kinase (PI3K), a lipid kinase that drives AKT signaling to govern cell growth and survival. PI3Ks are heterodimers, composed of catalytic (p110α; PI3Kα) and regulatory (p85) subunits. Catalytic units include the ABD, RBD, C2, helical, and kinase domains, whereas the regulatory unit comprises the SH3, GAP, nSH2, iSH2, and cSH2 domains. Mutations mostly cluster between the kinase domain and other domains within the catalytic subunit (Huang, Mandelker et al. 2007). The family of receptor tyrosine kinase, together with the MAP kinase and PI3K cascades, forms part of the obsolete growth factor signaling pathway governing tumor cell growth and survival (Samuels, Diaz et al. 2005). Due to complexity and diverse activation of PI3K signaling, such as activating mutations or amplification of *PIK3CA,* or upstream of RTK, loss of *PTEN* or activating mutations of *RAS* in human cancers (Courtney, Corcoran et al. 2010), developing the effective therapeutic agents against PIK3CA might be more challenging (Zhao and Vogt 2008). Hereby, either single agents or combination with other therapeutic agents against to PIK3CA are under development (Courtney, Corcoran et al. 2010).

3.4. Activating mutations at *EGFR*

This finding was followed by the identification of activating point mutations and small insertions/deletions in *EGFR,* an oncogene encoding a receptor tyrosine kinase, which is present more frequently in East Asian individuals with non–small-cell lung cancer (NSCLC) (25%) than in Caucasian people (10–15%) and occurs most frequently in lung adenocarcinomas (Lynch, Bell et al. 2004; Paez, Janne et al. 2004; Pao, Miller et al. 2004). Activating mutations were initially identified in 3 kinase domain exons (18, 19, and 21), encoding G719S and G719C in exon 18 and L861Q in exon 21; the most common mutations are small in-frame deletions in exon 19 and the leucine-to-arginine substitution mutation L858R. L858R mutation causes constitutive activation of the tyrosine kinase of EGFR. Oncogenic mutation of *EGFR* activates downstream signaling pathways of EGFR, which are implicated in tumor cell growth, proliferation, and survival. This discovery led to the development of the selective EGFR TKIs erlotinib and gefitinib. Inhibition of EGFR by EGFR inhibitors blocks the activity of tyrosine kinase, and hence the activation of the downstream cellular pathways. Individuals with lung adenocarcinoma harboring the G719S and L858R mutations are sensitive to gefitinib or erlotinib. Although patients harboring these mutations have a high response rate to the EGFR inhibitors gefitinib and erlotinib, the duration of the response is not long, and patients relapse after about a year of treatment (Pao and Chmielecki 2010).

One of the mechanisms by which resistance to erlotinib or gefitinib develops in 50% of relapsed patients is acquisition of a resistant mutation in exon 20 (T790M) in *EGFR* (Kobayashi, Boggon et al. 2005; Pao, Miller et al. 2005) or activating mutation in *KRAS* (Pao, Wang et al. 2005). A second mutation in *EGFR* (T790M) is also found rarely in the germline to be associated with an inherited susceptibility to lung cancer (Bell, Gore et al. 2005; Vikis, Sato et al. 2007). This mutation has been shown to decrease the affinity of EGFR to gefitinib in the L858R mutant by increasing the affinity of EGFR to ATP (Yun, Mengwasser et al. 2008). This resistant mutant led to the development of promising new agents as second-generation EGFR inhibitors (Li, Shimamura et al. 2007; Li, Ambrogio et al. 2008; Zhou, Ercan et al. 2009). Another mechanism by which resistance to erlotinib or gefitinib develops is amplification (20%) or mutation (Y1230H) in *MET*, an oncogene encoding receptor tyrosine kinase (Bean, Brennan et al. 2007; Engelman, Zejnullahu et al. 2007). Overexpression of HGF, a specific ligand of MET, is another mechanism by which resistance to EGFR inhibitors develops (Yano, Wang et al. 2008).

Gefitinib and erlotinib are first-generation, reversible EGFR inhibitors. Currently being developed are second-generation irreversible EGFR inhibitors, which inhibit EGFR kinase activity even when the T790M mutation is present. Neratinib (HKI-272) (Li, Shimamura et al. 2007; Wong, Fracasso et al. 2009; Sequist, Besse et al. 2010) and afatinib (BIBW 2992) (Eskens, Mom et al. 2008; Li, Ambrogio et al. 2008; Yap, Vidal et al. 2010) are dual inhibitors against EGFR and HER2, and PF-00299804 is a multi-inhibitor against EGFR, ERBB2, and ERBB4 (Engelman, Zejnullahu et al. 2007). For *MET* gene amplification, the MET inhibitor PHA-665752 has been developed (Engelman, Zejnullahu et al. 2007). Recently, new EGFR inhibitors (WZ4002, WZ3146, and WZ8040) have been reported that suppress the growth of *EGFR* T790M-containing cell lines by inhibiting phosphorylation (Zhou, Ercan et al. 2009). Erlotinib has a statistically significantly higher response rate than chemotherapy (83% vs 36%) (Friedrich 2011). In fact, some activating mutations, like those of *KRAS*, may not be drug targets but may rather govern the resistance to selective inhibitors of EGFR (Allegra, Jessup et al. 2009). Activating mutations of *EGFR* are also present in glioma, breast, endometrial and colorectal carcinomas. *KRAS* mutations at G12 and G13 are associated with resistance to erlotinib or gefitinib in *EGFR* mutated lung adenocarcinoma parients (Pao, Wang et al. 2005) and metastatic colorectal carcinoma (Allegra, Jessup et al. 2009).

Shortly after the discovery of *EGFR* mutations, somatic activating mutations of *ERBB2* were found in 2–4% of patients with lung adenocarcinoma. *ERBB2* is a receptor tyrosine kinase, one of the members of ERBB family, and the only one that does bind to any known ligand but activates downstream signaling pathways by homo- or hetero-dimerization with other ERBB family members. Small in-frame insertion mutations span exon 20 of the kinase domain of *ERBB2*, and these are analogous to the mutations in the paralogous exon 20 in the *EGFR* gene that confer resistance to erlotinib or gefitinib. ERBB2 is a receptor tyrosine kinase that heterodimerizes or homodimerizes with EGFR and other members of the ERBB family, ERBB3 and ERBB4, to activate downstream signaling pathways (Hynes and Lane, 2005)..

3.5. Activating mutations at *JAK2*

The discovery of the somatic gain-of-function mutation (V617F) in Janus kinase 2 (*JAK2*) in >90% of individuals with polycythemia vera, 50% of individuals with primary myelofibrosis, and 60% of those with essential thrombocytopenia (Levine, Wadleigh et al. 2005), all of which are Philadelphia chromosome -negative myeloproliferative neoplasms, generated interest in developing JAK2 inhibitors. The JAK kinases (JAK1, JAK2, JAK3, and JAK4) were first identified in 1989 (Wilks 1989). Structurally, all members of the JAK family contain seven distinct domains: JAK homology (JH) domains 1 to 7 (JH1–7). The tyrosine kinase domain (JH1) is located at C-terminus of the protein and is responsible for the kinase activity. The pseudokinase domain (JH2) has no kinase activity, but deletion of the JH2 domain leads to increased kinase activity. JH3 and JH4 are similar to the SH2 domain, and their roles are still unclear (Wilks, Harpur et al. 1991; Lindauer, Loerting et al. 2001; Giordanetto and Kroemer 2002; Saharinen and Silvennoinen 2002). JH5, JH6, and JH7 are located at the amino-terminus of the protein and play a role in binding the JAK molecule to the cytokine receptor and in maintaining receptor expression at the cell surface (Huang, Constantinescu et al. 2001). JAK2 is a nonreceptor tyrosine kinase that mediates signals between cytokine receptors and downstream targets.

An activating mutation of *JAK2*, a valine-to-phenylalanine substitution at position 617 (V617F) (Scott, Tong et al. 2007), leads to constitutive activation of STAT5. The JAK inhibitors INCB01824, TG101348, and lestaurtinib (CEP701), which inhibit JAK1 and JAK2, results in a marked reduction (>50%) in massive splenomegaly (Verstovsek, Kantarjian et al. 2010).

3.6. Activating mutations at *c-KIT*

Other kinase activating mutations have been found in the oncogene c-*KIT* in gastrointestinal stromal tumors (GIST), acral or mucosal melanoma, endometrial carcinoma, germ cell tumors, myeloproliferative diseases, and leukemias, which is the mutations cause constitutive activation of *c-KIT* (Malaise, Steinbach et al. 2009). c-KIT is a transmembrane cytokine receptor tyrosine kinase that is expressed on the surface of hematopoietic stem cells. Most GIST patients who harbor *c-KIT* mutations have a response to imatinib mesilate (80%). This raises the question of whether imatinib or nilotinib (TKIs) may elicit clinical responses in *KIT*-mutant melanoma or endometrial carcinoma or in other cancers that harbor *KIT* mutations. Acquired resistance to imatinib commonly occurs via secondary gene mutations in the *c-KIT* kinase domain in GIST. For example, the V560G mutation in *KIT* is sensitive to imatinib, although the D816V mutation is resistant to imatinib (Mahadevan, Cooke et al. 2007).

3.7. Mutations at *IDH1 and IDH2*

IDH1 encodes a nicotinamide adenine dinucleotide phosphate (NADP)+-dependent enzyme that converts isocitrate to 2-ketoglutarate in the cytoplasm. Somatic mutations were found to be present in *IDH1* and *IDH2* in 88% of individuals with secondary glioblastomas, 68% of those with grade II glioma (lower grade diffuse astrocytomas), 78% of those with grade III anaplastic astrocytomas, and 69% of those with grade III anaplastic oligodendrogliomas (Dang, Jin et al. 2010; Dang, White et al. 2010) as well as 31% of patients with myeloproliferative neoplasm (Green and Beer 2010) and 10% of those with acute myeloid leukemia (AML) (Dang, Jin et al. 2010; Yen, Bittinger et al. 2010). Mutations in *IDH* were first reported to be activating mutations, but subsequent studies of mutations at arginine R132 (in *IDH1*) and at R140 or R172 (in *IDH2*) in the enzyme showed a gain of new function and the ability to convert alpha-ketoglutarate to 2-hydroxyglutarate (Dang, White et al. 2009). Mutations that have been reported in *IDH1* and *IDH2* are summarized in Table 1. Mutations in these metabolic enzymes uncover novel avenues for the development of anticancer therapeutics, but specific inhibitors are needed for the mutated forms R132, R140, or R172. It is not clear what the role of this mutation is in cancer and whether it is crucial for tumorigenesis, although the 2-hydroxyglutarate metabolite is a biomarker that can be measured in whole blood and used to select targeted therapy (Yen, Bittinger et al. 2010).

3.8. Fusion genes

Another recent breakthrough was the discovery of translocations or other chromosomal rearrangements between ETS transcription factors (*ERG*, *ETV1*, and *ETV4*) in >40% of prostate cancers (Tomlins, Rhodes et al. 2005; Tomlins, Laxman et al. 2007; Berger, Lawrence et al. 2011) and the fusion of anaplastic lymphoma kinase (*ALK*) with other genes in NSCLC (Soda, Choi et al. 2007; Choi, Soda et al. 2010). Echinoderm microtubule-associated protein-like 4 (*EML4*) is fused to *ALK*, which leads to a fusion-type tyrosine kinase between the N-terminus of *EML4* and the C-terminus of the *ALK* that is a chimeric oncoprotein and is found in 3–5% of NSCLC tumors (Soda, Choi et al. 2007; Choi, Soda et al. 2010). The inversion on chromosome 2p [inv(2)(p21p23)] leads to formation of the *ELK4-ALK* fusion oncogene. The chromosomal inversion occurs in different locations, and multiple *EML4-ALK* variants have been reported; all involve the intracellular tyrosine kinase domain of *ALK* (exon 20) but different truncation of *EML4* (exon 2, 6, 13, 14, 15, 17, 18, or 20), TFG, and *KIF5B*; the most common inversion is in exon 13 of *EML4* (Hernandez, Pinyol et al. 1999; Choi, Takeuchi et al. 2008; Takeuchi, Choi et al. 2009). The amino-terminal coiled-coil domain within EML4 is necessary and sufficient for the transforming activity of *EML4-ALK* (Soda, Choi et al. 2007). This fusion tyrosine kinase may activate downstream signaling pathways of ALK, such as RAS/RAF. This recent discovery of the genetic rearrangement between ALK and the aforementioned genes has led to the development of another targeted agent, crizotinib (PF-02341066), for the treatment of NSCLC. Crizotinib, a TKI that was initially designed as an inhibitor of MET, is currently used to inhibit both tyrosine kinases, MET and ALK in NSCLC. *ALK* rearrangement has been found mostly in younger and more likely to be never or light smoker lung adenocarcinomas and is more frequent in the Asian population than in the American or European population (Sasaki, Rodig et al. 2010). Patients who developed resistance to BRAF inhibitors were found to be harboring the C1156Y (46.6%) and L1196M (15.1%) mutations in the *ALK* gene (Choi, Soda et al. 2010) and also the F1174L mutation (Sasaki, Okuda et al. 2010).

3.9. Activating mutations at *FLT3*

FLT3 encodes a receptor tyrosine kinase that is involved in stem cell development and differentiation, stem and/or progenitor cell survival, and the development of B-progenitor cells, dendritic cells, and natural killer cells in the bone marrow (Small, Levenstein et al. 1994). Two common mutations have been found in AML: internal tandem duplication (ITD) in-frame mutations of 3–400 base pairs in the juxtamembrane region, and point mutations in the tyrosine kinase domain (TKD) D835 (7%). Mutations in the ITD and TKD lead to constitutive activation of tyrosine kinase (Abu-Duhier, Goodeve et al. 2001), and this finding led to the design of the first-generation FLT3 inhibitors lestaurtinib (CEP701) (Smith, Levis et al. 2004), midostaurin (PKC412A) (Stone, DeAngelo et al. 2005), sunitinib

(SU11248)(O'Farrell, Foran et al. 2003), sorafenib (BAY43-9006), and tandutinib (MLN518), followed by the second-generation FLT3 inhibitors KW2449 (Pratz, Cortes et al. 2009) and AC220 (Zarrinkar, Gunawardane et al. 2009).

4. Future directions

Drugs targeting some of these mutations are now either undergoing clinical testing or have protocols in the approval process. The discovery of base mutations through systematic DNA sequencing has provided decisive genetic evidence that these same pathways play crucial roles in tumorigenesis and maintenance and has also opened up new avenues for the deployment of targeted therapeutics. We are just starting to understand the genetic mechanisms that lead to the development of cancer and play a role in treatment. Hence, we are still at the beginning of the road map to targeted therapy. We still need to discover all activating mutations or other chromosomal rearrangements, inactivating mutations, and epigenetic alterations in the genome that drive cells to tumorigenesis for each type and subtype of cancer, and we need to identify resistant and sensitive mutations to find the correct targets for the development of new selective therapeutic agents, and use combination of selective therapeutic agents.

Author details

Musaffe Tuna* and Christopher I. Amos
Department of Genetics,
The University of Texas MD Anderson Cancer Center, Houston, Texas, USA

5. References

Abu-Duhier, F. M., A. C. Goodeve, et al. (2001). Genomic structure of human FLT3: implications for mutational analysis. *Br J Haematol* 113(4): 1076-7.

Alitalo, K., M. Schwab, et al. (1983). Homogeneously staining chromosomal regions contain amplified copies of an abundantly expressed cellular oncogene (c-myc) in malignant neuroendocrine cells from a human colon carcinoma. *Proc Natl Acad Sci U S A* 80(6): 1707-11.

Allegra, C. J., J. M. Jessup, et al. (2009). American Society of Clinical Oncology provisional clinical opinion: testing for KRAS gene mutations in patients with metastatic colorectal carcinoma to predict response to anti-epidermal growth factor receptor monoclonal antibody therapy. *J Clin Oncol* 27(12): 2091-6.

Bachman, K. E., P. Argani, et al. (2004). The PIK3CA gene is mutated with high frequency in human breast cancers. *Cancer Biol Ther* 3(8): 772-5.

Balss, J., J. Meyer, et al. (2008). Analysis of the IDH1 codon 132 mutation in brain tumors. *Acta Neuropathol* 116(6): 597-602.

* Corresponding Author

Baselga, J., D. Tripathy, et al. (1999). Phase II study of weekly intravenous trastuzumab (Herceptin) in patients with HER2/neu-overexpressing metastatic breast cancer. *Semin Oncol* 26(4 Suppl 12): 78-83.

Bean, J., C. Brennan, et al. (2007). MET amplification occurs with or without T790M mutations in EGFR mutant lung tumors with acquired resistance to gefitinib or erlotinib. *Proc Natl Acad Sci U S A* 104(52): 20932-7.

Bell, D. W., I. Gore, et al. (2005). Inherited susceptibility to lung cancer may be associated with the T790M drug resistance mutation in EGFR. *Nat Genet* 37(12): 1315-6.

Berger, M. F., M. S. Lawrence, et al. (2011). The genomic complexity of primary human prostate cancer. *Nature* 470(7333): 214-20.

Bleeker, F. E., S. Lamba, et al. (2009). IDH1 mutations at residue p.R132 (IDH1(R132)) occur frequently in high-grade gliomas but not in other solid tumors. *Hum Mutat* 30(1): 7-11.

Bos, J. L., D. Toksoz, et al. (1985). Amino-acid substitutions at codon 13 of the N-ras oncogene in human acute myeloid leukaemia. *Nature* 315(6022): 726-30.

Branford, S. (2007). Chronic myeloid leukemia: molecular monitoring in clinical practice. *Hematology Am Soc Hematol Educ Program*: 376-83.

Broderick, D. K., C. Di, et al. (2004). Mutations of PIK3CA in anaplastic oligodendrogliomas, high-grade astrocytomas, and medulloblastomas. *Cancer Res* 64(15): 5048-50.

Brose, M. S., P. Volpe, et al. (2002). BRAF and RAS mutations in human lung cancer and melanoma. *Cancer Res* 62(23): 6997-7000.

Burgess, M. R., B. J. Skaggs, et al. (2005). Comparative analysis of two clinically active BCR-ABL kinase inhibitors reveals the role of conformation-specific binding in resistance. *Proc Natl Acad Sci U S A* 102(9): 3395-400.

Campbell, I. G., S. E. Russell, et al. (2004). Mutation of the PIK3CA gene in ovarian and breast cancer. *Cancer Res* 64(21): 7678-81.

Capon, D. J., P. H. Seeburg, et al. (1983). Activation of Ki-ras2 gene in human colon and lung carcinomas by two different point mutations. *Nature* 304(5926): 507-13.

Castaigne, S., C. Chomienne, et al. (1990). All-trans retinoic acid as a differentiation therapy for acute promyelocytic leukemia. I. Clinical results. *Blood* 76(9): 1704-9.

Chapman, M. A., M. S. Lawrence, et al. (2011). Initial genome sequencing and analysis of multiple myeloma. *Nature* 471(7339): 467-72.

Chapman, P. B., A. Hauschild, et al. (2010). Improved survival with vemurafenib in melanoma with BRAF V600E mutation. *N Engl J Med* 364(26): 2507-16.

Choi, Y. L., M. Soda, et al. (2010). EML4-ALK mutations in lung cancer that confer resistance to ALK inhibitors. *N Engl J Med* 363(18): 1734-9.

Choi, Y. L., K. Takeuchi, et al. (2008). Identification of novel isoforms of the EML4-ALK transforming gene in non-small cell lung cancer. *Cancer Res* 68(13): 4971-6.

Collins, S. and M. Groudine (1982). Amplification of endogenous myc-related DNA sequences in a human myeloid leukaemia cell line. *Nature* 298(5875): 679-81.

Courtney, K. D., R. B. Corcoran, et al. (2010). The PI3K pathway as drug target in human cancer. *J Clin Oncol* 28(6): 1075-83.

Curtin, J. A., K. Busam, et al. (2006). Somatic activation of KIT in distinct subtypes of melanoma. *J Clin Oncol* 24(26): 4340-6.

Dang, L., S. Jin, et al. (2010). IDH mutations in glioma and acute myeloid leukemia. *Trends Mol Med* 16(9): 387-97.

Dang, L., D. W. White, et al. (2009). Cancer-associated IDH1 mutations produce 2-hydroxyglutarate. *Nature* 465(7300): 966.

Davies, H., G. R. Bignell, et al. (2002). Mutations of the BRAF gene in human cancer. *Nature* 417(6892): 949-54.

de Muga, S., S. Hernandez, et al. (2010). Molecular alterations of EGFR and PTEN in prostate cancer: association with high-grade and advanced-stage carcinomas. *Mod Pathol* 23(5): 703-12.

Engelman, J. A., K. Zejnullahu, et al. (2007). PF00299804, an irreversible pan-ERBB inhibitor, is effective in lung cancer models with EGFR and ERBB2 mutations that are resistant to gefitinib. Cancer Res 67(24): 11924-32.

Engelman, J. A., K. Zejnullahu, et al. (2007). MET amplification leads to gefitinib resistance in lung cancer by activating ERBB3 signaling. *Science* 316(5827): 1039-43.

Eskens, F. A., C. H. Mom, et al. (2008). A phase I dose escalation study of BIBW 2992, an irreversible dual inhibitor of epidermal growth factor receptor 1 (EGFR) and 2 (HER2) tyrosine kinase in a 2-week on, 2-week off schedule in patients with advanced solid tumours. *Br J Cancer* 98(1): 80-5.

Esteller, M. (2007). Cancer epigenomics: DNA methylomes and histone-modification maps. *Nat Rev Genet* 8(4): 286-98.

Fernandes, M. S., M. M. Reddy, et al. (2009). BCR-ABL promotes the frequency of mutagenic single-strand annealing DNA repair. *Blood* 114(9): 1813-9.

Friedrich, M. J. (2011). NSCLC drug targets acquire new visibility. *J Natl Cancer Inst* 103(5): 366-7.

Garnett, M. J. and R. Marais (2004). Guilty as charged: B-RAF is a human oncogene. *Cancer Cell* 6(4): 313-9.

Giordanetto, F. and R. T. Kroemer (2002). Prediction of the structure of human Janus kinase 2 (JAK2) comprising JAK homology domains 1 through 7. *Protein Eng* 15(9): 727-37.

Goldman, J. M. and J. V. Melo (2008). BCR-ABL in chronic myelogenous leukemia--how does it work? *Acta Haematol* 119(4): 212-7.

Gravendeel, L. A., N. K. Kloosterhof, et al. (2010). Segregation of non-p.R132H mutations in IDH1 in distinct molecular subtypes of glioma. *Hum Mutat* 31(3): E1186-99.

Green, A. and P. Beer (2010). Somatic mutations of IDH1 and IDH2 in the leukemic transformation of myeloproliferative neoplasms. *N Engl J Med* 362(4): 369-70.

Hanahan, D. and R. A. Weinberg (2011). Hallmarks of cancer: the next generation. *Cell* 144(5): 646-74.

Hayes, M. P., W. Douglas, et al. (2009). Molecular alterations of EGFR and PIK3CA in uterine serous carcinoma. *Gynecol Oncol* 113(3): 370-3.

Hernandez, L., M. Pinyol, et al. (1999). TRK-fused gene (TFG) is a new partner of ALK in anaplastic large cell lymphoma producing two structurally different TFG-ALK translocations. *Blood* 94(9): 3265-8.

Hochhaus, A., P. La Rosee, et al. (2011). Impact of BCR-ABL mutations on patients with chronic myeloid leukemia. *Cell Cycle* 10(2): 250-60.

Huang, C. H., D. Mandelker, et al. (2007). The structure of a human p110alpha/p85alpha complex elucidates the effects of oncogenic PI3Kalpha mutations. *Science* 318(5857): 1744-8.

Huang, L. J., S. N. Constantinescu, et al. (2001). The N-terminal domain of Janus kinase 2 is required for Golgi processing and cell surface expression of erythropoietin receptor. *Mol Cell* 8(6): 1327-38.

Huang, M. E., Y. C. Ye, et al. (1988). Use of all-trans retinoic acid in the treatment of acute promyelocytic leukemia. *Blood* 72(2): 567-72.

Hutchins, G., K. Southward, et al. (2011). Value of mismatch repair, KRAS, and BRAF mutations in predicting recurrence and benefits from chemotherapy in colorectal cancer. *J Clin Oncol* 29(10): 1261-70.

Hynes, N. E., H. A. Lane (2005). ERBB receptors and cancer: The complexity of targeted inhibitors. *Nat Rev Cancer* 341: 5(5):341-54.

Kang, S., A. G. Bader, et al. (2005). Phosphatidylinositol 3-kinase mutations identified in human cancer are oncogenic. *Proc Natl Acad Sci U S A* 102(3): 802-7.

Kobayashi, S., T. J. Boggon, et al. (2005). EGFR mutation and resistance of non-small-cell lung cancer to gefitinib. *N Engl J Med* 352(8): 786-92.

Konopka, B., A. Janiec-Jankowska, et al. (2011). PIK3CA mutations and amplification in endometrioid endometrial carcinomas: relation to other genetic defects and clinicopathologic status of the tumors. *Hum Pathol* 42(11): 1710-9.

Koptyra, M., R. Falinski, et al. (2006). BCR/ABL kinase induces self-mutagenesis via reactive oxygen species to encode imatinib resistance. *Blood* 108(1): 319-27.

Lee, J. C., I. Vivanco, et al. (2006). Epidermal growth factor receptor activation in glioblastoma through novel missense mutations in the extracellular domain. *PLoS Med* 3(12): e485.

Lee, J. W., Y. H. Soung, et al. (2005). PIK3CA gene is frequently mutated in breast carcinomas and hepatocellular carcinomas. *Oncogene* 24(8): 1477-80.

Levine, R. L., M. Wadleigh, et al. (2005). Activating mutation in the tyrosine kinase JAK2 in polycythemia vera, essential thrombocythemia, and myeloid metaplasia with myelofibrosis. *Cancer Cell* 7(4): 387-97.

Li, D., L. Ambrogio, et al. (2008). BIBW2992, an irreversible EGFR/HER2 inhibitor highly effective in preclinical lung cancer models. *Oncogene* 27(34): 4702-11.

Li, D., T. Shimamura, et al. (2007). Bronchial and peripheral murine lung carcinomas induced by T790M-L858R mutant EGFR respond to HKI-272 and rapamycin combination therapy. *Cancer Cell* 12(1): 81-93.

Lindauer, K., T. Loerting, et al. (2001). Prediction of the structure of human Janus kinase 2 (JAK2) comprising the two carboxy-terminal domains reveals a mechanism for autoregulation. *Protein Eng* 14(1): 27-37.

Loeffler-Ragg, J., M. Witsch-Baumgartner, et al. (2006). Low incidence of mutations in EGFR kinase domain in Caucasian patients with head and neck squamous cell carcinoma. *Eur J Cancer* 42(1): 109-11.

Lugo, T. G., A. M. Pendergast, et al. (1990). Tyrosine kinase activity and transformation potency of bcr-abl oncogene products. *Science* 247(4946): 1079-82.

Lynch, T. J., D. W. Bell, et al. (2004). Activating mutations in the epidermal growth factor receptor underlying responsiveness of non-small-cell lung cancer to gefitinib. *N Engl J Med* 350(21): 2129-39.

MacConaill, L. E., C. D. Campbell, et al. (2009). Profiling critical cancer gene mutations in clinical tumor samples. *PLoS One* 4(11): e7887.

Mahadevan, D., L. Cooke, et al. (2007). A novel tyrosine kinase switch is a mechanism of imatinib resistance in gastrointestinal stromal tumors. *Oncogene* 26(27): 3909-19.

Malaise, M., D. Steinbach, et al. (2009). Clinical implications of c-Kit mutations in acute myelogenous leukemia. *Curr Hematol Malig Rep* 4(2): 77-82.

Mauro, M. J., M. O'Dwyer, et al. (2002). STI571: a paradigm of new agents for cancer therapeutics. *J Clin Oncol* 20(1): 325-34.

Metzger, B., L. Chambeau, et al. (2011). The human epidermal growth factor receptor (EGFR) gene in European patients with advanced colorectal cancer harbors infrequent mutations in its tyrosine kinase domain. *BMC Med Genet* 12: 144.

Montagut, C., A. Dalmases, et al. (2012). Identification of a mutation in the extracellular domain of the Epidermal Growth Factor Receptor conferring cetuximab resistance in colorectal cancer. *Nat Med* 18(2): 221-3.

Muller, M. C., J. E. Cortes, et al. (2009). Dasatinib treatment of chronic-phase chronic myeloid leukemia: analysis of responses according to preexisting BCR-ABL mutations. *Blood* 114(24): 4944-53.

Murugan, A. K., J. Dong, et al. (2011). Uncommon GNAQ, MMP8, AKT3, EGFR, and PIK3R1 mutations in thyroid cancers. *Endocr Pathol* 22(2): 97-102.

O'Farrell, A. M., J. M. Foran, et al. (2003). An innovative phase I clinical study demonstrates inhibition of FLT3 phosphorylation by SU11248 in acute myeloid leukemia patients. *Clin Cancer Res* 9(15): 5465-76.

O'Hare, T., D. K. Walters, et al. (2005). In vitro activity of Bcr-Abl inhibitors AMN107 and BMS-354825 against clinically relevant imatinib-resistant Abl kinase domain mutants. *Cancer Res* 65(11): 4500-5.

Paez, J. G., P. A. Janne, et al. (2004). EGFR mutations in lung cancer: correlation with clinical response to gefitinib therapy. *Science* 304(5676): 1497-500.

Pao, W. and J. Chmielecki (2010). Rational, biologically based treatment of EGFR-mutant non-small-cell lung cancer. *Nat Rev Cancer* 10(11): 760-74.

Pao, W., V. Miller, et al. (2004). EGF receptor gene mutations are common in lung cancers from "never smokers" and are associated with sensitivity of tumors to gefitinib and erlotinib. *Proc Natl Acad Sci U S A* 101(36): 13306-11.

Pao, W., V. A. Miller, et al. (2005). Acquired resistance of lung adenocarcinomas to gefitinib or erlotinib is associated with a second mutation in the EGFR kinase domain. *PLoS Med* 2(3): e73.

Pao, W., T. Y. Wang, et al. (2005). KRAS mutations and primary resistance of lung adenocarcinomas to gefitinib or erlotinib. *PLoS Med* 2(1): e17.

Parsons, D. W., T. L. Wang, et al. (2005). Colorectal cancer: mutations in a signalling pathway. *Nature* 436(7052): 792.

Passamonti, F., C. Elena, et al. (2011). Molecular and clinical features of the myeloproliferative neoplasm associated with JAK2 exon 12 mutations. *Blood* 117(10): 2813-6.

Peraldo-Neia, C., G. Migliardi, et al. (2011). Epidermal Growth Factor Receptor (EGFR) mutation analysis, gene expression profiling and EGFR protein expression in primary prostate cancer. *BMC Cancer* 11: 31.

Prahallad, A., C. Sun, et al. (2012). Unresponsiveness of colon cancer to BRAF(V600E) inhibition through feedback activation of EGFR. *Nature* 483(7387): 100-3.

Pratz, K. W., J. Cortes, et al. (2009). A pharmacodynamic study of the FLT3 inhibitor KW-2449 yields insight into the basis for clinical response. *Blood* 113(17): 3938-46.

Reddy, E. P., R. K. Reynolds, et al. (1982). A point mutation is responsible for the acquisition of transforming properties by the T24 human bladder carcinoma oncogene. *Nature* 300(5888): 149-52.

Reitman, Z. J. and H. Yan (2010). Isocitrate dehydrogenase 1 and 2 mutations in cancer: alterations at a crossroads of cellular metabolism. *J Natl Cancer Inst* 102(13): 932-41.

Robinson, M. J. and M. H. Cobb (1997). Mitogen-activated protein kinase pathways. *Curr Opin Cell Biol* 9(2): 180-6.

Saharinen, P. and O. Silvennoinen (2002). The pseudokinase domain is required for suppression of basal activity of Jak2 and Jak3 tyrosine kinases and for cytokine-inducible activation of signal transduction. *J Biol Chem* 277(49): 47954-63.

Samuels, Y., L. A. Diaz, Jr., et al. (2005). Mutant PIK3CA promotes cell growth and invasion of human cancer cells. *Cancer Cell* 7(6): 561-73.

Samuels, Y. and K. Ericson (2006). Oncogenic PI3K and its role in cancer. *Curr Opin Oncol* 18(1): 77-82.

Samuels, Y., Z. Wang, et al. (2004). High frequency of mutations of the PIK3CA gene in human cancers. *Science* 304(5670): 554.

Sasaki, T., K. Okuda, et al. (2010). The neuroblastoma-associated F1174L ALK mutation causes resistance to an ALK kinase inhibitor in ALK-translocated cancers. *Cancer Res* 70(24): 10038-43.

Sasaki, T., S. J. Rodig, et al., (2010). The biology and treatment of EML4-ALK non-small cell lung cancer. *Eur J Cancer* 46(10): 1773-1780.

Scott, L. M., W. Tong, et al. (2007). JAK2 exon 12 mutations in polycythemia vera and idiopathic erythrocytosis. *N Engl J Med* 356(5): 459-68.

Sequist, L. V., B. Besse, et al. (2010). Neratinib, an irreversible pan-ErbB receptor tyrosine kinase inhibitor: results of a phase II trial in patients with advanced non-small-cell lung cancer. *J Clin Oncol* 28(18): 3076-83.

Shimizu, K., D. Birnbaum, et al. (1983). Structure of the Ki-ras gene of the human lung carcinoma cell line Calu-1. *Nature* 304(5926): 497-500.

Slamon, D. J., B. Leyland-Jones, et al. (2001). Use of chemotherapy plus a monoclonal antibody against HER2 for metastatic breast cancer that overexpresses HER2. *N Engl J Med* 344(11): 783-92.

Small, D., M. Levenstein, et al. (1994). STK-1, the human homolog of Flk-2/Flt-3, is selectively expressed in CD34+ human bone marrow cells and is involved in the proliferation of early progenitor/stem cells. *Proc Natl Acad Sci U S A* 91(2): 459-63.

Smith, B. D., M. Levis, et al. (2004). Single-agent CEP-701, a novel FLT3 inhibitor, shows biologic and clinical activity in patients with relapsed or refractory acute myeloid leukemia. *Blood* 103(10): 3669-76.

Soda, M., Y. L. Choi, et al. (2007). Identification of the transforming EML4-ALK fusion gene in non-small-cell lung cancer. *Nature* 448(7153): 561-6.

Soverini, S., S. Colarossi, et al. (2006). Contribution of ABL kinase domain mutations to imatinib resistance in different subsets of Philadelphia-positive patients: by the GIMEMA Working Party on Chronic Myeloid Leukemia. *Clin Cancer Res* 12(24): 7374-9.

Stoklosa, T., T. Poplawski, et al. (2008). BCR/ABL inhibits mismatch repair to protect from apoptosis and induce point mutations. *Cancer Res* 68(8): 2576-80.

Stone, R. M., D. J. DeAngelo, et al. (2005). Patients with acute myeloid leukemia and an activating mutation in FLT3 respond to a small-molecule FLT3 tyrosine kinase inhibitor, PKC412. *Blood* 105(1): 54-60.

Stransky, N., A. M. Egloff, et al. (2011). The mutational landscape of head and neck squamous cell carcinoma. *Science* 333(6046): 1157-60.

Tabin, C. J., S. M. Bradley, et al. (1982). Mechanism of activation of a human oncogene. *Nature* 300(5888): 143-9.

Takeuchi, K., Y. L. Choi, et al. (2009). KIF5B-ALK, a novel fusion oncokinase identified by an immunohistochemistry-based diagnostic system for ALK-positive lung cancer. *Clin Cancer Res* 15(9): 3143-9.

Tanaka, Y., Y. Terai, et al. (2011). Prognostic effect of epidermal growth factor receptor gene mutations and the aberrant phosphorylation of Akt and ERK in ovarian cancer. *Cancer Biol Ther* 11(1): 50-7.

Taub, R., I. Kirsch, et al. (1982). Translocation of the c-myc gene into the immunoglobulin heavy chain locus in human Burkitt lymphoma and murine plasmacytoma cells. *Proc Natl Acad Sci U S A* 79(24): 7837-41.

The Cancer Genome Atlas Network (2008). Comprehensive genomic characterization defines human glioblastoma genes and core pathways. *Nature* 455(7216): 1061-8.

The Cancer Genome Atlas Network (2011). Integrated genomic analyses of ovarian carcinoma. *Nature* 474(7353): 609-15.

Teng, Y. H., W. J. Tan, et al. (2011). Mutations in the epidermal growth factor receptor (EGFR) gene in triple negative breast cancer: possible implications for targeted therapy. *Breast Cancer Res* 13(2): R35.

Thomas, R. K., A. C. Baker, et al. (2007). High-throughput oncogene mutation profiling in human cancer. *Nat Genet* 39(3): 347-51.

Tiacci, E., V. Trifonov, et al. (2011). BRAF mutations in hairy-cell leukemia. *N Engl J Med* 364(24): 2305-15.

Tomlins, S. A., B. Laxman, et al. (2007). Distinct classes of chromosomal rearrangements create oncogenic ETS gene fusions in prostate cancer. *Nature* 448(7153): 595-9.

Tomlins, S. A., D. R. Rhodes, et al. (2005). Recurrent fusion of TMPRSS2 and ETS transcription factor genes in prostate cancer. *Science* 310(5748): 644-8.

Van Raamsdonk, C. D., V. Bezrookove, et al. (2009). Frequent somatic mutations of GNAQ in uveal melanoma and blue naevi. *Nature* 457(7229): 599-602.

Van Raamsdonk, C. D., K. G. Griewank, et al. (2010). Mutations in GNA11 in uveal melanoma. *N Engl J Med* 363(23): 2191-9.

Vennstrom, B., D. Sheiness, et al. (1982). Isolation and characterization of c-myc, a cellular homolog of the oncogene (v-myc) of avian myelocytomatosis virus strain 29. *J Virol* 42(3): 773-9.

Verstovsek, S., H. Kantarjian, et al. (2010). Safety and efficacy of INCB018424, a JAK1 and JAK2 inhibitor, in myelofibrosis. *N Engl J Med* 363(12): 1117-27.

Vikis, H., M. Sato, et al. (2007). EGFR-T790M is a rare lung cancer susceptibility allele with enhanced kinase activity. *Cancer Res* 67(10): 4665-70.

Vogel, C. L., M. A. Cobleigh, et al. (2002). Efficacy and safety of trastuzumab as a single agent in first-line treatment of HER2-overexpressing metastatic breast cancer. *J Clin Oncol* 20(3): 719-26.

Weisberg, E., M. Sattler, et al. (2010). Drug resistance in mutant FLT3-positive AML. *Oncogene* 29(37): 5120-34.

Wellcome Trust Sanger Institute Catalog of Somatic Mutations in Cancer [online], http://www.sanger.ac.uk/perl/genetics/CGP/cosmic?action=gene&ln=BRAF]

Wilks, A. F. (1989). Two putative protein-tyrosine kinases identified by application of the polymerase chain reaction. *Proc Natl Acad Sci U S A* 86(5): 1603-7.

Wilks, A. F., A. G. Harpur, et al. (1991). Two novel protein-tyrosine kinases, each with a second phosphotransferase-related catalytic domain, define a new class of protein kinase. *Mol Cell Biol* 11(4): 2057-65.

Wong, K. K., P. M. Fracasso, et al. (2009). A phase I study with neratinib (HKI-272), an irreversible pan ErbB receptor tyrosine kinase inhibitor, in patients with solid tumors. *Clin Cancer Res* 15(7): 2552-8.

Xing, M., W. H. Westra, et al. (2005). BRAF mutation predicts a poorer clinical prognosis for papillary thyroid cancer. *J Clin Endocrinol Metab* 90(12): 6373-9.

Yan, H., D. W. Parsons, et al. (2009). IDH1 and IDH2 mutations in gliomas. *N Engl J Med* 360(8): 765-73.

Yano, S., W. Wang, et al. (2008). Hepatocyte growth factor induces gefitinib resistance of lung adenocarcinoma with epidermal growth factor receptor-activating mutations. *Cancer Res* 68(22): 9479-87.

Yap, T. A., L. Vidal, et al. (2010). Phase I trial of the irreversible EGFR and HER2 kinase inhibitor BIBW 2992 in patients with advanced solid tumors. *J Clin Oncol* 28(25): 3965-72.

Yeang, C. H., F McCormick, et al. (2008). Combinatorial patterns of somatic gene mutations in cancer. *FASEB J* 22(8):2605-22.

Yen, K. E., M. A. Bittinger, et al. (2010). Cancer-associated IDH mutations: biomarker and therapeutic opportunities. *Oncogene* 29(49): 6409-17.

Yun, C. H., K. E. Mengwasser, et al. (2008). The T790M mutation in EGFR kinase causes drug resistance by increasing the affinity for ATP. *Proc Natl Acad Sci U S A* 105(6): 2070-5.

Zarrinkar, P. P., R. N. Gunawardane, et al. (2009). AC220 is a uniquely potent and selective inhibitor of FLT3 for the treatment of acute myeloid leukemia (AML). *Blood* 114(14): 2984-92.

Zhao, L. and P. K. Vogt (2008). Helical domain and kinase domain mutations in p110alpha of phosphatidylinositol 3-kinase induce gain of function by different mechanisms. *Proc Natl Acad Sci U S A* 105(7): 2652-7.

Zhou, W., D. Ercan, et al. (2009). Novel mutant-selective EGFR kinase inhibitors against EGFR T790M. *Nature* 462(7276): 1070-4.